FOSTERING CREATIVITY
IN REHABILITATION

PHYSICAL MEDICINE AND REHABILITATION

Additional books in this series can be found on Nova's website
under the Series tab.

Additional e-books in this series can be found on Nova's website
under the e-book tab.

FOSTERING CREATIVITY IN REHABILITATION

MATTHEW J. TAYLOR, PH.D.
EDITOR

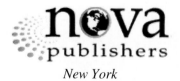

nova publishers

New York

NOTICE TO THE READER

The Publisher has taken reasonable care in the preparation of this book, but makes no expressed or implied warranty of any kind and assumes no responsibility for any errors or omissions. No liability is assumed for incidental or consequential damages in connection with or arising out of information contained in this book. The Publisher shall not be liable for any special, consequential, or exemplary damages resulting, in whole or in part, from the readers' use of, or reliance upon, this material. Any parts of this book based on government reports are so indicated and copyright is claimed for those parts to the extent applicable to compilations of such works.

Independent verification should be sought for any data, advice or recommendations contained in this book. In addition, no responsibility is assumed by the publisher for any injury and/or damage to persons or property arising from any methods, products, instructions, ideas or otherwise contained in this publication.

This publication is designed to provide accurate and authoritative information with regard to the subject matter covered herein. It is sold with the clear understanding that the Publisher is not engaged in rendering legal or any other professional services. If legal or any other expert assistance is required, the services of a competent person should be sought. FROM A DECLARATION OF PARTICIPANTS JOINTLY ADOPTED BY A COMMITTEE OF THE AMERICAN BAR ASSOCIATION AND A COMMITTEE OF PUBLISHERS.

Additional color graphics may be available in the e-book version of this book.

Library of Congress Cataloging-in-Publication Data

ISBN: 978-1-63485-118-3

Library of Congress Control Number: 2014953200

Published by Nova Science Publishers, Inc. † New York

CONTENTS

Foreword   ix
      Alfonso Montuori, PhD

Introduction   xiii

Part I: Creativity – Past and Present   1

Chapter 1   Historical Review of Creativity in Rehabilitation and
               Today's Need for Creativity   3
               Matthew J. Taylor, PT, PhD

Chapter 2   The Need for Creativity from the Patient's Perspective   15
               Matthew Sanford, MA

Part II: A New Understanding of Creativity   21

Chapter 3   A New Understanding of Creativity   23
               Matthew J. Taylor, PT, PhD
               and Alfonso Montuori, PhD

Chapter 4   Creativity and Evidence-Based Medicine   47
               Matthew J. Taylor, PT, PhD

Chapter 5   Systemic Limitations on Creativity in Academia
               and Professional Associations   59
               Staffan Elgelid, PT, PhD, GCFP

Chapter 6   The Role of Relationship and Creativity   71
               Ginger Garner, PT, ATC

Chapter 7   Creativity, Struggle and Sustainability   89
               Cheryl Van Demark, PT, MA

Chapter 8   The Implementation of Creativity   99
               Matthew J. Taylor, PT, PhD

Part III: Case Reports from Creators in Rehabilitation   111

Chapter 9   Occupational Therapy   113
               Arlene Schmid, PhD, OTR

Chapter 10   Physical Therapy   119
                  Mary Lou Galantino, PT, PhD, MS, MSCE

Chapter 11   A Fractured Path   127
                  Sara M. Meeks, PT, MS, GCS

Chapter 12   Speech and Language Pathology   137
                  Michelle Garcia Winner, SLP, MA-CCC

Chapter 13   Nursing   147
                  Carey S. Clark, PhD, RN, AHN-BC

Chapter 14   Nutrition   153
                  Beverly Price, RD, MA, E-RYT

Chapter 15   Art Therapy   161
                  Renée van der Vennet PhD, LCAT,
                  LMHC, ATR-BC, CGP

Chapter 16   Recreational Therapy   171
                  Marieke Van Puymbroeck, PhD, CTRS, FDRT

Chapter 17   Music Therapy   175
                  Robin Rio MA, MT-BC

Chapter 18   Dance/Performance Rehabilitation   187
                  Staffan Elgelid, PT, PhD, GCFP

Chapter 19   Women's Health   197
                  Diana Munger, PT, DPT

Chapter 20   Social Work   205
                  Jennifer Collins Taylor MSW
                  and Charles Trull PhD

Chapter 21   Psychology   215
                  Sari Roth-Roemer, PhD

Chapter 22   Guided by the Muse into the Uncertain   223
                  Cheryl Van Demark, PT, MA

Chapter 23   Career Transitions and New Horizons   229
                  Jerry Gillon, PT, ATC, OCS

Chapter 24   The Work Begins   235
                  Matthew J. Taylor, PT, PhD

Chapter 25   Domain Practices to Prime for Creativity   243
                  Matthew J. Taylor, PT, PhD

Chapter 26   Improvising New Actions   251
                  Matthew J. Taylor, PT, PhD

Chapter 27   Recreating the Larger Rehabilitation Community:
            Small Offices to Institutions   **257**
            Matthew J. Taylor, PT, PhD

Editor's Contact Information   **265**

Index   **267**

FOREWORD

"The more commonplace claim that we don't now have systems to create health is also correct… Here is the rub: the new way, the way to health, may be vastly further from the current design of care than we may at first wish it to be, or believe it to be."

~ Donald Berwick, MD, CEO and founder of the Harvard-based Institute for Health Improvement, 2014.

In the first decades of the 21st century, there seems little doubt that the world is in the throes of a remarkable transformation (Morin & Kern, 1999; Ogilvy, 1989; Slater, 2008). Dr. Berwick's comments regarding the current design of care being vastly further from the future design are a clarion wake up call for all of you involved in rehabilitation. The rehabilitation professions are under pressure to innovate in order to deliver services to a growing market of increasingly savvy consumers no longer limited to their conventional care choices and increasingly responsible for paying for their services. In the past, innovation and creativity have not been on the curriculums of these professions. The schools continue to produce graduates doing what has been done before and current providers are admonished by their professional organizations to practice only what has high-level research evidence to support the practice. Meanwhile veteran professionals, as both employees and owners, find themselves faced with the acute need to innovate in order to survive and thrive. This book will be an important first step in filling this critical void in knowledge and application of how to best transform both the individual and the organizations that are responsible for rehabilitation professions' futures.

It appears rehabilitation is in need of rehabilitation based on my conversations with Matt and the dynamics in the larger healthcare arenas. This need of rehabilitation for rehabilitation is very clear and just one of so many human systems (government, education, healthcare in general, etc.). Included in this list of systems which are in need of rehabilitation are the delivery and theoretical foundations of conventional medical rehabilitation professions. But even in this state of need, I am particularly intrigued to hear that the American Physical Therapy Association's new vision statement is "Transforming society by optimizing movement to improve the human experience." Clearly others are sensing the need to bring forward a new and more powerful role for rehabilitation beyond the individual patient experience. This need for a bigger and bolder vision can be better understood by broadening our habitual lens of perception to include the context of our larger society.

When one adopts that larger societal view it would be easy to become overwhelmed. The complexity of modern life is further complicated by the pluralism of perspectives. That milieu lends an increasing sense of uncertainty in life which can feel like being tossed in a blender of the accelerated rate of change across the planet. We are arguably in the middle of the Future Shock discussed by Toffler (1984). For the sociologist Zygmunt Bauman, "solid" modernity has become "liquid" modernity: Everything is fluid, changing; there is no predictability, no certainty, no stability; and human beings have to become flexible, adaptable, and capable of working under conditions of great uncertainty (Bauman, 2005). Sardar argues that we are in postnormal times, an "in between period where old orthodoxies are dying, new ones have not yet emerged, and nothing really makes sense" (Sardar, 2010). Certainly in rehabilitation the sheer volume of information, increased productivity and documentation demands, profound technology changes, dwindling reimbursements and high rates of professional burnout are symptomatic of a postnormal experience.

In this period of transition, this postnormal age, creativity is changing, too. The way we understand creativity is changing, the way we practice and express our creativity is changing, and this new creativity is in turn influencing how we might best rehabilitate rehabilitation.

Creativity has not only been a topic of popular interest—always somewhat mysterious— but also the subject of much mythologizing and misinformation (Berkun, 2007; Melucci, 1994; Montuori & Purser, 1995). Too often creativity has been taken to be a call for "anything goes" and a long, slippery slide back to potions and conjuring. As you will read later, the new understanding actually demands more rigor and discipline then the current dominant processes, not less. The emphasis is shifting from the modern individualistic focus oriented toward "eminent" or uncontroversial creatives (Gardner, 1994) producing exceptional products (Einstein, Picasso, Mozart, Feynman, etc.), toward a more collaborative, "everyday," ecological understanding and practice of creativity.

The emerging creativity moves from the rarefied realm of the genius in the arts and science to everyday life. This new focus is on generative interactions in a variety of mundane or everyday activities and contexts, rather than on the individual lone genius working on a major contribution. Consequently this book is not about some expectation that the reader generate a revolutionary new technique in their field (although that is not outside the realm of potential outcomes!). Creativity can permeate our everyday lives and can be tremendously useful in strengthening our adaptive responses to the rapid change characterizing these times. It involves a reenchantment of the everyday moments as well as an acknowledgment of the creativity that is possible in rehabilitation. Fostering creativity invites you to reinvent how you think, act in the world, and embody that change in the very process of reinvention of yourselves and your professions.

For the rehabilitation practice owners and directors taking up this text, rest assured that in business, creativity and innovation are now core competencies. For those of you who are students in your training program, you well know that at the personal level, the notion of self-creation has already taken root: whereas at the beginning of the 20th century, our lives were shaped if not entirely determined by our race, class, and gender, in the 21st century, the notion that individuals can "create" their own lives is the subject of serious philosophical, sociological, and psychological reflection as well as the stuff of wildly popular television shows such as Oprah and many independent movies (Montuori & Donnelly, 2013). Matt has laid out a format that will appeal to a broad spectrum of the rehabilitation community remaining firmly rooted in the traditions, embracing the emerging science of creativity, and bolding point toward better futures for the professions and society at large.

In closing, I would like to invite you to consider a musical analogy I often employ from my experience as a jazz saxophonist. My passion for creativity and the process of group creativity is rooted in my days as member of a band in England, as well as my ongoing play today to include my marriage to the incredible jazz vocalist Kitty Margolis. I can envision creativity in rehabilitation being like what happens in powerful jazz performance. There is a delightful mix of soloists, group interaction and a sense of fun for both the band and the audience. The more rooted the members are in the foundational skills of their instrument and the more open they are to the unexpected and changed up riffs of the other members, the more freely they create and respond as each song becomes its own new version. So too for you, I invite you to riff anew with each new patient, class or student while grounded on your "chops" of excellence from your profession's foundational knowledge base. Together with your colleagues an entirely new rendition will emerge and I look forward to kicking back and enjoying the music you make to change our society in the vastly different way that Dr. Berwick foresees.

References

Bauman, Z. (2005). *Liquid life*. London: Polity Press.

Berkun, S. (2007). *The myths of innovation*. Sebastopol, CA: O'Reilly.

Gardner, H. (1994). *Creating minds: An anatomy of creativity as seen through the lives of Freud, Einstein, Picasso, Stravinsky, Eliot, Graham, and Gandhi*. New York: Basic Books.

Melucci, A. (1994). *Creativita: miti, discorsi, processi: [Creativity: myths, discourses, processes.]*. Milan, Italy: Feltrinelli.

Montuori, A., Donnelly, G. (2013). Creativity at the opening of the 21st century. *Creative Nursing*, *Volume 19, Issue 2*, 58-62.

Montuori, A., Purser, R. (1995). Deconstructing the lone genius myth: Towards a contextual view of creativity. *Journal of Humanistic Psychology, 35*(3), 69–112.

Morin, E., Kern, B. (1999). *Homeland earth: A manifesto for the new millennium*. Cresskill, NJ: Hampton Press.

Ogilvy, J. (1989). This postmodern business. *The Deeper News, 1*(5), 3–23.

Sardar, Z. (2010). Welcome to postnormal times. *Futures, 42*(5*)*, 435–444.

Slater, P. (2008). *The chrysalis effect*. Brighton, United Kingdom & Portland, OR: Sussex Academic.

Toffler, A. (1984). *Future shock*. New York: Bantam.

Weeks, J. (2014). Hooking up: Don Berwick, integrative medicine and his call for a radical shift to 'health creation' *The Huffington Post*. Retrieved July 7, 2014 from http://www.huffingtonpost.com/john-weeks/don-berwick-integrative-m_b_4781105.html

Alfonso Montuori, PhD
Professor
California Institute of Integral Studies
San Francisco, CA, US

INTRODUCTION

Julie* perches on the edge of the chair, leaning forward, fidgeting side to side, spine collapsed, knees braced together, and her large, red-rimmed, hazel eyes look up to me silently pleading. She's just recounted her story of bilateral mastectomies with reconstruction efforts gone wrong. This catastrophe was followed by bowel surgery producing persistent pelvic pain that is now generating increasing back and knee dysfunction. Subsequently, she can no longer dance, hike, or participate her other forms of physical and social outlets. Her longtime lover recently left, forcing her to move from her home to a small apartment followed by months of sleepless nights. To make matters worse, she's a health professional who has sought relief of her pain and depression from seminars and colleagues to no avail. A friend thought I might be able to help. I sit quietly, gently returning her gaze, watching the protests and clamor for action arise within me, but I keep returning to the deep silence behind her eyes realizing I don't know THE solution, but I do care so very much. And from this blank canvas of silence and 'not knowing' that we are both resting in ... we begin to create together.

[*A pseudonym representing an amalgamation of various patients seen by the author.]

We have all sat with a complex patient like Julie and experienced a moment of "not knowing". The challenges differ by our specific profession, but the "not knowing" experience is shared across rehabilitation. I suspect I am not alone in having that experience with the "simple" diagnosis patient as well who fails to adhere or respond to their treatment plan. This book will explore these invitations to be creative that "not knowing" signals each of us, both as individual professionals and collectively as entire professions. My purpose in creating this textbook goes far beyond just addressing those moments of "not knowing." I have experienced a growing fire of realization in my 33 years as a physical therapist and an integrative health educator that the rehabilitation professions are in need of rehabilitation. Not in some gloom and doom, "the sky is falling" rant, but because the rehabilitation of rehabilitation is part of a much larger process of growth and evolution of human systems. This process of evolutionary change will require much of both Julie and me, as well each of us and every patient, colleague or student we encounter. Before we begin, allow me to first further describe the purpose of this textbook, the challenges it will address, and the benefits we hope to provider for all of us.

The purpose of this textbook has many facets built around my desire for our rehabilitation professions to make the next leap in development to better serve our communities and our own health. While rather dry writing, creating a list of objectives is a comfortable and familiar way to quickly communicate these purposes much like a continuing education flyer.

Rehabilitation professionals that read this textbook and utilize the exercises should be able to:

1) Describe and discuss creativity as it applies to rehabilitation, its historical context, present-day misunderstandings, and how to harness the creative process in their practice and profession.
2) Confidently share the importance of creativity at both local and larger scales within their profession to inspire further investigation and conversation about generating better futures.
3) As either graduate students or experienced professionals, identify and appreciate their own unique creativity and the creativity of the patients or students they serve.
4) Point to specific examples of colleagues expressing their creativity in rehabilitation based on the shared case reports.
5) Demonstrate and perform the practices that build the skills needed by providers and patients to prime the creative process and enact it in their unique circumstance.

What do I see as the problems that require so much attention to creativity? In my travels as a national continuing education provider, I have the occasion to hear and see first-hand the challenges many of us face in delivering rehabilitation services and education. Many of the larger system effects in our society have squelched our curiosity and passion, while reducing real income and too often dehumanizing what should be the very human, very creative experience of rehabilitation for both the consumer and provider. Specifically, this textbook addresses the following challenges and offers the potential benefits of:

1) Re-igniting the passion and curiosity that have been squelched by productivity loads, information glut, reimbursement models and so forth.
2) Through creative change preserve and increase real income in the face of school debt, inflation and after-hour work requirements that are not compensated.
3) Restore a sense of sacred and human interchange to interactions that now feel superficial and profane compared to an initial vocational calling.
4) Generate a personal and collective resiliency for our own health and well-being to accommodate the continued accelerated pace of change in society.
5) Re-invigorate both academia and professional organizations through active participation to take bold and well-grounded steps in creating new delivery systems for care and education.
6) Making EBM a catalyst for substantive and dramatic change and evolution rather than small incremental adjustments to our knowledge base.

The title of this book, "Fostering Creativity in Rehabilitation," was selected because the words point to key principles required to achieve these lofty goals and purposes. How do we, begin to foster, or in its original meaning, "nourish," our innate human capacity to adapt and create these results? The word "rehabilitate," which we all share in common, holds a vision of what is possible in the rehabilitation of rehabilitation. Rehabilitate has many meanings, but my favorite is the non-medical definition of "To make fit to live in again." Anyone who has rehabbed a house fully knows there is no end point. So too, once we begin demolition of our old patterns of thought and behavior, we will have taken up an unending process of emergence and adaptation, regularly seasoned with surprises and unexpected challenges just like that old house project.

At the heart of this rehabilitation adventure is creativity, which invites us to surrender to the process of re-imagining and birthing what is to come forward in the future as our professions. We will explore creativity in detail in the Chapters 1 and 3. For now, consider that first and foremost, creativity is a state or quality of being human, not a technique or artistic gift limited to a few. Like all living creatures, humans have the fundamental life capacity to respond and adapt to stimuli in their environment. In effect creativity is what we are, not something we do or a skill we add to our treatment tool box. This principle applies of course to us and the people we serve. So the outcomes of this creative expression can further defined as:

> ...the ability to transcend traditional ideas, rules, patterns, relationships, or the like, and to create meaningful new ideas, forms, methods, interpretations, etc.; the process by which one utilizes creative ability (Dictionary.com).

As one pattern gets torn down and rebuilt, new forms will emerge requiring new methods, just like tearing out a wall requires rewiring and changes in traffic flow of the old house. In this book we will explore together how we foster this creative essence in ourselves and in the process, also rehabilitate our beloved professions. The labor is our creative response-ability to the environment and circumstances we find ourselves in today. Not someone else's responsibility, not another person's with more knowledge, nor some other profession telling us who we shall be. No, it is ours!

I invite you to join me and the other creative collaborators of this book, as well as the many others at large that creating the future of rehabilitation. Use this text as it best suits your needs. After reviewing the skeleton of this four-part book below, decide where you wish to begin your contribution and dive in. Most of all, have fun again. We are not here long, so be sure what you do is worthy of your unique, creative essence.

Part I "Creativity – Past and Present" The first chapter sets the context for this point in history with our current strengths and challenges. This includes a critical examination of the assumptions that drive our current circumstances in rehabilitation. Through this process of reflection and questioning we undertake a crucial portion of the practice of clinical mastery. The current science of today calls into question many of these foundational assumptions about human health, illness and change. There is also a broader description of the present and foreseen challenges from our perspective that justifies this call to greater creativity in rehabilitation. Significant creativity will be needed in order meet those needs while providing each of us with fulfilling and financially sustainable careers.

The second chapter of Part I is written from the voice of the consumer to broaden our understanding for the need to radically recreate our services. Matthew Sanford, M.A., is an award-winning author whose non-profit Mind Body Solutions has been advocating this need for creativity on our part for many years. Matt writes from the heart and soul of each of our patients, grounded in his own experience rehabilitating from a spinal cord injury at the age of thirteen and now an international yoga teacher. This passionate and urgent articulation of patients' values will enrich our appreciation for this call to greater creativity.

Part II "A New Understanding of Creativity" When I began my doctoral studies in 2001, I was surprised to learn that much of what I knew about creativity was at best misleading, and in many instances just plain wrong. It has been my experience in teaching and reading popular literature that these inaccurate depictions of creativity continue to be the case in our culture. Consequently the first chapter, "A New Understanding of Creativity," is written in collaboration with my doctoral advisor and dissertation chair, Alfonso Montuori, PhD. He is an expert in social creativity and a sought-after consultant by organizations wanting to keep up with the rapid pace of change in today's postnormal environment. This chapter's inquiry into creativity will form the seed bed for your ongoing personal and professional development as you progress through the remainder of the book. The pop-culture portrayal equating creativity as making vision boards, lone genius worship, and attending brainstorming sessions will be replaced. In its place is an evidence-based, engaging description of how creativity is the very nature of being human and not some skill to merely develop like a better golf swing. This transdisciplinary summary of creativity sets the stage for the Chapter 4, "Creativity and Evidence-based Medicine," on how creativity and evidence-based medicine (EBM) relate to one another. This fresh look at EBM and creativity reveals how EBM actually invites each of us to be creative rather than rigid in practice. This perspective is of course is in sharp contrast to the all-too-often perceived dry, lifeless endurance test of EBM. The chapter is key as it keeps our creative efforts in the chapters ahead grounded in this critical practice standard.

Chapter 5, "Systemic Limits on Creativity from Academia or Professional Associations," investigates the why there seems to be so little new that comes from our respective schools and professional associations. Ideally creative initiatives would be cascading from our respective schools and professional associations that are charged with developing our knowledge base and advancing our collective professional agendas. Unfortunately a whole host of systems factors has produced just the opposite effect with slow, glacial change and adoption of new developments in the field. Staffan Elgelid, PT, PhD, a Swedish-born associate professor of physical therapy, shares his global experience and diverse professional background in this chapter. This critical reading is not just for academicians and students, but every clinician as it will address not only our frustrations with the limited bureaucratic changes from both groups, but will challenge each of us to engage our professions at a more powerful and effective level in the exercises in Chapter 27.

The next two chapters address very important topics that are often glossed over in discussions about creativity. Chapter 6, "The Role of Relationship and Creativity," examines the important impacts of relationship dynamics and how they can either suppress or foster creative emergence. The author, Ginger Garner, PT, DPT, ATC, is an entrepreneur and advocate for mothers, and she shares her important understanding of how relationship affects each of us and our patients. A major historical factor for our rehabilitation professions is the stifling influence of a power-over, or dominator relationship in medicine that has led many to become passive and lose their sense of agency and power to rehabilitate. Our collective shift to a more partnering relationship with others both as individuals and disciplines is described as crucial for the new creative responses we will spawn and implement.

Threads of the partnering process naturally dovetails with the following Chapter 7, "Creativity, Struggle and Sustainability," by Cheryl Van Demark, PT, MA, on the very real considerations of both struggle and sustainability in the creative process. The very real labor of birthing something new is a reality any innovator will acknowledge. She addresses supportive ways of sustaining the creative initiatives for bringing new rehabilitation methods into fruition. Part of this process is the understanding of how both local and larger systems influences offer roadmaps for our future generative efforts to take root and flourish despite the struggle of creativity.

Chapter 8, "The Implementation of Creativity," is the last chapter in Part II. This chapter links the more conceptual qualities of Part II to the very lived, concrete experiences of the innovators in Part III. The new ideas for how to rehabilitate rehabilitation is the easy part of creativity. The execution of these ideas into new behaviors, action, policies and institutions then requires implementation into engagements in society. This discussion of implementation will be shared in the individual case reports of creative efforts that are shared in Part III. Think of the chapter as a way that offers each of us a traveler's guide for what stepping up as a creator in rehabilitation entails and use it as a useful toolkit of effective strategies to adopt and potential potholes to avoid.

Part III "Case Reports from Creators in Rehabilitation" In Part III issues that thwart innovation and call for change within each specific profession are described by the authors. Written in a variety of ways based on the contributing author's preference, each chapter addresses open-ended, interview questions. The rehabilitation professionals' case reports share how they began, how they overcame some challenges, and in other cases how they were overcome by challenges. From their experience they also offer inspiration and insight about the future needs of their specific profession. I strongly recommend readers review all the chapters, not only the one or two most pertinent to their practices because readers will gain additional insight by reading across professions to glimpse new or related experiences from the other rehabilitation chapters.

The final two chapters of Part III focus on the creative experience in different ways. Chapter 22, "Stepping Off into the Uncertain," is very personal story of Cheryl Van Demark's creative process in a remote, conservative in a relatively challenged socioeconomic area. Her story is a must-read for anyone hearing that internal voice of "Well, it wouldn't be possible in my situation." We then move to Chapter 23, "Career Transitions and New Horizons" by Jerry Gillon, PT, ATC, OCS. The rehabilitation professions are mature enough now that many of us have or will soon transition our careers in new ways by changing focus or retiring. This moment creates an incubator of talent and innovation of professionals wanting to stretch and serve in new ways that can potentially yield many new ways of offering rehabilitation. Jerry's experience as a long-time private practice clinician led him to discover the deleterious effect of lifeless, inflammatory food on his patients' rehabilitation efforts. His is an inspiring story of a stepped down clinical schedule, coupled with his new bread baking business that now nurtures his community with quality, healthful baked bread. This chapter is a warm invitation to all of us to innovate our personal career trajectories to heal ourselves and our communities on new levels.

Part IV Action Steps to Foster Creativity The book closes with a workbook of practices to prime us for creativity. These chapters are designed to experientially foster both personal and organizational creative expression of our shared vocational call to ease the suffering of others. These practical chapters are useful in every creative endeavor from our small, ordinary human interactions to igniting major cultural change. The action-based steps reflect the emerging science that continues to reveal an ever increasingly embodied, interconnected world of consciousness and ongoing creativity.

Chapter 24, "The Work Begins," takes you through preparatory exercises for creativity from your unique embodied social context and will help you establish the critical skill of creating silence and the accompanying space that such silence generates. This space allows the coming forward of what's next for you personally, or when done together with others, what is next for the entire group. Chapter 25, "Domain Practices to Prime for Creativity," will offer a structure for more fully engaging your personal canvas of circumstance, embodiment and how that will influence your inquiry and enactment of creation. Chapter 26, "Improvising New Actions," The techniques in these chapters are utilized by the full spectrum of human activity from Fortune 50 company executives to the fallen patient on the floor trying to get up. Presently not valued by our culture, these skills are sorely needed to honor and utilize this important practice of emergence to foster creativity. Out of these practices comes the emerging future of rehabilitation.

These many changes will often require the rehabilitation of institutions and organizations as a whole. The final Chapter 27, "Recreating the Larger Rehabilitation Community from Small Offices to Institutions," has exercises for how you and your groups can foster processes for taking new possibilities into the intervention, classroom, home or boardroom. Here we learn to seize our creative power and engage our world to truly begin to transform society and rehabilitation.

CONCLUSION

In our rapidly changing and evolving global society, new ways of remaining or creating cultural relevance are essential for our earlier definition of creativity, "creating meaningful new ideas, forms, methods, interpretations." Our creative journey requires our partnering with all of the layers of connectivity between the many evolving systems today. This weaving together demands that we expand our awareness of our audiences and ourselves in order to deftly address the needs, desires, and hopes of all as we make our world more "fit to live in again" for today and the many tomorrows that will follow. That expanded awareness begins next in Chapter 1, "Historical Review of Creativity in Rehabilitation and Today's Need for Creativity."

EDITOR'S NOTE

The reader will notice that our text includes not only numerous references to the literature, but also an abundance of cross-references to chapters and sections in this book. There is a good reason for this abundance of references. A central characteristic of the systems view of creativity is its nonlinearity: creativity is complex – i.e., highly nonlinear – networks; and there are countless interconnections between the biological, cognitive, social, and ecological dimensions of creativity. This conceptual framework integrates these multiple dimensions as it reflects creativity's inherent nonlinearity. In our struggle to communicate such a complex network of concepts and ideas within the linear constraints of written language, we felt that it would help to interconnect the text by a network of cross-references. Our hope is that the reader will find that, like the web of creativity, this book itself is also a whole that is more than the sum of its parts (Capra, Luisi, 2014).

REFERENCES

Capra, F., Luisi, P.L. (2014). *The systems view of life: A unifying vision.* New York: Cambridge University Press.

Creativity (n.d.). In *Dictionary.com.* Retrieved March 30, 2014 from http://dictionary. reference.com/browse/creativity

PART I: CREATIVITY – PAST AND PRESENT

In: Fostering Creativity in Rehabilitation
Editor: Matthew J. Taylor

ISBN: 978-1-63485-118-3
© 2016 Nova Science Publishers, Inc.

Chapter 1

HISTORICAL REVIEW OF CREATIVITY IN REHABILITATION AND TODAY'S NEED FOR CREATIVITY

Matthew J. Taylor, PT, PhD
Director, Matthew J. Taylor Institute, Scottsdale, AZ, US

ABSTRACT

This chapter reviews the history of our modern understanding of creativity and how that limited understanding shapes our attitudes and beliefs about creativity. The philosophical and cultural biases through today have left society with anything but a robust and effective understanding of what creativity is and how to foster it. A considerable discussion of how creativity has emerged in rehabilitation documents a long list of shortcomings and needs within the rehabilitation professions. The context established in the chapter opens the way to explore what patients need and points to the utility of developing a new understanding of creativity from beyond the current limitations.

INTRODUCTION

Julie was introduced in the Introduction as our fictitious, complex patient. Merely add in additional diagnoses based on your professional focus and she will guide us through this book. My bias as editor is that however imperfect our patients' attempts are at healing, people don't want to suffer. My vocation as a rehabilitation professional is to serve Julie with every ounce of skill and ingenuity to allow her to ease her own suffering and enhance her quality of life. I have had the privilege to attend one of the best physical therapy programs in the U.S., enroll in countless quality continuing education programs, gain an advanced training in a mind/body profession and obtain a transdisciplinary doctorate focusing on chronic pain. I remain overwhelmed by the immensity of the suffering that arrives in my little clinic each day. How shall we serve our Julies in the face of limited resources of funding, staffing, reimbursement changes and access limitations? As with any journey, we need to begin by knowing where we are and how we got here. Let us begin together for Julie, ourselves and our professions...

"... there is good reason to inquire about creativity, a reason beyond practicality, for practicality is not a reason but a justification after the fact. The reason is the ancient search of the humanist for the excellence of man: the next creative act may bring *humans* to a new dignity."

~ Jerome Bruner's "On Knowing: Essays for the Left Hand"

(Popova, 2014)

We need creativity in rehabilitation today because there are many processes in place that are steadily stripping away dignity in our professions for both our patients and us. The following chapter is critical for our clinical mastery and the insights will be key to facilitating creative responses to address these indignities. While it may be tempting to jump ahead, please bear with this reflection and orientation. We begin with a short history of creativity and how it has been viewed in society until today. The next section then situates how creativity in rehabilitation has been nested within that larger cultural perspective. The effect of that environment has left us with where we find ourselves today. While much of what is being done in rehabilitation has been adequate and is good, there are a great deal of shortcomings and challenges that exist which need to be addressed in order to rehabilitate rehabilitation. Our ability to articulate these challenges from this chapter's context will generate new associations that will prime the pump of creativity that can guide us along our journey.

A BRIEF HISTORY OF PERSPECTIVES ON CREATIVITY

First, what is creativity and why does it deserve this much attention? Creativity takes us back to our first biology class where we discovered the characteristics of living things. The ability to respond and adapt to our environment is one of those basic qualities that separate us from non-living things. Those organisms that are most successful go on to live another day and reproduce to extend the generations of that particular species. So too may we as rehabilitation professionals. Those of us that respond and adapt to our environments effectively will be the ones who carry our professional genetic line so to speak.

As healthcare changes, demographics shift, technology encroaches, information grows exponentially, and business systems affect delivery practices, how will we both collectively and individually remain relevant and robust? Much of what we considered our domain of knowledge just a decade ago is now available for free on the internet or being offered by other professions encroaching on our historical scopes of practice. It is difficult to imagine how even much more this will be the case in the next ten years. What will be our response? Is it a threat or an invitation? Today I can consult with your patients via telemedicine for their condition if you can't get the results they want, provided they have an internet connection, webcam and a bank card. That brings the topic home in a hurry, doesn't it? But fear shouldn't be our motivation to explore creativity. Rather, the celebration of the vast untapped potential for each us to be more engaged in bringing forward the best future for rehabilitation, ought to be our impetus. So the celebration begins by examining the historic course of events that brings us to today.

Creativity is a current hot topic in the popular media and business press. By the number of books and blogs on creativity one would think the topic is something that is well studied and understood. As it is, neither is correct. This chapter and chapter 3 will orient us to what is understood about creativity and how it applies to rehabilitation, but this book is not an exhaustive treatise on the topic for reasons that will soon be evident. Consider the following synopsis of the fascinating history of our human inquiry into our ability to create.

After five years of formal study and 13 years total, I could make a strong case that understanding creativity is a very complex proposition. Montuori and Purser (1997) offered an excellent detailed review that allows us to glimpse the enormity of the task of truly understanding creativity vs. the glib, upbeat quips on the topic from our current media and experts. Despite its age, the article remains relevant today. Our current understanding of creativity has been shaped by three powerful forces:

1. Cultural biases and limitations;
2. The methodologies employed by the cultures; and,
3. The epistemological (how we come to know reality) factors that ground those methodologies.

Prior to investigating each factor, consider a simple question as an illustrative case in point. What accounts for the incredible creativity in music generated by the Beatles during the 60's? Easy enough, after all we aren't talking about spinothalamic tracts or the Kreb's cycle, right? Well, be careful...

1. First, there were and probably still are millions, even billions of people on the planet who wouldn't consider them creative to this day;
2. If you do think they were creative, most would want to look back at their early history, musical inclinations/exposures, favorite artists, early bands, etc. ;
3. Gladwell broke it down even further in Outliers (Gladwell, 2008) describing the many thousands of hours of tour time the band spent together in Europe prior to becoming popular;
4. Gladwell also spread the lens wider to include the other factors of mass marketing, technology recording, the instruments and advancement of the radio, TV and phonograph in creating financial streams that fueled new travel, movies and other exposures for the members as individuals and collectively;
5. There is of course also the influence of psychedelic drugs, the Maharishi's relationship, and the girlfriends/wives of the band members;
6. And what of the interactions between the members themselves, the power structures and relationships with recording companies, the cataclysmic shift in morality within society and the Vietnam war?

This only a short, partial list of factors that would grow exponentially when we begin to bring in other ways of inquiry beyond our dominant habits of inquiry. This same cascading unfoldment of fascinating questions and new relationships is available for every aspect of our rehabilitation practice as well. So below is the skeleton of understanding to allow us to look boldly anew at everything we do in rehabilitation. Pay close attention to your own experience while reading, noting any strong emotional responses, distastes, sense of curiosity, puzzlement, physical tension, altered breathing patterns, etc.

Cultural Biases and Limitations

Our current understanding about creativity is often taken for granted as thorough and objective. We literally can't see or haven't examined our assumptions, as is generally the case when describing fundamental paradigms of reality. One significant artifact of this process is that until recently most research on creativity has failed to place attention on the social dimensions of creativity. There has been very little investigation of why creativity should be seen largely as an individual and not a social phenomenon. Likewise, there has been little work done and little debate addressing the very notion of such a split, and its philosophical, social, and methodological implications in healthcare and rehabilitation specifically. The majority of the literature surveyed on creativity originates in the United States, a culture which orients strongly to individualism, and whose method of study has largely been reductionistic (Sampson, 1983, 1993). These cultural factors have played a powerful role in shaping our understanding. Therefore our perspective of creativity has largely left out cultural differences in the study of creativity, and the differences in self-concept as considerations of the creative person, process, and product. In rehabilitation, ours is primarily a North American perspective that is based on:

a. The self as the fundamental unit of creativity;
b. A limited consideration of the effects of community, tradition, and shared meaning upon the self;
c. A bias away from sociological and philosophical principles in discussions;
d. A self-concept that prevents an understanding of the many cross-cultural variations in self-concepts;
e. Despite a cultural emphasis on freedom of choice and autonomy, there is an unawareness of the subtle but pervasive pressures to conform to be like everyone else at work, at school and at conferences with colleagues.

We have focused on individual factors rather than attempting to change and understand social circumstances, in part because of the above normal times perspectives. Collectively we have generally been unwilling to explore the extent to which we are shaped by our culture. In the case of the encouragement and promotion of creativity, we find most publications still focused on the individual, whether as self-help or training others.

Ironically our very wish to escape our social circumstance is itself a product of cultural conditioning of individualism. We can see this manifest itself in clearly pre-established roles which have taken on mythical status in North-American culture, such as the myth of the lone genius (Montuori, Purser, 1997).

But we get ahead of ourselves discussing the replacement of that myth, as a new understanding of creativity is for chapter 3. First, consider how closely linked our methods of inquiry are to these cultural biases.

The Methodologies

On this topic of creativity, methodologies are the actions of how we come to know what something is. Our methodologies include the biases of our culture and the related epistemology below. Chapter 4 has a thorough description of what amounts to reductionistic methods based on our normal times worldview (i.e. there's one way reality is and we need only break down things to their smallest pieces to understand and predict reality).

The process of trying to simplify and ferret out responsible variables to predict creativity looks absurd alongside our brief example of the Beatles. So it would be in the clinical research to find answers for patients like Julie. Yet we ask such questions in earnest time and time again. What are the variables that account for your personal creativity or absence of it? How do you know? Can you compare it to others in a homogenous group of peers to confirm your assessment? Apologies for continuing to push to the obvious shortcomings by example, but it is this very shortfall that invites our renewed and new exploration of the topic. It is also interesting to note that much of the focus in research on group creativity has been on brainstorming, an artificial procedure, rather than on natural everyday interactions; as if brainstorming sessions were the only time people as individuals grudgingly get together to 'generate ideas.' Over and over the limitations of our normal times epistemology bumps up against the uncertainties of our complex, post-normal times.

The Epistemology

So we find ourselves looking in the house of mirrors asking, "How do we come to know what our creativity is in face of the post-normal times that exist?" Our methods of inquiry and cultural biases have come up short and limited in discovery. It appears we need a new epistemology in order to gain a more functional and deeper understanding of creativity. Montuori and Purser suggested that multiple forms of inquiry may be the way forward, with the insights and shortcomings of each, holding potential for new questions and perspectives. Chapter 3 offers an extended discussion of what that might look like.

Such flexibility in inquiry would require individual and collective awareness of our habits of mind in studying creativity. That same flexibility is also the skillset that can unleash creativity in rehabilitation, to include the big professional questions, but also the ordinary creativity of everyday encounters. Chapter 4 and the exercises in Part IV offer greater detail into both the theory and practice of this reflective and introspective aspect of our clinical mastery.

As promised at the start of the chapter, this book cannot address the full realm of creativity, let alone just the epistemological foundations. However, with this basic historical understanding, we can consider what our processes of inquiry have generated to fuel the popular, but far from complete, descriptions of creativity in Western culture.

A.) Silos of Inquiry - Montuori and Purser (1997), using psychology as an example, offered this partial list of the silos of inquiry that now exist in and between our normal time divisions of knowledge:

1.) Psychology alone considers:
    a.) Psychometrics
    b.) Psychohistory
    c.) Social constructionism
    d.) Cognitive psychology
    e.) Systems theory
    f.) Phenomenology
2.) Anthropological perspectives
3.) Organizational
4.) Sociological inquiry into creativity, and,
5.) Historical examinations of creativity

Every one of these methodological slants places limiters which leave something out of its inquiry, something which it considers 'noise'. Montuori and Purser argue this very noise can be the source of new learnings as it opens up new avenues of inquiry; avenues which create not just more questions but different kinds of questions, questions which may well not have been addressed previously (Ceruti, 1986). For most rehabilitation processes, this would also include almost exclusive focus of both the creative individuals and their social recognition at the expense of the social environment and interaction. In Chapter 3 we explore that given our largely North-American understanding of creativity has been socially constructed, we need to in these post-normal times broaden our understanding of the phenomenon we call creativity. This includes understanding the larger systems of thought which has produced this creativity construct. Such a clinical mastery practice of expanding our perspectives is a way of opening us up to further inquiry into the theory, practice, and popular understanding of creativity and specifically, rehabilitation practice.

While our culture does have some examples of highly interactive and collaborative creative processes, we have to repeatedly ask to what extent disciplinary categories and cultural biases have obscured our understanding and appreciation of creative processes. For example, collaborative or group enterprises, are often viewed by our dominant culture as inevitably leading to dependence and a subsequent loss of autonomy (Slater, 1991).

Such blind spots also have many of the techniques listed below being based on the assumption that time has to be set aside to collaborate creatively in a structured manner, since by bias, this process of creativity apparently does not happen spontaneously. From our North-American individualist perspective, group interactions are viewed as either neutral or a hindrance to the individual and hence to creativity. Clinical interactions with patients are rarely recognized as opportunities to generate creativity. Consequently we've overlooked the potential for creativity in our daily 'interruptions' bedside or in the activities of our ordinary day.

B.) What is Creativity? - One of the greatest preoccupations not only of our time but of our civilization is the question of what is creativity?

These ponderings date back to the dawn of recorded thought. What understanding do we have about what happens in creativity? While there's no way or reason to try to include the many approaches available, all of which are presented here with the above biases. It wasn't until the early twentieth century that our answers to the question began to take the shape of something more structured and systematic than metaphysical musings. Again most formal study has been in North America and here are the more prevalent descriptions we will hear variants of described in modern discussions (Popova, 2014).

1. Graham Wallas's model that outlines four stages of the creative process — preparation, incubation, illumination, and verification from 1926;
2. James Webb Young published a five-step technique for producing ideas in 1939; a.) Gathering raw material; b.) Digesting the material; c.) Unconscious processing; d.) The a-ha moment; and, e.) Idea meets reality;
3. Arthur Koestler's *famous "bisociation" theory of how creativity works* from 1964; a.) Creativity operates like a slot machine; b.) It relies on the mind's pattern-recognition machinery; and, c.) Creativity requires the combining of raw material into new ideas;
4. A number of derivative modern ideas such as Steve Johnson's, "Chance favors the connected mind." He points to recurring environmental patterns that produce a slow hunch, not a Eureka, but via collisions of smaller hunches over time to incubate and collide. This includes creating spaces for ideas to bump into each other and make use of the ability to borrow other hunches.

This short list and the many other derivatives that are being touted, to include brain imagery studies are all the steady advancement of descriptions that have a very mechanical approach of proper ingredients, slow or fast, to try to explain creativity or at least how new ideas come along. Certainly these descriptions all have useful components, but from a post-normal time perspective, they still yearn for that predictable, prescriptive certainty that falls well short of fully holding the mystery and messiness of creativity. Consider the traits Barron below found for creative individuals and organizations. No more conformity and certainty here!

C.) Traits of Creatives - Frank Barron (1980) discovered 5 broad traits of creatives through his research that distinguish creative individuals and organizations. These traits are a convenient summary of how the evidence has demonstrated that both organizations and individuals that exhibit these traits are apparently in opposition with the values of the normal times perspective. Keeping with the post-normal times perspective however, creatives tend to have the paradoxical ability to include both polarities of each of these traits at various times, as is detailed in chapter 3. Within each of these traits lie opportunities to discover and develop our individual and collective tools for generating creative strategies. Creative individuals and organizations tend to exhibit:

1. An independence of judgment rather than conformity;
2. A tolerance for ambiguity rather than a need for certainty;
3. A preference for complex thinking rather than polarized, simplistic oppositional thinking;
4. Androgynous behaviors with clarity on gender attributes and roles rather than a masculine preference (See Garner chapter 6);
5. A preference for complexity of outlook and a tolerance for asymmetry rather than symmetric, constrained possibilities.

As Elgelid will detail in chapter 5, both our professional associations and academic structures presently may espouse such values. In practice however they continue to be largely operated from the opposite polarities with some of the outcomes listed below in how creativity has emerged in rehabilitation.

HOW CREATIVITY IN REHABILITATION HAS EMERGED

Our rehabilitation professions are fairly nascent in the broader course of human history, especially in terms of autonomous function and identity. Our respective professions' emergences each reflect an adaptation to various needs within society and healthcare specifically. In our developmental processes, each profession has staked its position through definitions, scopes of practices, and many levels of standardization of care and regulation. All of this started during Sardar's normal times where boundaries and certainties were both the goal and perspective. The tensions of the current post-normal times have mental health professionals paying attention to somatic experience and bodily position, physical therapists employing cognitive behavioral techniques, nutritionists teaching mindfulness, and occupational therapists declaring, "Well of course!" to all of it and more. This tension both beguiles and fuels the potential for future creativity if we can hold our regard for the past and tradition, AND get comfortable with assuming Barron's traits of creativity above. In our brief traditions, we worked to bring forward the best of normal times order, structure and certainty. While there have been notable exceptions, chapters 4, 5 and 6 go into more detail about the following general list of how creativity has been managed or emerged:

1. In a power hierarchy, most professions at least originally were ancillary and subordinate to medical doctors and were expected to follow their orders for care. Anything new fell within dictated limitations and regulatory processes vetted any new practices or movements toward autonomy.
2. Reimbursement models have and continue to drive participation and care dictating to providers and consumers what will be reimbursed as rehabilitation services. Both providers and consumers have tended to limit their possibilities of care then to whether payers will cover types and quantities of treatment. If it isn't covered, it isn't made available or even if it is, it is often declined by the consumer.
3. Research money decisions and school departmental organizational dynamics reflect the normal times of what is investigated, tested and taught by whom. Turf wars over who does what continue today despite public declarations of interprofessional collaboration.
4. Each profession tends to teach from what Montuori defines as "reproductive" education as the dominant pedagogy. That is, students are instructed in what is known, what is to be done and how it is to be done. Students then pass if they can reproduce that knowledge as instructed and perform the behaviors of treatment as delineated in clinical education settings. There is generally not room or credit given for innovation, deviation or adaptation.

5. EBM has been skewed to imply only interventions with high level research evidence are acceptable as treatment. Clinical mastery and patient values have been subordinate to research evidence.

6. Numerous examples of new developments from either grass roots emergence or foreign import of ideas exist, but generally have undergone long, rather tortuous periods of adoption into practice, often at great peril to personal and professional reputations of the early pioneers of the practices. In normal times, change has been viewed with skepticism and caution, especially if it demanded substantial restructuring of foundational systems of control and process. Fluid, flexible and swift have not been words associated with rehabilitation professions' collective or individual approaches to creative change.

This drive for safety and predictability from the normal times mode of change has left us in our present circumstance. We are awash in increasing productivity loads, information glut, and strangling reimbursement systems. There is a sense of loss of depth of meaning and sacredness of care that generates a sense of making profane our vocations, and a loss of resiliency to the accelerated pace of change in post-normal times just when we need it most. We conclude with the heavy list of needs prior to turning our sites on addressing how we create a better future. Note what you can add to the lists as you read through this section.

WHAT NEEDS EXIST IN REHABILITATION TODAY

What is most lacking in our current circumstance in rehabilitation echoes back to Bruner's quote at the top of the chapter. Succinctly, the drawback of our process of creativity is that in many instances it is stripping both the consumer and the provider of dignity. Consider the following outcomes and how it impacts human dignity for the all of the involved parties. Today we are challenged with:

- Passive patients wanting to be fixed and wanting the cost covered by someone else. How do we foster active patients engaged in the ordinary creativity demands of their days in regards to their rehabilitation? The process has left the patient with minimal response-ability and generally passive vs. being co-creators of their own health. We need to deeply mine "ordinary creativity" in the patient/provider relationship as well as the teacher/student interactions.

- The normal times ontology and subsequent epistemology has left us with mountains of data and information but failed to deliver on the clinical prediction models that were promised. Related to this and the first challenge, we are left as the experts to fix the broken patient. Now that we know the simplification of realism and its methodologies can't fully address the complex realities of the modern rehabilitation patient, how do we proceed clinically and as separate disciplines in building our body of expertise?

- In addition to the vulnerabilities of being unable to address complexity, the old view of predictability falls far short, and in fact is incapable of addressing paradox. For instance, how do we build off the early creativity of pain education that can hold the two apparent opposing truths that pain can be due to tissue damage AND is an output of the brain?

- Our education systems are replete with "reproductive education"... we look to others for ideas and then try to reproduce what they instructed. The new understanding around creativity will mark the end of reproductive learning and the beginning of generative learning as will be discussed further by Elgelid in Chapter 5. How well has that new technique worked when you returned home? How do we ignite generative learning where the past is understood in the immediate context to create new knowledge and behaviors at that unique moment?

- Doing to and just doing anything for Julie has been the focus in the past. The values of silence, sensing being, and presence have been ignored or devalued. How do we instill (pun intended) the practice and positive valuation of these crucial ingredients of creativity?

- Transdisciplinary perspective is required to negotiate post-normal times. Mere interprofessionalism or interdisciplinary approaches sustain boundaries and thwart creativity despite good intentions and many creative efforts to name what needs to happen. Without the paradigmatic flexibility to examine our post-normal circumstances, we're bound to be left in the same box we talk about getting out of when creativity is considered.

- How do we stack up individually and collectively re: Barron's traits of creativity when we spurn independent judgment, seek conformity and uniformity, despise ambiguity and uncertainty, teach symmetry and engage in oppositional debate and dichotomous interactions? How will we shift from those deep habits of our culture and traditions?

- How do we balance the very real financial compensation concerns of the system for providing a living wage AND address the also very real affordability and accessibility concerns of the present systems of delivery? A post-normal response brings forward Berwick's quote in the Preface about, "...the new way, the way to health, may be vastly further from the current design of care than we may at first wish it to be, or believe it to be."

- How do we care for ourselves as professionals, suffering high levels of burnout, compassion fatigue, chronic pain related conditions and a general loss of verve for our vocation? Any new system must include care of the providers as well as the patients.

- The march of the providers to today's newest guru of care reveals an inherent distrust in the provider's sense of their own creative agency. This spills over to the clinic where we blame the patient, student or technique when the desired outcome fails to emerge in the post-normal environment. How do we restore trust in our role and the patient's role as part of the creative inquiry beyond looking just to others as experts?

- Timidity and obedience rule the day. Stay the course, don't ruffle feathers and by all means be a compliant, I mean, adherent patient. When do we become bold and audacious? How will we transform society like the APTA vision statement about transforming society? Our well-trained passive memberships are in need of a new calling or re-ignition of their vocation rather than tighter controls and more regulation.

- We sit with an impending tidal wave of care needs of an aging boomer population with long lists of challenges and by all reports insufficient personnel and resources to attend to those needs. Is doing more of what we're doing the way out? Really?
- Professionally and personally we need to re-examine and update our ontological (what can be known) and epistemological (how we can come to know) as well axiological (what is worth knowing) assumptions. This is hard, emotionally distressing work that is too easily avoided or glossed over. Trying to address all of these needs without this foundational work is destined to failure as any new wine of creativity is going to require new wineskins to hold the newly rehabbed rehabilitation.

CONCLUSION

An often overlooked fact about creativity is that destruction is the first step to creativity. We have to ruin the blank canvas to begin to paint a better picture with Julie and others like her in the future. The new rehabilitation will need to be able to hold the many paradoxes of the postnormal era. This postnormal era requires us to be able to answer questions with "and". i.e., "We provide quality care AND meet bottom-line needs." This is to include more rich examination while incorporating the spiritual aspect of our vocation, or calling, to be integrated with our practice behaviors and concepts. It's no longer ok to stay distant, professional. The post-normal clinical master sustains appropriate boundaries AND falls in love with every patient (doesn't mean you have to like every patient). The blurring of boundaries between disciplines will also accelerate as transdisciplinary education continues to become more valuable and available. This will include then an embodied clinical mastery and contextualized integral understanding of health. We can't afford more isolation in the silos of the respective disciplines. Below are our goals as we now hear from Matthew Sanford on how our patients need us to step up the task ahead.

1. Re-ignite our passion and curiosity that has been squelched by productivity loads, information glut, reimbursement models and so forth.
2. Through creative change, preserve and increase real income in the face of school debt, inflation and after-hour work requirements that are not compensated.
3. Restore a sense of sacred and human interchange to interactions that now feel superficial and profane compared to an initial vocational calling.
4. Generate a personal and collective resiliency for our own health and well being to accommodate the continued accelerated pace of change in society.
5. Re-invigorate both academia and professional organizations through active participation to take bold and well grounded steps in creating new delivery systems for care and education.
6. Make EBM a catalyst for substantive and dramatic change and evolution rather than small incremental adjustments to our knowledge base.

REFERENCES

Barron, F. (1990). *No rootless flower: Towards an ecology of creativity*. Cresskill, NJ: Hampton Press.

Ceruti, M. (1986). Il vincolo e la possibilita`. Milano, Italy: Feltrinelli. English Translation (1994). Constraints and possibilities. *The evolution of knowledge and knowledge of evolution*. New York: Gordon & Breach.

Gladwell, M. (2008). Outliers: The story of success. New York: Little, Brown and Company. Montuori, A., Purser, R. (1997). Le dimensioni sociali della creatività. Pluriverso, 1, 2, 78-88.

Popova, M. (2014). How to master the art of "effective surprise" and the 6 essential conditions for creativity. Brian Pickings. Retrieved 4/21/2014 from http://www.brainpickings.org/index.php/2014/04/21/jerome-bruner-on-knowing-left-hand-creativity/?utm_content=buffer5f5fe&utm_medium=social&utm_source=twitter.com&utm_campaign=buffer
http://www.brainpickings.org/index.php/about/

Sampson, E. (1983). *Justice and the critique of pure psychology*. New York: Plenum Press.

Sampson, E. (1993). *Celebrating the other: A dialogic account of human nature*. Boulder, CO: Westview Press.

Slater, P. (1991). A dream deferred: America's discontent and the search for a new democratic ideal. Boston: Beacon.

In: Fostering Creativity in Rehabilitation   ISBN: 978-1-63485-118-3
Editor: Matthew J. Taylor   © 2016 Nova Science Publishers, Inc.

Chapter 2

THE NEED FOR CREATIVITY FROM THE PATIENT'S PERSPECTIVE

Matthew Sanford, MA

Director, Mind Body Solutions, Minnetonka, MN, US

ABSTRACT

Sanford shares his experience both as a patient and an international leader in changing rehabilitation. This carefully crafted chapter moves gracefully from private story to specific examples and moving descriptions of why creativity is needed in rehabilitation. The need is there for both patients and caregivers. As he illustrates, the one informs the other, while each then comes to discover something powerful. That something is mind-body awareness within the healing therapeutic relationship. Sanford transports the reader to a new understanding of what lies at the heart of true rehabilitation from the perspective of one who awakens each morning to the harsh realities of a mind-body injury. The progression of rehabilitation to embrace this important advancement will require creativity and an embodied practice by rehabilitation professionals.

INTRODUCTION

Lying in bed after nearing a month in intensive care, I attempt to feel my whole body. I feel something, a tingling, a hum. This is strange because I am a thirteen-year-old boy who has just survived a devastating car accident that claimed the lives of my father and sister and put me through a shredder of sorts. I was in a coma for three and one half days. I broke my neck at C-1, my back at T-4, broke both my wrists, filled a lung with fluid, and injured my pancreas such that I could not eat for nearly sixty days. I went from a one hundred nineteen pound, very athletic young boy to seventy-nine pounds. The thoracic injury severed my spinal cord and rendered me completely paralyzed from the chest down. The year was 1978.

Some thirty-six years later, I am paraplegic yoga teacher and author of *Waking: A Memoir of Trauma and Transcendence* (Sanford, 2006). I founded the non-profit Mind Body Solutions, an organization dedicated to transforming the lives of people living with trauma, loss, and disability by unlocking the connection between mind and body. I train yoga teachers from around the world how to adapt yoga for people of all abilities, but I also train healthcare professionals how to integrate mind-body principles into their care practices to benefit both themselves and their patients. Although my life's work begins with my personal story, the vast majority of us will all be patients at one time or another. The distinction between patient and caregiver is ultimately illusory. Both are in need of healing.

The thirteen-year-old boy tells doctors that he can feel something in his legs. His doctors give him a concerned look. They "know" that this is not possible because his spinal cord is severed, so he is "not feeling" what he thinks he is feeling. They have good hearts. They are good people who want the best for him. And yet, they are limited by their conceptual paradigm. "Matthew, those sensations are not real," they say. "You are like a person who has had a leg amputated that thinks his leg is still there." Then he looks under the covers. "Those sensations are phantom feelings like what an amputee feels," the doctor continues, "mental memory that will fade with time." The thirteen-year-old boy lies there as the adults around him impose their picture of reality.

In many ways, this encounter with the doctors begins my path toward yoga, toward training healthcare professionals, not because they did something wrong but because we can do better. We have a medical and rehabilitation system that is in need of rehabilitation. The system is producing patients who are overly dependent on their caregivers, who do not "comply" with treatment plans, and who do not take an active enough role in their own healing process. On the flipside, we have caregivers who are also suffering, who are increasingly constrained by a cumbersome healthcare system, and who are losing connection to the very thing that started them in their professions: the desire to help others.

How do we change this? How do we access the strength, resilience, and engagement of both patients and caregivers alike, improving the outcomes for both within a healthcare delivery system that is unlikely to undergo substantial structural change? We have to get creative enough to think more at a grassroots level. We can shift the healing relationship – something we can affect as individuals – in a way that nourishes both patients and caregivers. The challenge is to deepen the connection between patient and caregiver while maintaining professional boundaries Breakthroughs in science and technology can improve healthcare only so far. In a changing healthcare landscape where patient-satisfaction is becoming an increasingly more powerful driver, improvements must come in the fundamental relationship that is the bedrock of quality healthcare: the patient-caregiver dynamic. This will require our creativity, both as patients and as caregivers.

The strategy that underpins my work is deceptively simple. We should increase the teaching, sharing, and practicing of mind-body awareness within the healing/therapeutic relationship. This approach is ultimately based upon a simple insight about human nature. The way to access the strength, resiliency, and engagement in human beings is not strictly physical. It's not strictly mental. Rather these attributes reside within the mind-body relationship, that is, where the mind intersects with the body within human consciousness. I know this sounds philosophical, but I mean it literally. The key to improving outcomes for both patients and caregivers is to improve our ability to rehabilitate the mind-body relationship more directly, not just rehabilitate the body and then the mind separately. If we do this, we can better access strength, resiliency, and engagement in both patients and caregivers.

This ultimately means reworking our conception of what and how we are rehabilitating. We must confront some misconceptions about how best to approach the mind-body relationship, ones that are implicit within the way we work with patients. To oversimplify, our paradigm currently separates mind from body and treats the body physically and lets the rest fall into the realm of psychology. We already know such a split is a false dichotomy. We already know that the mind affects the body and the body affects the mind. Unfortunately, the definitions of our professional disciplines reinforce this false dichotomy, i.e. we separate the physical health professions from mental health ones. This does not mean that a physical approach to the body is bankrupt or a psychological approach to the mind is misguided. Clearly, they have important and critical value. It does mean, however, that more attention must go to the rehabilitation of mind-body relationship directly.

What does it mean to rehabilitate the mind-body relationship directly? This question raises more issues than can be adequately covered in this chapter. For now, suffice to say, I mean what it feels like to live in one's body, however changed or damaged that body is. This does not mean how one feels about one's body or condition. I literally mean the experience of 'presence' within the body, the quality and distribution of the sensation of 'presence.' So to oversimplify, we should rehabilitate how it feels throughout the body as one is moving in addition to working for the functional return of that movement. For example, let's consider someone living with rheumatoid arthritis in the hands. In addition to helping maintain hand functionality, there would be attention and practice giving to keeping the mind equally distributed throughout the body, even when experiencing pain when using the hands. This means getting better at rehabilitating the subtlety of experienced sensation within the mind-body relationship, not just overt action. To facilitate this, the caregiver must also transform. When both patient and caregiver work together to experience the subtlety of mind-body interaction, they become more engaged and resilient.

We typically do not think about rehabilitation this way. We default to a paradigm that separates mind from body and treats each separately. Back to the thirteen-year-old boy. The problem with the "phantom feeling" story runs much deeper than the fact that the doctors didn't listen to or honor my experience. The problem is that they didn't believe me; they were entrenched in their dichotomous paradigm. The unfortunate result of their guidance was that I believed in what they said rather than in my own experience. This is perhaps the most profound level of disengagement: I no longer trusted in what I was feeling. In the doctors' defense, they were in a tough spot. They had been trained to conceptualize my injury on two major axes: the physical injury and the psychological/emotional injury. The physical injury was irreparable. They could not fix it and I was never going to walk again. They felt badly. For the psychological and emotional injury, they believed that acceptance of my condition was integral to my recovery. So I was told stories of phantoms and ghosts and convinced of their truth. This caused me to stop listening to my own body below my point of injury and pushed me further away from my body.

But I do not experience the injury in the manner in which the paradigm conceptualizes it. The fundamental axis of the injury that I actually experience every day is a mind-body injury. My mind no longer possesses direct and effective connection with much of my body. For example, my mind cannot voluntarily access my legs to initiate muscular action. Thus my legs sit idle. Of course, there is a physical cause of my paralysis – my spinal cord severed. Of course, there are psychological and emotional repercussions to living with a paralyzed body – in many respects living with paralysis is incredibly hard and often quite disappointing. No one in his or her right mind would dispute these things. But the medical model has confused the cause and consequence of my injury with the actual experience of my injury. I live with is a mind-body disconnection, not just a physical injury with psychological and emotional repercussions.

This mistake of this conceptualization has far-reaching implications, more than can be fully addressed in a chapter. One is that the thirteen-year-old boy confronted a rehabilitation model that focused almost exclusively on compensation. The short story was that I was guided to make my upper body really strong and learn to drag my paralyzed body through life. To help me feel whole, I was encouraged to explore all the things I could still do, especially recreational, for example, adapted sports like basketball, skiing, swimming, horseback riding and the like.

But what about feeling whole within the only body I will ever have? What was the rehabilitation for that? There was none. This was because the doctors, rehab professionals, and their conceptual framework defined my injury from their perspective, from their knowledge base and experience. They didn't think about my situation through the lens of what I actually experience. I do not mean my thoughts, emotions, and other psychological expressions. I also do not mean that they were not caring and compassionate, because they were. I mean they did not consider the impact of my injury in my mind-body relationship itself. Thus, they missed the true, experienced nature of my injury.

The consequence was that I did not fully engage in my recovery until I started practicing yoga some twelve years after my accident. Up until then, I tried to fit into my life by learning to willfully overcome my paralyzed body. This is not a good recipe for maximizing long-term outcomes. It took practicing yoga for me to rehabilitate my mind-body relationship, for me to realize that my mind can still inhabit my whole body, for me to realize that there is a level of sensation that runs throughout my whole body that precedes my paralysis. This does not mean that I am walking again or that I can now engage muscles where I previously could not. It simply means that now I have rehabilitated my physical injury, my psychological and emotional injury AND my mind-body injury to the greatest extent possible.

I hope that it is clear that my comments do not apply only to spinal cord injuries. Recovery from any illness or injury also requires a return to one's body. Under duress, our coping mechanism is to disassociate from the body. Coming home to one's body is a central feature of any meaningful healing process. This is true whether a patient is recovering from catastrophic injury, life-threatening illness, trusting a knee after a ligament tear, living with chronic pain and on and on.

Truth be told, this is true for caregivers also. The pace of healthcare, the rules, the electronic documentation, the pressure not to make a mistake, the hours, always being asked to do a little more, to see just one more patient – all these demands are causing many caregivers to lose contact with the essence of their profession, to lose connection with their family life, their patients, with how to have fun, and on and on. The caregiver needs healing too.

The shared exploration of mind-body interaction, the integration of mind-body practices into the healing relationship is a simple, attainable solution to a very complicated problem. Here's what I know from being a patient: the more connected I am to my body when I leave the healthcare system, the better I will take care of it, the more engaged I will be in my healing process, and consequently, the less likely I am to end up back in the system. Here's what I know from training healthcare professionals: the more connected they are to their bodies, the more present they are with their patients and in their own lives. This means they listen better; they interact better; and they have better, more compassionate boundaries. They are more engaged, more satisfied, less stressed, and more dedicated to their professions.

There are a myriad of reasons why infusing mind-body awareness into the healing relationship is a practical and elegant solution for our healthcare system. To touch on a few: It deepens the connection between patient and caregiver. In order to share and teach mind-body awareness with patient, caregivers must practice mind-body awareness themselves – this requires that caregivers develop a self-care practice but the motivation is to better serve their patients. Mind-body realization teaches important and profound skills for the caregiver, for example, how to sit in the presence of suffering and stay grounded or how to give and receive simultaneously. Increasing mind-body awareness within the healing relationship does not change *what* caregivers are doing, but rather *how* they are doing it. This creates all sorts of advantages. Because it is a process improvement, not an additional technique, it is not a separate modality that must receive special new coding and reimbursement. Mind-body awareness is something that caregivers can practice while they are working, not just when they are interacting with patients. They can also practice at home with friends and family. Integrating mind-body practices seamlessly into their work does not take more time. It is a different way of living, not another thing to do. Deepened mind-body awareness doesn't create more 'time' in the day. It can, however, create more 'space.' Mind-body awareness can deepen the connection with patients without compromising professional boundaries. It increases one's strength, resiliency, and engagement. This is good for both patients and caregivers alike.

I want to end with a brief sketch of what increased mind-body awareness might look like in practice. Principles of mind-body awareness have be explored and revealed by various Eastern practices, especially yoga, ones that can be very helpful in the process of recovery and rehabilitation. For example, an experiential distinction between the subtle body and the gross physical body opens a new world of wholeness for patients living with a wide variety of deficits. Subtle body awareness is affected through more than muscular action. Alignment and precision create an effortless level of mind-body integration. For example, as a paraplegic, I can feel more on the 'inside' of my legs when I sit up straighter in a precise manner and lift my chest. The same is true for people who are not paralyzed. Bringing one's upper thoracic spine gently forward into the body spreads subtle body awareness through the limbs. (Again, this is true for everyone if one learns how to key into subtle sensation.) Think of what this means for someone living with an impaired or missing limb. Or imagine telling someone who has trouble standing up to lift the tailbone up through one's mouth while simultaneously pushing down through one's inner heels. (This makes standing up much less strenuous.) Or what if we taught patients what balance feels like as a sensation as a precursor to teaching balance as a physical accomplishment? This would translate to helping hemiplegic patients feel the sensation of balance directly throughout their bodies before making them stand on squishy surfaces and throwing balls at them to catch.

But how might this impact the patient-caregiver dynamic? Teaching and sharing at subtler levels of the mind-body relationship is more experientially based rather than knowledge based. In short, the subtlety is shared before it can be effectively taught. This means patient and caregiver must explore the mind-body relationship together. In my book *Waking: A Memoir of Trauma and Transcendence*, I qualitatively describe this process of learning to feel vibrantly through my paralyzed body as a process of listening to and then working with the 'silence" I experience within the mind-body relationship. By this I meant the parts of me that were not as tangible, that were less under my direct control. It took the practice of yoga for me to realize this level of subtlety. Such exploration was not possible in my rehabilitation experience because the emphasis was place exclusively on doing and outward action, rather than also feeling inwardly and deepening my inward experience. Working with and rehabilitating the 'silence' within the mind-body relationship, that is, more inward sensation and awareness, changes the tone of the patient-caregiver dynamic. This book is full of ideas and methods for caregivers to explore the subtlety of silence within the mind-body relationship. The journey is worth it.

The implications of rehabilitating subtle mind-body awareness, however, move well beyond rehabilitation. Imagine patients in acute care with serious conditions. Think of all the fears and unknowns under which they are suffering, both consciously and unconsciously. Then imagine nurses coming in and helping patients calm down by putting weight on their laps, whether with sandbags or even blankets to help create the sensation of grounding. Or imagine rather than a sleeping pill, a nurse lightly grounds a patient's ankles by touching them because the nurse knows (because she has felt it in her own body) that calming joints calms the mind and thus helps one sleep. There are countless examples.

Finally, imagine any caregiver, whatever the discipline, who knows how to lift out of her ankles and activate her feet in a way that brings renewed energy to her spine while she is standing. Or a caregiver who knows how to exhale out tension while he is washing his hands between patients. Or how about caregivers who learn to pause momentarily between patients using mind-body techniques so they can be fresher in their next patient encounters? Or how about caregivers that know in both mind and body how to give care without giving away their energy? Or most importantly, caregivers that can come home from an intensely chaotic day of giving and still have energy to give to their families.

Such a dynamic is good for everyone.

REFERENCE

Sanford, M. (2006). *Waking: A memoir of trauma and transcendence*. Emmaus, Pennsylvania: Rodale Press.

PART II: A NEW UNDERSTANDING OF CREATIVITY

In: Fostering Creativity in Rehabilitation
Editor: Matthew J. Taylor

ISBN: 978-1-63485-118-3
© 2016 Nova Science Publishers, Inc.

Chapter 3

A NEW UNDERSTANDING OF CREATIVITY

Matthew J. Taylor, [1] *PT, PhD*
and Alfonso Montuori, [2] *PhD*

[1] Director, Matthew J. Taylor Institute, Scottsdale, AZ, US
[2] Professor, California Institute of Integral Studies, San Francisco, CA, US

ABSTRACT

The first two chapters established the background and need for creativity in rehabilitation. This chapter answers what is creativity? What comprises creativity? What interactive processes prime creativity? And, what optimizes and sustains creativity? The new understanding is built upon the new postnormal times philosophical underpinnings described for rehabilitation professionals. The ethical aspect of creativity is also introduced informing an understanding rooted in compassion and an intention to relieve the sufferings of others and the providers. Also included is the articulation of the importance of ordinary creativity as well as correcting a number of other modern misconceptions of creativity. The chapter concludes with a discussion of the implications of this new understanding.

INTRODUCTION

The predicaments of Julie and our many complex patients demand a response of humility from the rehabilitation community. If the second half of the 20th century was tinged with a hubris that we could get to certainty in outcomes, these post-normal times of the early 21st century should have brought us all down a peg or two on "knowing" what to do for Julie. Things have changed through the history of rehabilitation, often for the good, but acknowledging the many present day complex health challenges will demand that we create a "new way, the way to health...vastly further from the current design of care" of Berwick's as quoted in the Preface. This chapter invites us into a fresh new understanding of our creativity and the surprising promise of concepts such as "silence" and "being" that can complement our action-oriented noise of "doing" and "doing to" that we surveyed in the first chapter.

> "Creativity is not a talent,
> It is a way of operating."
> ~ John Cleese

How do we begin to operate creatively and also find a balance between doing and being in silence as mentioned above in Julie's saga? As we will discover, creativity isn't a talent or aptitude we train like a muscle. So let us dive deep into a new understanding that should both perturb and delight us, if it's truly new. As we do so, bear in mind the lists of challenges from Chapters 2 and 3, and note how this new understanding begins to point to exciting possibilities for our future. Will it be hard work? Labor? You bet, but then each of us wouldn't be reading this as a rehabilitation professional if hard work was a real barrier.

In Chapter 1 there was a thorough discussion of the history of creativity, a summation of the past research and a detailed review of how that history has affected rehabilitation. The context created in that first chapter is important to maintain as we begin this chapter's exercises for arriving at a new understanding of creativity. Most of us, as rehabilitation professionals, would probably be surprised to learn that there are even several journals now published that focus on creativity. So there is considerable recent research and that will be summarized later in this chapter to support this new understanding for those of us that appreciate the scholarly rigor of published evidence. However, this exercise of new understanding is intentionally presented in an unfamiliar manner without the normal "literature review first" in order to prime a more active engagement of our whole being, rather than just our conceptual mind. So please humor us and take on the beginner's mind of not knowing what creativity is at this moment. Consider instead this new way to understand ourselves and the privilege it is to be creators by our very nature.

THE NEW UNDERSTANDING EXERCISE BEGINS...

Creativity is...? In both the Introduction and Chapter 1 we visited standard definitions that varied around the accepted general definition, "to bring something new and adaptive into the world." However, consider for the moment, what if the most accurate and honest answer is, we aren't certain? That would be a bit of let down in a book dedicated to creativity! But that's post-normal times and the acknowledgement of uncertainty. Consider the exercise of holding that uncertainty for now. Might it not generate a fresh attitude of humility regarding predictability and control in light of our post-normal times appreciation for the complex systems that contribute to health and rehabilitation? So beware of immediately grasping for some final answer regarding what creativity is and isn't in this exercise. As we proceed, hopefully we will comfortably arrive with a richer, more fluid appreciation of creativity. Whatever creativity is--and Torrance (1988, p.43), a leading researcher, argues that "it defies precise definition"--it seems to be a complex, multifaceted phenomenon (Montuori & Purser, 1997).

Recall that in normal times the main focus of traditional scientific methods was to reduce the phenomena under study to its single elementary units and find the general laws which govern those units. In studying creativity, as noted in Chapter 1, this methodological slant led to a focus on what was perceived to be the smallest identifiable variable, e.g. the individual, at the exclusion of 'external' factors such as the social environment. Now a post-normal inquiry invites us to employ numerous ways of knowing beyond just that reductionistic approach.

Another way to come to a new understanding is to review what something, in this case creativity, doesn't appear to be at this point in time. We do this through an analysis of negation. Analysis as a form of inquiry is ancient, to include the Vedic scholars in yoga, who named the inquiry a Sanskrit expression, neti neti. Neti neti means "not this, not this", or "neither this, nor that". The assumption in this exercise is that by sweeping away our past limited or inaccurate understandings, we make space for a new and, hopefully, more functional and fluid understanding of what, in this instance, creativity might be. So we will begin with a neti neti assessment, then build out a new framework of understanding from a post-normal times constructivism process of multiple perspectives to include a neurophysiological framework. These perspectives will reshape how each of us can begin to foster creativity at multiple levels and the many new implications this understanding has for each of the ensuing chapters and exercises.

THE NETI NETI PROCESS

The following neti neti process is a part of our clinical mastery. This process of reflection and introspection regarding our assumptions about creativity begins by dismissing those that have been found to be inadequate or false. David Burkus's "The Myths of Creativity" (2014) is an accessible summary of much of the recent research where he described 10 myths of creativity, some of which are included in our more extensive list below. So here goes neti neti.

Creativity isn't:

- A skill or talent that you develop or learn.
- Limited to a few people.
- An abandonment of convention or a spirit that anything goes in clinical care.
- Expressed in isolation or the sole domain of a lone genius.
- A thing you do.
- A pattern of brain activity.
- Contrary to evidence-based medicine.
- Easy or simple.
- Something we do 'to' patients.
- Threatening.
- Generally taught in rehabilitation curriculums.
- Haphazard, spontaneous, useless or impractical.
- Isn't a new fad or "hot topic."
- A moment of "Eureka!" that happens in a flash, or that was brought to us from something outside ourselves.
- A certain type or breed of creative individual; there is no evidence supporting a creative gene or personality type.
- Wholly original or without context.
- Limited to expertise.
- Usually driven by external incentives, and can actually be negatively affected by external incentives.
- The result of brainstorming, or at least brainstorming is not sufficient by itself.

- Without personal or interpersonal conflict, and unruffled cohesion can be a sign that nothing new is emerging.
- Due to an absence of constraints or limitations.
- Innovation of something new or better necessarily. Put another way, new or better isn't necessarily creative.
- Just a matter of whether there is, or is not, competition or collaboration.

Pause to consider which of those assumptions had been part of your understanding about creativity. Note any thoughts, emotions or somatic responses to reviewing the list once more. Taking the time to reflect and notice is the literal exercise of clinical mastery vs. just reading the list and moving on without reflection. Once you have completed the exercise, then we move on to see what the new space for understanding of creativity might begin to include that wasn't part of our previous understanding and practice.

THE NEW UNDERSTANDING

Our attempt to define creativity is a bit like trying to define other broad phenomena, such as life, love, God, time, and death, etc. This new post-normal understanding renders a single sentence definition essentially impossible, and to be practical we need to constrain the description to match our interests as rehabilitation professionals. So bear with a fairly extended exploration that will conclude with a short summary definition. We will get there by building out the many layers of expression on this now relatively blank canvas of understanding of creativity post-neti neti.

In the process there will be four core questions that we will visit non-linearly, but always seeking insight and new perspective through their interrelationships:

1) What is creativity?
2) What comprises creativity?
3) What interactive processes prime creativity?
4) What optimizes and sustains creativity?

To visit these questions, there will be the following component sections which are:

1) A short ontological description (what can be known);
2) A somewhat extended epistemological (how do we come to know) exploration. Both of these first two explorations are key to a transformational shift in our understanding (otherwise we're still in the normal times paradigm);
3) New to many of us "objective medical professionals" will be the addition of a brief axiological investigation (what is worth knowing);
4) Transition to a vocational affirmation grounded in a shared value of compassion as rehabilitation professionals;
5) Explore the broader process of ordinary creativity throughout all aspects of life;
6) Investigate (or similar verb) the implications of this new understanding.

Ontology and Epistemology

Aside from being really fun words to say aloud, these two philosophical terms describe the bedrock of our clinical mastery practices and all of EBM. Reflecting on *what can we know* (ontology) and *how can we come to know* (epistemology) are very functional definitions of these two terms. How we answer these two questions determines what operating system we are functioning under per Cleese's quote at the start of this chapter. A useful analogy is to think of the past differences between the two biggest computer operating systems (PC vs Mac) as a way to appreciate this important issue. Less so today, but still with significant differences, you might be word processing, gaming, creating graphics, managing music files, etc., and your experience will be substantially shaped and influenced by which operating system you are using. Not only was the functioning different, but the status, aesthetics and fun-factors will color your experience as well. So too, with our personal and collective ontologies and epistemologies in these post-normal times. What then grounds our new understanding of creativity?

The normal times ontology was that there was one way reality is and our job was to discover that one reality in order to accurately represent it for control and predictability. Chapters 1 and 4 include broader discussions of that perspective and its limitations. This worldview trickled down to our rehabilitation practices as a representational epistemology; if we could just collect all the right ingredients of care that matched the situation before us and apply them to the clinical situation, Julie would be better. Complex human interactions, such as mine with Julie, are just one of the many places where this way of coming to know breaks down as we have seen in the examples and will continue to explore in ensuing chapters.

The post-normal way of *coming to know* is one of constructivism. This new approach acknowledges, with humility, that every perspective is limited and, therefore, fallible. Subsequently, our responsibility (and privilege) is to *construct* multiple ways of describing a reality that is dependent on who is inquiring and with what tools. This multiplicity of descriptions generates, for someone operating in the old normal times view, a very frustrating plurality of reality!

A great example of this within rehabilitation is the exploration of the reality of pain. If you have followed the rapid shift in understanding about pain in the past decade, you are witnessing this very plurality. What can we know about pain? Turns out, it depends. Pain was a nociceptive input from the periphery. Wait, no it's the output of the brain and composed of a matrix of factors collectively known as a neurotag. Oops, no the immune system seems inextricably influential. But then, social isolation generates a similar response…Can you feel it? The normal times tension for, "Just tell me what it is!" Creativity shares the same slipperiness and fluidity. What can be known depends on who and how they are looking at it and then the description they construct of its reality. There no longer seems to be just one way pain, or creativity, or any aspect of what reality is, that can fully encompass all possible understanding. There will be exercises in Part IV to fully explore your personal ways of *coming to know*, as well as opportunities to practice trying on new lenses.

For now, in answer to what can be known about creativity, we must humbly state we are not certain. However, we do know that both *who*, and how and why the *who*, looks at creativity will all influence our understanding of its reality. That leads us to consider then the *who* and how of the epistemology of creativity.

Extending our pain example, we can see the understanding shift has been based on who and what tools they used (How can we *come to know*?). The electrophysiologist saw it one way, but that shifted with the functional anatomist and new staining and imaging technology, but it shifted in the hands of the neurophysiologist in clinical trials, and yet that morphed from the finding of the immunologist's discoveries using different tools. And who knew when the social psychologist examined social exclusion and isolation, with everyone else's' tools, there would be an even different reality that social exclusion creates a similar brain output like that of chronic pain? This epistemological morphing based on who and how one looks has left many of our colleagues and institutions figuratively frozen in uncertainty with what to do next about any number of complex challenges in each of our respective disciplines. There's almost a palpable pull for someone to just please tell us how *it* [fill in your challenge] really is.

This clamor for certainty is both the ontological and epistemological angst of normal times in the face of the post-normal times plurality. Here we find the lynchpin to creativity. Do we choose to hold on to the old normal times and do more of what has been done, or do we adapt to practice a metaperspective of constructing many possible realities? This bifurcation point is fundamental to how we will act in the future. Presuming we want to create better futures for Julie and ourselves by shifting to post-normal times inquiry, a deeper look into this new epistemology will further illuminate our new understanding of creativity. In short, dealing with Julie's complex circumstance requires casting aside the simplistic, linear thinking of the past. In its place we put on the complex, systems thinking/sensing/being/acting of the post-normal times in which we live.

Complex Being

In the normal times perspective this section would be titled "Complexity Thinking" or how to think complexly as an epistemological approach. However, the post-normal times plurality needs to be inclusive of the entire being. One aspect of our being is thinking, but we are also informed by sensing/acting/attention. Through these metaperspectives of inquiry beyond thinking, we will come to experience every aspect of our lives in a richer, deeper fabric of possibility than the normal times, thought-centric existence. First let's consider the following exploration of complex being from what else, but a plurality of perspectives.

We began with Julie's complex circumstances and challenges. It is only fitting that to truly gain understanding (and then act creatively) we need to better understand complexity and what being complex entails. Complexity is understood, according to Morin (1983), as difficulty and uncertainty, as a challenge. As Ceruti (1986, 1989) has shown so clearly, developing an awareness of complexity is tied to a shift from a representational epistemology to an epistemology of construction. Complex being requires that we be able to not only construct the many new understandings, but also have the skill of deconstruction of both the old and every new understanding. What are the ways we would have approached Julie? What are new ways we might construct with her? Can we reflect sufficiently to both build and tear down ways of being with her in each moment? Seems terribly, and appropriately, complex at this point. That's why Part IV is included in order to re-discover the simplicity within complexity. But first, let us explore this complexity and how simplicity and complexity can co-exist despite being diametrically opposed in normal times thinking.

In order to order understand complexity we must adopt a systems-theoretical view. A complex understanding begins to emerge as we examine and understand the many systems that make up the phenomena under study, as well as those other systems which form smaller parts within the phenomena. No longer breaking down just to the smallest circles of relationships that make up the part, the systems view also spreads our awareness in an ever expanding wider circles of influence and relationship beyond the part itself. We plumb not only Julie's internal systems of existence, but now also look at those external to her, to include most importantly, ourselves as provider. For instance if Julie is obese, physically unattractive and covered in tattoos, how does our systems of relationship around those superficial visual issues influence how we assess and interact with her? Suddenly Julie's circumstance is woven with our's in a larger whole. Without awareness of these systems influences within ourselves, the creative possibilities for treatment remain constrained by not only her personal limitations of perspective, but also our own. Quite literally her rehabilitation is woven into our ability to be with her without diminishing her opportunities to heal in light of our personal systems influences. Creativity in rehabilitation is no longer a removed, objective (sic) provider with expertise doing fixes to patient with broken parts. Quite literally from a systems view we come to see the interaction as "the whole is more than the sum of its parts" in every encounter.

The complexity of being doesn't allow us to rest in this familiar set of relationships based on past systems-based health. Complexity, it turns out, is inclusive rather than exclusive. From this epistemology of complexity, there emerges what in normal times would be the inconsistencies of exclusivity. Out of this complexity perspective there arises at the same time relativity, relationality, diversity, alterity, duplicity, ambiguity, uncertainty, antagonism, and the union of all of these notions which can be complementary, competitive, and antagonistic. (Morin, 1983, p.190, translation by AM).

Therefore it's no surprise to discover that the systems view also emphasizes the equally valid corollary, that a system is also less than the sum of its parts, because any system also imposes certain constraints on its parts (Morin, 1983; Wilden, 1980). These constraints inhibit the part, and allow it only limited expression of its full capacities (i.e. while you might have a fashion suggestion for Julie, the system probably discourages you from fully utilizing your fashion sense as a rehabilitation professional).

Societies impose constraints on individuals, as do groups and any form of social organization, including marriage and family. Individuals also impose constraints on their own "parts" in choosing careers, spouses, and in making other decisions which may inhibit some of their potentials for healing, while opening up others (Ceruti, 1986; Morin, 1992). Julie and you are constrained in many ways, and that is reality. But according to systems theory in the post-normal times, we need to keep in mind that a system is *BOTH* more *AND* less than the sum of its parts (Morin, 1983). Focusing on one half of that statement (i.e. *either* less *or* more), does violence to the complexity of the system(s) of the rehabilitation opportunity. Enhancing our ability to hold both statements as true is another clinical mastery skill we will pursue for good reason.

By holding two opposing thoughts, we can glimpse the positive implications of developing a systems view. When we realize that, along with imposing certain constraints, interactions among individuals in a larger system can also trigger emergent properties, which could not be predicted through knowledge of the single individual parts. This phenomena of the whole as also more than just the sum of its parts is because of the appearance of emergent properties. Systems can open up possibilities for parts which the parts in and of themselves might not be able to have. Being part of a research group, a musical or theater group, or a community rehabilitation group, opens up possibilities while/AND at the same time creating constraints. For instance, you note that one of Julie's tattoos is of the elephant-headed Hindu deity Ganesha. Last night your social system had a friend drag you to a silly yoga class where the teacher went on and on about Ganesha as the remover of obstacles and barriers. That system influence now allows you to ask Julie what obstacles she would ask Ganesha of her spiritual system to remove and how you two might work with Ganesha to make that happen. Had there been no silly yoga class last night, then no deep binding rapport with Julie, from her tatted and otherwise foreign world, today in the clinical encounter. The many circles of systems between the two of you met and out of it emerged a new way forward that couldn't have been predicted from your individual "parts."

This example illustrates the powerful and considerable expansion of our scope of awareness when we broaden our lens. We begin to see rehabilitation as a phenomenon that can in simple circumstances emerge creatively. This emergence takes place in time and space, across different settings, between different cultural perspectives, and immediately taking on quite different forms from the ones we are accustomed to in our 20th-century rehabilitation discourse. Had you just focused on her posture for instance, not seeing her broader self via her tattoo, that simplification would have isolated and therefore hid the relational shared nature to her larger system (relations not only with the environment, but with other systems, with time, and with you the observer/conceptualizer/provider.) Now with this broader lens you discover what might possibly renew her hope and engagement in rehabilitation.

This complex being also invites us to re-examine our understanding of causality. What if Julie now begins to improve dramatically? Who or what is the cause? The friend, the yoga teacher, Ganesha, you, or Julie? Morin (1992) describes complexity as a recognition of complex causality, or in our example "more specifically an eco-auto-causality, where auto causality means recursive causality in which the organizing process elaborates the products, actions, and effects necessary for its creation or regeneration, and where autocausality needs causality from outside" (pp.130-131). In other words, post-normal times understands complexity entails a shift in our description of phenomena, which at minimum in our example recognizes 1.) Mutual (friend, you, teacher, Ganesha, and Julie), 2.) Recursive (your ability to relate to Ganesha, propose incorporating Ganesha therapeutically, and Julie's agreement to investigate that way), and, 3.) circular causality (Julie becomes interested in identifying new barriers, you gain additional insights into those barriers and offer additional strategies to what were previously hidden obstacles to both of you for her healing). Our new understanding of complexity then emerges out of the inclusion of the systems of relationships as a constitutive part of the creativity we want to understand.

We can take our example deeper by analogy, because this same 'identity crisis' of causality may be said to afflict our understanding of human beings in general. For when we view patients only as single actors and not as parts of larger social entities, depending on our perspective and methodology as the rehabilitation professional, we have diminished the emergent systems properties of complex being. If, however, we understand that we all have certain 'blind spots' in the broader discourse and practices of care, and that these blind spots become all the more clear when viewed from a complex systems perspective, then this is where we can individually and collectively, begin to relax into the tension of a post-normal times perspective as new insights and practices emerge.

As we appreciate these basic principles of systems theory, it becomes apparent that if we do not look at the whole of a patient's system beyond the familiar health systems history review, we cannot see the connections between its various components, and thus the system's configuration. Much like what happens if we look at only part of a picture, we cannot possibly see the whole picture's configuration. Our willingness to expand our awareness as part of our clinical mastery allows us to draw from a more complex perspective. Potter and Eisler (2014) stated that the study of relational dynamics makes it possible for us to see social configurations: connections between different parts of social systems beyond our habituated and limited world view. New possibilities then emerge that were not visible through the lenses of our conventional social categories such as ancient/modern, Eastern/Western, religious/secular, rightist/leftist, technologically developed/undeveloped, or capitalist /communist. It will be essential that we learn to be comfortable with the normal times discomfort of constant lens shifting as we will always find ambiguity and diversity in the complexity that is inherent in any unified system. Each system that comprises our rehabilitation experiences is paradoxically both unity and diversity, in fact, also a unity in the diversity too. We so deeply want to know wholly, and yet limit that knowing if we ignore or miss the many layers of diversity. Part IV will take you deeply into exploring these phenomena experientially. To complete this epistemological discussion, a bit more on systems and complexity remains to be introduced into how it affects our understanding of creativity.

As we incorporate the complexity of being practices ahead, how does it affect our new understanding of creativity within rehabilitation? Systems theory argues that we must understand any system in the context of 1.) Its environment, 2.) Its relation with time, and, 3.) Its relationship with the observer (Emery, 1969; Morin, 1983). The methodological problem might seem to be how does one possibly hold all of these systems in awareness in addition to our already overwhelming load of information from our conventional rehabilitation knowledge base? This concern is an indication that the normal time perspective of having to have all the right parts to fix before being able to begin has slipped back into our worldview. Fortunately we don't have to be able to hold every possible aspect of the system to practice as a complex being. Emergent systems properties, and that slippery lack of causality, provide us relief from what otherwise would be overwhelming in the old view! Rather, a systemic or contextual approach stresses the importance of giving regular consideration to the many relationships between our varied daily settings. This includes the EBM practices outlined in chapter 4 and the process of 'system definition' in this section whereby we outline our multiple methods of inquiry for any new clinical challenge. Beyond that, we employ a practice of "silence and being" vs. "doing" to discover the emerging future possibilities. Just a bit more systems discussion first before the silence and being.

In Chapter 1 we discussed the history and evolution of the concept of creativity and of creativity research and practices as we know them today. As we introduce the concept of creativity into rehabilitation, we want to keep in mind the very deep biases that limit our current understanding as evidenced by the long list of neti's earlier in this chapter. Montuori and Purser (1997) emphasize that this is particularly relevant in an age when we speak of both creative genius and creative accounting, when the word creativity is used in discussions of advertising, finance, art, science, and, now rehabilitation.

So we will remain vigilant about how the intellectual and cultural traditions affect not just the discourse about what creativity is, but what the emergence of creativity is and how it might be fostered. We need to expand the discourse on creativity in many directions and avoid limiting our understanding of creativity to what is dispensed by popular media and experts dishing the biased results of those popular traditions. An additional benefit of holding a complexity perspective is that when we explore these historical and social issues, we also find ourselves inevitably confronted with issues of power and domination: Who, if anyone, sets the agenda for creativity in rehabilitation, how does the agenda set trends, and who determines who and what shall be considered creative or not in the rehabilitation professional circles? Chapter 6 by Garner fully develops this concern as it has had, and will continue, to have far reaching consequences on what rehabilitation looks like in the future.

These and many more questions about creativity in rehabilitation need to be addressed from a plurality of perspectives. As we reviewed in chapter 1, questions about creativity presently fall somewhat awkwardly between a number of different disciplines outside of rehabilitation, and according to Montuori and Purser (1997) are generally ignored for lack of an appropriate category or methodology. When rarely discussed in a rehabilitation discipline, the discussion often appears without any reference to the work done in other disciplines. Clinical mastery demands we begin regularly examining the assumptions underlying any such inquiry and discussion of creativity. This demand means the historic assumptions that undergird much of the present day creativity discussion now need to address the recent critiques of individualism (e.g. Bellah, Madsen, Sullivan, Swidler & Tipton, 1985; Sampson, 1993) and reductionism (e.g. Laszlo, 1991; Morin, 1992), arising in a variety of disciplines outside of rehabilitation. Our willingness to examine this epistemology behind the subject of creativity will prove to be a very fertile area in which to study the implications of these critiques, and may finally generate a greater awareness of interdependence such as the above example of Julie's situation.

There are early signs of such a broader view of creativity (often called innovation) in rehabilitation, but as Elgelid points out in chapter 5, that discussion needs to be radically expanded in our academic, regulatory, and professional associations. Part of the current movement toward more interprofessionalism should be to capture the emergence of a social focus on creativity research and bring it into our strategic and operational processes. By placing emphasis on the social dimensions of creativity in rehabilitation, an important new trend could develop in rehabilitation that touches on many crucial issues in psychology, the social sciences, and philosophy, enriching our professions beyond our normal times, science-only operations.

For both experienced professionals and new students, our clinical mastery will deepen through the further study of creativity in its social and historical contexts. That study will allow us to address many current limiting conceptual polarizations between self and society, sociology and psychology, individualism and collectivism, isolation and community, reductionism and holistic or systemic approaches to rehabilitation (Wilden, 1980; Hampden-Turner & Trompenaars, 1993). Potter and Eisler (2014) have extended discussions on how this deeper examination applies to interprofessionalism and mirrors those discussions that are made on creativity research. This suggests the need for approaches which are interdisciplinary, historical, ecological, systemic, critical, and aware of cultural and gender differences (Barron, 1972; Helson, 1990; Montuori, 1989; Runco & Albert, 1990). This richer fabric of complexity prepares us for our next consideration: what is worthy of inquiry as we generate our future professions?

Axiology and Compassion

In normal times, the inquiry for knowledge was based on *the more information and data the better* in order to get closer to having the entire representational map of reality. In post-normal times, there is a greater appreciation for not only *is the knowledge constructed within contexts and dependent on the inquirer* (gone is the illusion of objectivity), but that we have a responsibility to also determine *what is worth knowing* given we are constructing our reality. This question brings us to the concept of axiology, the branch of philosophy that deals with values, or put simply, what is worth knowing? Axiology is a new term to most clinicians as it addresses the very subjective practice of acknowledging what we choose to inquiry about in reality always involves us as the inquirers. This is in direct opposition from the normal times, remote, objective inquirer. Knowing we will never have that complete realism map of normal time, and because we do have limited time and resources, we now need to decide what is worthy of our time? So, what is worthy of our time?

The answer to that question has direct implications to our creativity in rehabilitation. In normal times that question would have been relegated only to a few rare researchers with independent, unlimited funding sources. Everyone else was dependent on what bosses, funding sources and department chairs were interested, as Elgelid delineates in Chapter 5. The clinician got the trickle-down of information from those decisions (remember the reproductive education model...do what has already been done) and the patient was mute in the entire process. With a constructivism ontology and a complex being epistemology, inquiry takes place at all levels of action all of the time, including the patient, hence driving a patient-valued perspective. Out of this new approach, and in combination with the provider and all of the other factors illustrated in our Julie example, new possibilities emerge that would never be valued or considered in the old top-down models of a formal, partitioned understanding of inquiry limited to formal research settings.

So each moment is a decision point for us, no matter the circumstance, as to determining what deserves inquiry at that moment. The creativity operating system transforms the old black and white laboratory-only artificial division of inquiry into a new exciting, unending palette of creative choice through these moment to moment value-based decisions. Every situation is now an inquiry, be it with a patient, student, referral source, coworker, significant other, parent or child. The freedom of choice is exciting, but how do we make these momentary decisions time and time again without some exhausting, plodding process? That's where compassion becomes practical.

Compassion? In our post-normal times state of complex being, it is incumbent that in making value-based decisions on inquiry that our criteria reflect our and our patient's highest values. While these values can be myriad, when we as rehabilitation professionals consider what our calling to our respective vocation is/was, it almost certainly had a strong component of compassion at its core. Com = together + passion/pati = to bear with/suffer with, and speaks to our individual and collective yearning to make meaning and purpose out of our lives by sharing and alleviating suffering with and for others. In post-normal times, we don't have to keep this "subjective" aspiration in the closet anymore. In fact, it moves front and center as a primary filter for every interaction in our lives. Girded to the spiritual aspect of our complex being, when we act in accordance with compassion in our practice, we transform the profane, aloof, distanced healthcare business transaction into a meaningful, sacred vocational response to both our patient's and our own suffering. As Sanford so beautifully illustrates in chapter 2, our rehabbing rehab means we both arrive at the moment with some shared brokenness that becomes the common ground of exploration and creativity in the encounter. We no longer are masquerading as the distant, objective expert dispensing fixes to the broken with a power-over relationship. But how do we do this without getting all mushy and losing our professional boundaries, etc.? It turns out compassion, and its direct relationship with creativity, are far more powerful (and evidence-based!) than we have been told in the past.

Compassion has been the focus of a great deal of study during the past decade. The published findings have fascinating implications for both creativity and rehabilitation. The only known course on compassion in physical therapy advertises compassion as a "non-clinical skill" that affects outcomes. Such a classification represents the normal times parsing of one discipline from another. The course introduces techniques to be employed with patients and colleagues as augmentations rather than the complex, embodied and emergent process the evidence is demonstrating compassion to be. One possible conceptual bridge into a new post-normal times understanding is that compassion is at the center of our core competencies in rehabilitation, as well within our entire complex life outside of rehabilitation work. This proposed understanding is uncertain and open to shift across time. Particularly exciting is the understanding offers a contextual framework for us as rehabilitation professionals to expand our clinic mastery inquiries much differently than any past model and have those inquiries deeply rooted in our subjective social, ethical and political values.

Creativity has been defined as an emergent process, arising out of interactions of a given system and therefore unpredictable (Amabile, 1983; Montuori, 2011a; Sawyer, J.E. 2006; Sawyer, R.K. 1999). Paraphrasing Joan Halifax (2012) note how easily creativity mirrors her dynamic systems definition of compassion, "Compassion [Creativity] is not a discrete feature but an emergent and contingent process that is at its base enactive. Compassion [Creativity] is best primed through the cultivation of various noncompassion [noncreativity] factors. This article endeavors to identify the interdependent components of compassion [creativity]." In short, both compassion and creativity are composed of enactive (how we bring forth meaning via intimate interactions with our environment) emergent processes that arise out of the interaction of a number of noncompassion and noncreative processes. What is especially fascinating is that there are a great deal of shared processes between our value of compassion within our vocation and our present quest for greater creativity.

Both compassion and creativity are at their base dispositionally enactive. In the neti we discarded creativity as brainstorming new ideas. New ideas and innovations out of context and not able to be enacted with a perceived value are not creative. Additionally as illustrated in the Julie tattoo example, the creativity emerges and is contingent upon interaction with the environment and therefore enactive. This enactive view posits all living beings to be fundamentally sense-making creatures to include humans and human organizations. We (Julie and us) bring forth meaning in our intimate interactions with our environments (Thompson, 2007; Thompson, 2009). The term enaction, as originally proposed by Francisco Varela, Evan Thompson, and Eleanor Rosch, is grounded in the interactions between us as living organisms and our environments, and in our embodied action in the world. This constitutes our perception and thereby grounds our cognition. This new perspective transforms creativity and compassion from head-only conceptual realm to a fully embodied and engaged process that unfolds from our and our patients' complex being. Halifax's model offers even more substantiation for adopting this new emerging understanding of creativity.

Creativity can be considered to be a process that is grounded in interrelationality (incomplete in isolation), is mutual (does not arise out of isolation per neti process), reciprocal (affected by relational interaction), and asymmetrical (does not represent some equilibrium between, but has variable degrees of contribution). The Julie tattoo example wasn't creative without the relationship between you and Julie, your mutual interaction from both of your systems of experience, and while initiated and supported by you, only occurred because of "smaller" concurrence and participation by Julie. The word fostering in the title of this book captures this idea suggesting an aspect of cultivation and nurturing much like planting a seed. Initially the asymmetry may appear to be one direction (the one who plants and tends). But then, in the harvest, the other party's contribution may emerge in wholly unexpected and surprising ways much like a plant nourishing others or a sapling growing into a tree, offering a lifetime of aesthetic pleasure. Who is to say how Julie may enact in her life with a new found way to face her life challenges based on this hypothetical rehabilitation experience? Given that potential of surprise of possibility, let's explore the shared elements of factors that came together to allow this creativity to emerge from the compassionate relationship between you and Julie.

Again our new understanding is context sensitive to us as rehabilitation professionals. So understanding this isn't an exhaustive list of all known factors supporting creativity, can we fashion a practical, evidence and value based understanding for our use? Consider the following as just such an understanding.

Because creativity is so nebulous and complex, any explanation needs a skeleton or frame of reference. The bones of this system will draw on what Halifax described as three axes that each hold two domains for cultivating and sustaining compassion. These borrowed bones with some modification also make a great skeleton for creativity in rehabilitation. See the graphic as a starting point before the conceptual explanation of the skeletal relationship.

Halifax proposed the three interdependent experiential modes that appear to prime and optimize compassion from complex beings. We are adapting these axes to prime for creativity and the domains are behaviorally-based practices of noncreative activities that set in motion the potential for creativity to emerge. Because they are experiential, just reading about the practices by definition will be insufficient for creativity to be fostered, hence Part IV of the book will guide us through the practices influencing the domains. While the concepts are presented here in both a graphic and linear description, the three modes are understood to be nonlinear and coemergent even though writing constrains our description to a sequential format.

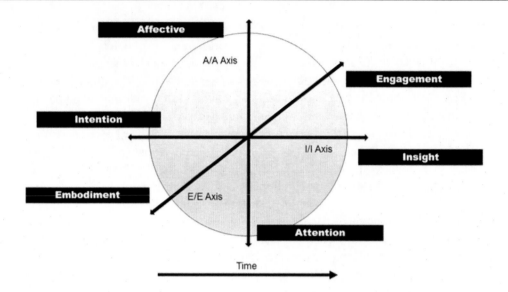

Figure 1. Domains to Prime Creativity.

The three axes create a skeleton that can hold the post-normal reality of the complex being. Together they contain the infrastructure for describing the ubiquitous marketing description of body-mind-spirit, the International Classification of Functioning model of body-mind-environment, and the hallmarks for fostering creativity in rehabilitation. The dynamism of the axes generates cascading levels of insight and possibility as one plays with the heuristic continuous cycles of relationship discovery. In order to begin that play, each domain will be briefly described with the details of each available in Halifax (2012). In Part IV of the book will be practical exercises to cultivate these axes and allow us to ground these conceptual descriptions experientially. For now, in order to sense a more direct clinical application, we will utilize the following short scenario with Julie.

After noticing your neighbor's cat used your rose bed by the garage for a litter box again, you listen to an argumentative talk show about inaccurately portraying climate change while driving your electric car to work. Consumed with the frustrations of the commute, you walk past your longtime receptionist with a dismissive "Hi" completely forgetting it is her birthday. That disappoints her and she in turn is terse with Julie upon her arrival and literally rolls her eyes when Julie asks for some insurance documentation. Julie's mom always rolled her eyes at Julie, more so after she had been drinking heavily. Have fun in your visit with Julie!

THE AXES

Figure 1 illustrates the three axes that may have prevented the above scenario for us and Julie, and definitely will now be needed to find our creative way to save this visit that has begun so poorly. Here's how the each axis comes into play in fostering creativity.

The Attentional/Affective (A/A) Axis

The practices along this axis enhance mental balance, to include concentration, emotional regulation and allocating mental processing resources. Our ability to direct and sustain attention on both our own and the other's (patient, student. colleague, etc.) mental state makes it possible to recognize the presence of suffering with a sustained, selective focus that is otherwise lost with misdirected attention or loss of affective balance. Returning to Julie, your distraction with the neighbor's cat and upsetting talk show produced an unintended affective imbalance in you and then in both the receptionist and now Julie. Had you been able to refocus on the moment and the affective needs of the receptionist as you entered your office, her interaction with Julie would have been different and wouldn't have triggered Julie's habitual response of emotional dysregulation. Her upset will now inhibit her ability to participate in session in an optimal therapeutic state to generate new creative possibilities for her therapy. The question then becomes will you finally re-orient yourself going into the session to re-direct your attention to both of your states, and not become emotionally dysregulated yourself when you realize Julie's affective state, etc., etc.? The goal is to be able to perceive in an unfiltered way the nature of the present suffering and also your own response to that suffering with attentional balance. This ability then grounds your cognitive control to be balanced in a nonjudgmental and nonreactive way for creative emergence.

And how do you sustain attention and become attuned to your and the other's affective state? Now we begin to jump between the bones of the axes. Attentional clarity and balance through mindful embodied practices (the E/E axis) results in decreased susceptibility to the effects of emotionally arousing events and task performance (Ortner, 2007). This embodied attention appears to prime our brain circuits that associate with empathy/affective attunement. One study demonstrated that mindfulness meditation practice from the E/E axis raises both their inner reality awareness (physical, emotional, and cognitive) and of the external reality with which they are engaged (Shapiro, Brown, Biegel, 2007). This balance is dependent on the awareness of the somatic expressions of emotions that offer insight (I/I axis) which then through our intention to practice compassionately redirect us to our or the other's affect, etc., etc., etc. Hopefully this illustrates in a small way the cycles of interaction.

Halifax (2012) goes on to describe how the practices in the A/A axis generate affective processes of kindness and equanimity. She defines kindness as genuine concern with a dispositional tenderness toward others. Equanimity, an emerging buzzword in mindfulness research, is defined as mental balance or a process of stability characterized by mental composure and acceptance of the present moment. Together kindness and equanimity create a foundation of regulated responses for sense making in social interactions, both clinical and ordinary. This balanced easel creates a steadiness for full creative expression in the uncertainty of our post-normal uncertain lives. With this foundation of broadened attentional base and enhanced ability to uncouple negative emotional reactions, we are able to access more resources and have clearer discernment. From that base we move on to further explanations of the other two related axes we have already articulated with the example above.

The Intentional/Insight (I/I) Axis

In describing the I/I axis, Halifax asks what processes beyond the A/A axis allow us to cultivate compassion and not fall into reactions of "avoidance, abandonment, numbness or moral outrage" that would inhibit our rehabilitation care? She proposes that our focused attention and ability to guide our mind with the intention to be compassionate generates insights about the suffering, the suffering's origins and how to transform suffering in a creative emergence. The double I's of intention and insight refer to our cognitive dimension of experience and as we've seen, interact in conjunction with the other axes. Reciprocally our intention and insight also prime our attention and affective balance. Again our complex being reveals that this weave of attentional, affective, cognitive and somatic domains are interlaced and intimately further associated with our social, cultural, and environmental fabric. Our ability to appreciate a broader palette of the full nature of the suffering (patients, students and us!) allows for the emergence of novel and effective insight, as well as action not otherwise available in our care. This I/I axis, or bone of insight and intention, warrants a bit more explanation.

Again this model of creativity is built on premise of the shared intention of rehabilitation professionals' to transform suffering for others and ourselves through creative service. This intention primes our creativity while being inseparable from our subjective professional and personal ethics. No more cold, distant separate compartment of "objective" care of the normal times that is not affected by our personal ethics and choices. The ongoing practices of the axes then raise our clinical mastery to allow us to deeply touch the other AND utilize objective discernment as tools available to best transform suffering. There always has been, and will continue to be, a dance of awareness and response to our aversive reactions to situations that arise out of our conditioning. As with Julie's tattoo, the practices of these axes provide the ability to override our otherwise habitual responses, engage in a more positive reappraisal, and then downregulate arousal or shift away from thoughts and behaviors that in past might have stymied a more creative engagement. This grounding intention to be open to the experience of the other while attending to our own experience sets the additional foundation for insights of how we best serve unselfishly.

Insight is the other domain of this I/I axis. The insight domain can be confused with our popular neti neti prior understanding of "thinking outside the box", the Eureka flash, and "lone genius" experiences. This new model of the interactions of the 3 axes, however, reveals the weave of how each domain informs and makes possible insight AND how insight then affects each of them in turn and not in isolation. All of these practices prime the ability to adapt meta-cognitive perspectives while nurturing mental pliancy and autonomy (Halifax 2012). This enhanced perspective taking includes cognitive attunement with the other, allowing us to understand the experiences of the other. It also sustains the related ability to support insight into distinguishing between one's self and the other, without which could lead to the traditional ethical concerns about keeping distant barriers, etc. This accurate sense making of the unfolding moments with the A/A foundation supports creative responses while diminishing the risk for conflated or habituated responses. All of which leads to possibly one of the most difficult aspects of this model of creativity, but as usual, paradoxically also the fun of surprise.

The difficult aspect is that within the post-normal times worldview we need to paradoxically try with all our might to affect suffering AND let go of our attachment to the outcome of our interaction. Reread that sentence and sit with it a moment. Anathema to the old mantra of predictability and control of outcomes, this perspective holds both as is further described in chapter 4 on EBM. For now, consider what Halifax defines as the perspective of therapeutic humility. Suddenly we are sliding down to the bones of the A/A axis noting the emotional response to such a perspective, while sustaining attention to the thoughts and insights that arise in the insight domain as we imagine trying to practice with such a paradoxical intention of humility. Inability or refusal to acknowledge any of these domain, as well as the embodied responses of the moment will affect our engagement as explained in the E/E axis below. The good news is that when we do utilize all of these bones of experience there emerges the opening for surprise within this presence emergence, where by suffering can be transformed in ways never predicted or anticipated. And so we let go as these interdependent bones of domains produce mental pliancy and discernment that prime enactive, context-sensitive creativity.

THE EMBODIMENT/ENGAGED (E/E) AXIS

As rehabilitation professions, these domains of the somatic or physical E/E axis may be the most familiar to most of us professionally, but not what we may have considered to be important in regards to our creativity. Emerging science is revealing how attention, practice, and behavior alter both function and structure of our very anatomy and physiology via neuroplasticity, epigenetic function and the exhibition of altruistic behaviors, including compassion. This experiential E/E axis celebrates these new facts and demands our engagement with these domains to foster the greatest emergence of possibility in our rehabilitation practices. What we sense, how we move, and why we move are essential to our effectiveness and our creative capacity not just at work, but in every aspect of our lives. The walls of separation between how we sit, breathe, sense and take action have come down. These new insights are an invitation to us for experiencing so many more rich, life enhancing intersubjective and interactive processes associated with creativity.

The embodied dimension of the intersubjective and interactive processes associated with creativity are based on the enactive experiences where body, mind and environment are contexts for each other. Our embodiment is the source of our felt sense of suffering, both the other's and our own. The empathy of the A/A axis arises out of our ability to literally sense the other's state through that affective attunement. Because of this grounding in our body sensation, it is incumbent we attend to our own embodied experience along this axis as we engage in our lives. This attention connects our interoceptivity and our own visceral experience as key to priming empathy. Without such attention, we end up guessing or worse yet, ignoring the deepest understanding of the suffering of the other and all of the potential insights from such an enactive relationship. This subjective embodied experience of our embeddedness in the world gives rise to our enaction via perception, cognition and the actions of our engagements via our bodies. Put more simply, it really is all connected. No longer is creativity a mental thinking up something new, but a moment of unfolding across all three axes with enormous implications. To be truly creative we must be able to enact that insight with our environment in useful and valued ways aligned with our ethics.

Our engagement domain takes us beyond wishing for better and invites the harder half of creativity (the idea being the easy half), which is executing the idea as we will explore in Chapters 7 and 8. The courage, perseverance and focus to see the old normal time view of creativity as just a novel idea through to the actual engagement in rehabilitation will need the skeleton of creative axes. The courage to face resistance from others, the ability to move in fear of the unknown, and the return to try again after numerous setbacks will all be enhanced by this model as you will read in Part III accounts of our colleagues. As we practice this creative being, we model for Julie, colleagues and peers an attractive and inviting new way of operating in the world. As each of us discovers how richly the world and our bodies prime new understanding, fresh new ways of operating will transform us and our rehabilitation world. And it's OK that we aren't certain how that "*vastly further from the current design of care*" emerges, we will be engaged and a vital part of the creativity that fosters the new design. For as Cleese and the others of Monty Python soothingly prophesied from their creative operating, "Blessed are the cheesemakers…."

A Pause

Pause just a moment and reflect on this new model of creativity in rehabilitation. Consider that this embedded neurophysiological explanation would have been just some New Age tale not too long ago. Now we can delight in the weave of the emerging science around neuroplasticity, training effects, environmental influences, epigenomics, and interpersonal neurobiology as we glimpse the evolving understanding of creative possibilities expanding in real time. This expansion of possibilities is much (just?) like how the known universe unfolds: Technology allows us to explore more deeply both inward and outward in life's creative emergence on every scale of perception available to us, from the far reaches of time and the edge of the known universe to the blinking bits of sub-atomic Higgs Boson particles and dark matter. Even better, this proliferation of creativity is no longer reserved for those peak brief experiences of a normal times understanding, but is readily available in every ordinary moment.

Ordinary Time

The concept of ordinary creativity bears a bit more emphasis. Our vocation to identify and relieve suffering through compassionate interaction is no longer constrained to specific clinical interventions. As complex beings, we understand every moment of our life as an invitation to creativity, even in the most ordinary moments. And each of these ordinary moments via the 3 axes will affect our rehabilitation experiences ultimately even if distant in time or location. The implications we discuss in the next section of this new understanding are truly radical in transforming how we act and engage our lives within and beyond our professional responsibilities. Ordinary creativity also has tremendous implications when we begin to explore the decades and centuries' old power dynamics around creativity in chapters 5 and 6.

How do our ordinary time responses apply to our creativity in rehabilitation? One way to envision this concept is the metaphor we have been using of life as a single fabric, to include all of what we do as rehabilitation professionals. Over 70 years ago, Angyal (1941) argued that what is needed to understand complexity is a shift from elementary single units to systems viewed as a unitas multiplex, or complex unity. The Latin root of the word complex, complexus, means different elements interlaced together to form a single fabric. In fact, another characteristic of complexity is its unity in diversity AND diversity within a unity. The fabric of life is composed of many threads. Tweak one thread and the entire fabric is affected; change the whole fabric, every thread is affected. Hopefully the vignettes around Julie have been an example to better appreciate this metaphor.

So this ordinary creativity enlivens every moment of our day as each thread of interaction does affect the whole fabric. Consequently the development of our ability to regulate our responses moment to moment is paramount to not block the emergence of creativity by our or someone we encounter's dysregulation, and thereby default to reactivity in habituated, uncreative behaviors.

This is a huge responsibility. At this point, retreating to the old normal times understanding of creativity may have some attraction! How do we sustain this heavy responsibility of creativity? How can we always be primed to respond creatively in every moment?

Short answer, we can't and won't. When we err, or on our reflection in silence come to insight of where we fell short, that is where the self-compassion practice emerges. We aren't in control, we won't be, and that is alright. Post-normal times embrace this uncertainty rather than flog us to press harder to reach control and perfection. Each time that we can smile softly at our limitations in our reflections and then re-commit to our intention of compassion, it is one more practice of affective regulation that over time transforms our anatomy and physiology via neuroplasticity to create a greater capacity for a creative response the next time. Literally our practices create the continuous quality improvement of our clinical mastery via our embodied response to failures. Now the responsibility of every moment becomes the gift to create within this marvelous virtuous loop of complex being. These virtuous loops have refreshing implications for our rehabilitation practice as well.

THE IMPLICATIONS OF THE NEW UNDERSTANDING

Any new understanding of the relationship between creativity and complex being ought to be rooted in at least one of the domains just described. The understanding should also be applicable to both extraordinary and ordinary creativity. The implications of this new understanding as rehabilitation professionals can be understood by briefly noting the research changes around creativity and then revisiting our neti neti practice from the beginning of this chapter. From there we will prepare to enact our innate creativity.

Research

There are strong indications that in the 21st century, the discourse and practices of creativity are changing dramatically (Montuori, 2011b; Pachucki et al., 2010). In the post-normal, non-deified cosmology, creativity is the fundamental nature of the universe—the process of creation itself, rather than the spark of a (C/c) creator. It is therefore a basic "every day, everyone, everywhere" human capacity. Creativity is described now as networked, ecological, historical, and relational process rather than an isolated phenomenon (Barron, 1995; Harrington, 1990; Kearney, 1988; Montuori, 1989; Montuori & Purser, 1999; Sawyer, J.E. 2006).

Additional research has demonstrated that our understanding of creativity is indeed paradoxical/cybernetic. In the characteristics of the creative person, process, product, and environment are found to be seemingly incompatible terms. For instance, creativity requires both order and disorder, rigor and imagination, hard work and play, idea generation and idea selection, times of introspection and solitude and times of interaction and exchange; the relationship is one of cybernetic "navigation" rather than exclusively either/or choice (Barron, 1995; Csikszentmihalyi, 1990; Hampden-Turner, 1999; Montuori, 2011a; Rothenberg, 1979). The exercises in Part IV allow for experiencing these paradoxes first hand.

Burkus's (2014) book is a good summary source of recent research. The most recent emerging research on, and practices of creativity can be summarized in the following propositions as facets of facilitating the gem of creative emergence, but now understood to not be just followed like a recipe to train one's creativity. These facets are derived from our initial neti neti practice, and the previous disclaimer sentence holds that these facets too are paradoxically neti neti!

Creativity isn't:

- A skill or talent, but an emergent process.
- Limited to a few, but a way each of us can operate.
- An abandonment of conventional care, but rests on our traditional rigorous disciplines.
- Expressed in isolation, but is imbedded in our many environments and dependent on interaction with others.
- A thing you do, but a process that emerges from the practice of other behaviors you practice.
- A pattern of brain activity, but the brain participates and changes in the process of creativity.
- Contrary to EBM, but the core of clinical mastery.
- Easy or simple, but worth the risk and effort compared to the boredom of the rote and safe.
- Something done to patients, but something that we do 'with' patients when we do a best practice of rehabilitation.
- Threatening, but is often stifled by institutions and systems processes.
- Taught in graduate rehabilitation programs, but should be.
- Haphazard or impractical, but the outgrowth of the creativity process must be deemed useful and practical to be truly creative.
- A new fad, but it's what Life has been doing since the Big Bang or whatever cosmological explanation you believe in first began.
- A Eureka moment, but requires a time of incubation, where ideas and relevant knowledge linger in the subconscious.
- A certain breed, expert or personality type, but some level of expertise matters, and often involves those on the fringes of the subject area who know enough to

understand but not enough to constrain their thinking or perspective. Those who continue at high levels of productivity are the ones who cultivate outsider mindsets by constantly learning new fields and applying those new lessons to old challenges.

- Wholly original or without context, but novelty comes from the combination or application of other knowledge, not the idea itself.
- Driven by external motivation, but is driven by intrinsic motivation, and unless an incentive is aligned with intrinsic desires, the incentive won't have an effect.
- The result of brainstorming, but requires various stages. Almost all fixed creative methods (from creative problem solving to design thinking) as described in chapter 1 describe a period of rapid idea generation, but then time where ideas are combined and externalized.
- Without conflict, but building in some conflict can facilitate a creative process and the presence of conflicting opinions and emotions can be a sign that new ideas are being brought forward.
- Due to an absence of limitations, but constraints can give structure to the challenge to enhance better understanding and insights.
- Just innovation or something new, but should be in line with ethics and add to the flourishing of life.
- Hiring some creative people or making providers or patients more creative, but appreciating the need to get better at recognizing the creativity in one another.
- Just the result of competition or collaboration. Competition and collaboration are variables, but not recipe ingredients to control outcomes.

It may be helpful to hold this new understanding of creativity as akin to a new operating system update on your computer or phone. It isn't so much that version 1.0 of creativity was wrong, but limited in function, just like that old computer system. As we roll out and create a 2.0 version of creativity, there are many new features to discover, but along the way probably more than a few glitches or awkward learning moments as well. That's going to be fine, as your axes of creativity are also your built-in and responsive tech support system. Rather than racing to flip through the manual, we now start by going to silence, practicing along the axes in the various domains, knowing the search is the process, not the problem. The normal times worldview will still creep back time to time wanting to just know how to do it or have "them" do it. That will create it's own set of somatic, embodied responses to cue you to reassess your thinking and subsequently your actions as you engage this new, slippery shifting way of being in the world. The word "radical" comes from the word *root*. Adopting this new creative operating system is a radical departure from our former understanding, and as such uproots or disturbs nearly all of the old roots. The implications are many and will continual to unfold daily as we move and sit still in our worlds. We need only know that the adoption of the new system will be both exhilarating and terrifying at once.

One tool we have in rehabilitation to soften this wild ride is an expression you have undoubtedly used with patients in the past. We often describe our work with patients as facilitating change/function/education etc. Interestingly, the word facilitate has as one of its definitions "to make magic." The creative powers of our new operating system will make seem "easy" what was before hard or impossible, but it isn't conjuring or trickery. Rather, by accessing the practices of the axes, we will participate more completely with the unfolding of life that in our post-normal times humility is appropriate and fulfilling both personally and professionally. The sharing of this process to rehabilitate our respective disciplines and share with and invite participation from our "Julies" will be radically transformed.

CONCLUSION

In summary our understanding of creativity has been shaped by our cultures, our beliefs in what and who we are, and our professional education's biases about how we deliver rehabilitation services and why. You were promised a new definition at the beginning of this chapter. Hopefully you can now appreciate what a tall order that was. As rehabilitation professionals, consider this one and change it as you wish:

> "Creativity in rehabilitation is our (your and the patient's) participation more fully in practices that facilitate the emergence of a renewed flourishing of our being at home in our circumstances."

Now before that "magic" appears, we need to explore what Govindarajan & Trimble (2013) describes as the other side of the innovation coin. The insight and new direction is the relatively easy side of the coin. Good ideas are everywhere according to Trimble. So while we are eager to start and that willingness to start is important, we first need to know more about the other bigger side of the coin: executing those ideas into enactment in our and our patient's world. The following chapters are like high-quality GPS maps of the terrain we are approaching. Time spent orienting returns substantial benefit before heading out on our adventure. Our first atlas is to discover how the new creativity transforms EBM to better guide our trip.

REFERENCES

Amabile, T. (1983). *The social psychology of creativity.* New York: Springer.

Angyal, A. (1941). *Foundations for a science of personality.* Cambridge, MA: Harvard University Press.

Barron, F. (1995). *No rootless flower: Thoughts on an ecology of creativity.* Creskill, NJ: Hampton Press.

Barron, F. (1972). Towards an ecology of consciousness. *Inquiry, 15,* 95-113.

Bellah, R., Madsen, R., Sullivan, W., Swidler, A., & Tipton, S. (1985). *Habits of the heart.* Berkeley, CA: University of California Press.

Burkus, D. (2014). *The myths of creativity.* San Francisco: Jossey-Bass.

Ceruti, M. (1986). *Il vincolo e la possibilita`.* Milano, Italy: Feltrinelli. English Translation (1994). *Constraints and possibilities. The evolution of knowledge and knowledge of evolution.* New York: Gordon & Breach.

Ceruti, M. (1989). *La danza che crea. [The creative dance].* Milano, Italy: Feltrinelli.

Eisler, R., Potter, T.M. (2014).Transforming interprofessional partnerships: A new framework for nursing and partnership-based health care. *Sigma Theta Tau,* Indianapolis, IN.

Emery, F. E. (Ed.). (1969). *Systems thinking: Selected readings.* London: Penguin Books.

Govindarajan, V., Trimble, C. (2013). *Beyond the idea.* New York: St. Martin's Press.

Halifax, J. (2012). A heuristic model of enactive compassion. *Curr Opin Support Palliat Care Vol 6* 2: 228-235.

Hampden-Turner, C. (1999). Control, chaos, control: A cybernetic view of creativity. In R. Purser & A. Montuori (Eds.), *Social Creativity (Vol. 2).* Cresskill, NJ: Hampton Press.

Hampden-Turner, C., Trompenaars, A. (1993). *The seven cultures of capitalism.* New York: Doubleday.

Harrington, D. (1990). The ecology of human creativity: A psychological perspective. In M. Runco, & R. Albert (Eds.), *Theories of Creativity.* (pp. 143-169). Newbury Park, CA: Sage.

Helson, R. (1990). Creativity in women: Inner and outer views over time. In M. Runco, & R. Albert (Eds.), *Theories of Creativity.* (pp. 46-58) Newbury Park, CA: Sage.

Kearney, R. (1988). *The wake of imagination: Toward a postmodern culture.* Minneapolis, MN: University of Minnesota Press.

Laszlo, E. (1991). *The age of bifurcation. Understanding our changing world.* New York: Gordon & Breach.

Montuori, A. (1989). *Evolutionary competence: Creating the future.* Amsterdam, Netherlands: Gieben.

Montuori, A. (2011a). Systems approach. In M. Runco & S. Pritzker (Eds.), *The encyclopedia of creativity (Vol. 2,* 414–421). San Diego, CA: Academic Press.

Montuori, A. (2011b). Beyond postnormal times: The future of creativity and the creativity of the future. Futures: *The Journal of Policy, Planning and Future Studies, 43*(2), 221–227.

Montuori, A. & Purser, R. (1997). Le dimensioni sociali della creatività. *Pluriverso, 1, 2,* 78-88.

Montuori, A., & Purser, R. (1999a). Introduction. In A. Montuori & R. Purser (Eds.), *Social Creativity (Vol. 1).* Cresskill, NJ: Hampton Press.

Morin, E. (1983). *Il Metodo. Ordine disordine organizzazione. [Method. Order disorder organization.]* Milano, Feltrinelli. [Eng. trans. (1992), *Method. The nature of nature.* New York: Peter Lang.

Morin, E. (1992). The concept of system and the paradigm of complexity. In M. Maruyama (Ed.), *Context and Complexity. Cultivating contextual understanding.* (pp.125-136) New York: Springer-Verlag.

Ortner, C.N.M., Kilner, S.J., Zelazo, P.D. (2007). Mindfulness meditation and reduced emotional interference on a cognitive task. *Motivation Emotion, 31,* 271–283.

Pachucki, M. A., Lena, J. C., & Tepper, S. J. (2010). Creativity narratives among college students: Sociability and everyday creativity. *Sociological Quarterly, 51,*122–149.

Rothenberg, A. (1979). *The emerging goddess: The creative process in art, science, and other fields.* Chicago: University of Chicago Press.

Runco, M. & Albert, R. (Eds.), (1990). *Theories of Creativity.* Newbury Park, CA: Sage.

Sampson, E. (1993). *Celebrating the Other. A dialogic account of human nature.* Boulder, CO: Westview Press.

Sawyer, J. E. (2006). *Explaining creativity: The science of human innovation.* Oxford, NY: Oxford University Press.

Sawyer, R. K. (1999). The emergence of creativity. *Philosophical Psychology, 12,* 447–469.

Shapiro, S.L., Brown, K.W., Biegel, G.M. (2007). Teaching self-care to caregivers: Effects of mindfulness-based stress reduction on the mental health of therapists in training. *Train Educ Prof Psychology, 1:*105–115.

Thompson, E. (2007). *Mind in life: Biology, phenomenology, and the sciences of mind.* Cambridge, MA: Harvard University Press.

Thompson, E., Stapleton, M. (2009). Making sense of sense-making: Reflections on enactive and extended mind theories. *Topoi , 28,* 23–30.

Torrance, E. P. (1988). The nature of creativity as manifest in its testing. In Sternberg, R. (Ed.), *The nature of creativity.* (pp.43-75). Cambridge: University Press.

Wilden, A. (1980). *System and structure: Essays in communication and exchange.* London: Tavistock.

In: Fostering Creativity in Rehabilitation
Editor: Matthew J. Taylor

ISBN: 978-1-63485-118-3
© 2016 Nova Science Publishers, Inc.

Chapter 4

CREATIVITY AND EVIDENCE-BASED MEDICINE

Matthew J. Taylor, PT, PhD
Director, Matthew J. Taylor Institute, Scottsdale, AZ, US

ABSTRACT

This chapter builds on the new understanding of creativity based on the complexity of being. It begins with a review of the development of evidence-based medicine (EBM) and the original intentions of the three components (clinical mastery, patient values and research evidence). A discussion of the current day shortcomings and misuses of EBM sets the stage for optimizing how EBM should be a powerful force of innovation in the future. Each component is revisited based on the new understanding with guidelines to foster creative emergence while honoring a best practice of rehabilitation. This analysis sets the stage then for the subsequent chapters that visit in details other practice aspects that affect creative emergence in rehabilitation.

INTRODUCTION

People like Julie are trapped in the conundrum of evidence-based medicine (EBM). Her unique, chronic, complex challenges by definition means there won't be any published research available with high level evidence to direct her care. Those same people who can't find answers in the conventional system often however begin to look elsewhere for relief and fall prey to all manner of modern snake oil and charlatanism. Julie has been unable to obtain the relief she seeks from the literature, her professional community, and the various individual providers. What is she to do next? This chapter explores this dilemma about the current limits of EBM as it exists and its exciting potential in light of our new understanding of creativity from the last chapter.

EBM should be a catalyst for substantive, dramatic change and evolution rather than just small incremental adjustments to our knowledge base. EBM has a tremendous potential to foster creativity in rehabilitation, especially to support someone with complex challenges such as Julie. Those two statements probably caused some of us to nod our heads in thoughtful concurrence, while others of us may have shook our heads side to side in dismay at the 'obvious' incongruity of pairing creativity with EBM. That polarization of opinion is the state of EBM today.

This chapter explores that polarization by beginning with a succinct history of the development of EBM which explains how we have such a dichotomy of perspectives about creativity and EBM. That history offers a valuable context to understand the misuses and shortcomings of EBM's current contribution to creativity within rehabilitation today. From that context we build a vision for how all three components of EBM can foster creativity while satisfying the best practice concerns of even our most conservative colleagues.

THE DEVELOPMENT OF EBM

In order to make sense of the current state of EBM, it is helpful to review how EBM developed over time. Before we dive into those details, the first thing to consider is the worldview or paradigm from which EBM emerged. In the Preface Montuori described Sardar's terminology for the larger social shift of worldviews presently underway. We are shifting from the age of predictability and surety that characterized the former normal times to what Sardar now describes as postnormal times. Postnormal times are a new worldview that acknowledges the uncertainty of reality, to include medicine, and the perils of forecasting future outcomes to include complex human circumstances such as Julie's.

The normal times perspective would insist there was one right answer to whether EBM does or does not foster creativity in rehabilitation, also referred to as the 'either/or' worldview. Either it does or doesn't, and those are the two choices. The postnormal perspective maintains that the answer to that question is probably 'yes' to both EBM fosters and thwarts creativity, or the 'and' worldview. If we understand that this tension exists between the two worldviews, then we hold the key to unleashing EBM's potential to foster creativity in the future.

As we proceed, notice during the following chapters when you read something that evokes a strong response of either approval or disapproval, and ask yourself, from which worldview am I considering this statement? Neither is right or wrong, but practicing the noticing and becoming aware of which view you are operating from is a powerful exercise to foster your creative expression.

The term "evidence-based medicine (EBM)" is relatively new with investigators from McMaster's University first using the term during the 1990s. EBM's philosophical origins however extend back to mid-19th century Paris and earlier (Gray, Muir et al., 1996). The concept and impetus for EBM can be attributed to an increasing awareness during the 1970's and 1980's of the very real weaknesses of standard clinical practices and their impact on both the quality and cost of patient care in the United States (Sackett, 1969; Sackett, Rosenberg, Gray, Haynes, Richardson 1996).

There were efforts from a number of areas of medicine to bring more certainty to clinical decision making that spurred this novel approach to practice. Clinical practice had historically been viewed as the "art of medicine" rather than the science. The clinical authority of expert opinion, experience, and authoritarian judgment were the foundation for decision making with little or no correlation to research findings or patient values. The use of scientific methodology, as in biomedical research and statistical analysis, were rare in the world of medicine to include rehabilitation. Knowledge during this era was shared through textbooks and eventually peer-reviewed journals that were not readily accessible to most clinicians. The original, or classic EBM was founded on the principle that uncertainty could be minimized by bringing the burgeoning new research knowledge together with clinical mastery and patient values in a new form of medicine.

Technology has had a large role in the advancement of EBM. Computers and database software today have allowed compilation of large amounts of data. This wasn't the case when the person credited with bringing EBM to the forefront, Dr. David Sackett, shared his early vision in the 1969 that clinical epidemiology was "the application, by a physician who provides direct patient care, of epidemiological and biometric methods to the study of diagnostic and therapeutic process in order to effect an improvement in health (Sur & Dahm, 2011). EBM was initially defined as "a systemic approach to analyze published research as the basis of clinical decision making." Then in 1996, the term was more formally defined by Sackett et al., who stated that EBM was "the conscientious and judicious use of current best evidence from clinical care research in the management of individual patients." The Index Medicus was the gold standard of resources for such evidence, but has since been replaced by the Internet and in 1993 the founding of the Cochrane Collaboration. This modern gold standard collaboration is committed to 10 principles: collaboration, building on enthusiasm of individuals, avoiding duplication, minimizing bias, keeping up-to-date, striving for relevance, promoting access, ensuring quality, continuity, and worldwide participation (Sur & Dahm, 2011). We will later evaluate how successfully these principles have been achieved. In hindsight, one thing we know for certain is that rehabilitation then by guesswork and opinion was not some romantic Eden of creativity as it may occasionally be imagined in nostalgic pinings for the early days of rehabilitation.

The Intention Behind the 3 Components of EBM

EBM in rehabilitation can be defined as the conscientious, explicit, and judicious use of current best evidence in making decisions about the care of individual patients, to include Julie. EBM is properly understood then as not just research evidence, but care equally informed by clinical mastery and patient values. The practice of EBM in rehabilitation means integrating individual clinical expertise with the best available external clinical evidence from systematic research. Individual clinical expertise (mastery) is the proficiency and judgment that we individual clinicians acquire through clinical experience and clinical practice. Increased expertise is reflected in many ways, but especially in more effective and efficient assessment and in the thoughtful identification and compassionate use of individual patients' circumstances, rights, and preferences in creating and carrying out their rehabilitation plan of care. Properly executed, EBM uses external clinical evidence to both invalidate previously accepted tests and treatments and replaces them with new ones that are more powerful, more accurate, more efficacious, and safer. In effect, creating better rehabilitation.

EBM is still very much evolving, Let us look at where we are today which still leaves such a division of appreciation for EBM among medical professionals despite the best early intentions.

CURRENT SHORTCOMINGS AND MISUSES OF EBM

Succinctly, along the way EBM has been co-opted by some to preserve the normal times yearning for certainty and predictability. Greenhalgh, Howick, and Maskrey (Greenhalgh, Howick, & Maskrey 2014) Maskrey, offered an extensive summary of this phenomenon with an excellent bibliography in their 2014 analysis. Seen through the normal times lens, EBM has come to be interpreted by some in a manner that produces a tired, unidirectional model of care that has left us with the circumstances described by Taylor and Sanford in the first two chapters. In that interpretation, the care provider is the expert and knows best, delivers the known best treatment and the passive patient consumes that expert service. No wonder EBM is sometimes described as "cookbook" rehabilitation given such a perception of EBM. Elgelid and Garner describe in detail how in some cases EBM has been used to preserve power, control reimbursement and impede creativity leading to what appears to be cookbook applications of EBM. These instances have led others to claim that it transforms the complex process of clinical decision making—which includes data gathering, years of rehabilitation knowledge, experience, and astute intuition—into an algorithmic exercise that is not individualized for specific clinical scenarios and therefore subject to error in patient care. This is most clearly seen in the over-reliance by many on the random control trial (RCT) studies. RCTs are not certainty (the normal time quest) but are simply a comparison of one treatment to another treatment, rather than some superior form of truth. Those same factions too often rely on these epidemiological tools, and when they do, their form of EBM does not incorporate the "soft" data that clinicians use to formulate diagnoses and treatments.

These "soft" data include type and severity of symptoms, and rate of growth of illness. Additionally, social and political contexts within which patients live are also not addressed in that form of EBM. Lastly, critiques of EBM cite the potential for abuse of the label "best available evidence." Health care policy makers and both government and private payers can coerce and justify reimbursement based on the "best available evidence" and marginalize practice that does not conform to these standards. For someone like Julie, there is no evidence to suggest what to do next, so treatment can be denied or terminated by the purchasers and managers to cut the costs of health care. At that point the model becomes a reflection of the power-over relationship of a dominator rather than partnership model of the payer over both the provider and the patient as further described in Chapter 6 by Garner.

Clinical Prediction Rules (CPRs) have been widely discussed and advocated in the literature in recent years as a further expression of the sought after certainty toward treatment choices. Not unexpectedly, as we move deeper into the postnormal times of complexity and uncertainty, the research is catching up to reflect the limitations of CPRs in conditions that are either chronic or complex. These limitations begin to bridge us into the post-normal understanding of EBM as we see that CPRs have utility in some instances, especially acute conditions, AND lack utility in many others where they have attempted to address more complex conditions across time. It is our collective wake up call to face these limitations of EBM after decades of failing to examine the assumptions behind the old normal times "objective" quantitative mantra of RCTs and CPRs. We in rehabilitation are not alone in witnessing the constant discoveries of uncertainties and complexities that describe reality for everything from physics to genomics. Epigenomics and multiverse theories of cosmology suggest to us that we ought to take on a more nuanced use of research evidence. While this dashes the initial hopes for more certainty in care models, once it can accepted, the acceptance clears the way to greater creativity. (To be clear, the founders however were calling for "minimizing uncertainty" and "judicious use" of evidence in contrast to the above co-opted, polarized adaptations of EBM.) With such uncertainty and complexity in these postnormal times, how then might we use EBM?

One area rich in potential is to consider the limited applications thus far of the other two aspects of EBM: clinical mastery and patient values. The present dominant use of EBM undervalues both of these aspects. Clinical mastery has been largely a heady, conceptual critical thinking-only process of reflection when it is consulted. Any other insight or direction derived from that introspective attention is held in suspicion as invalid or "non-scientific." This leaves no place for empathy, compassion or intuition which are literally described as "non-clinical" skills by some evidence backers in physical therapy that have only recently begun to acknowledge that those same skills are however important in outcomes. Scarcer yet, at least in the physical therapy world, has been the valuing of the therapist's felt, somatic responses during and after treatment as evidence to influence care. This would include that depth of silence of not-knowing in the introduction of Julie, as well as Sanford's Chapter 2 and our new understanding of creativity from Chapter 3. Suggestions for adopting these practices are in the final section of this chapter, but first some additional observations regarding the related shortcomings.

Ideally as rehabilitation professionals we should also be asking, "What evidence is practical and results in human flourishing?" To begin with this question first would be a sharp contrast to what so often happens with the minutia of data generated that lacks any practical application and value to the providers or consumers. The current EBM focus has been on the rank order of the quality of evidence—less on the application of evidence to a particular clinical scenario and its potential to enhance human experience. The third-leg of EBM, patient values, suggests this practicality and value be considered, and yet so many journals and conferences drill down to arcane or impractical results that leave clinical practice little changed. Elgelid expounds on some of these influences in Chapter 5.

Beyond a greater focus on patient values, EBM should also address whether the care supports the health and flourishing of the rehabilitation professional too. So often the business models of healthcare and reimbursement have generated a gulf between what we know is best practice as clinical masters and what the systems allow us to do (and this is even recognized by student novices at times). This gulf has very real impact on our own health and our risk for burnout and compassion fatigue. How to address these shortcomings is detailed in the next section regarding methods of incorporation of our flourishing and values for our creative expression.

But first, and finally, there's the issue of financial sustainability and right livelihood for our services. We as rehabilitation professionals can literally no longer afford to be irrelevant to the end-users as was outlined in detail Chapter 1. Practical creative clinical mastery is going to be key in pay for performance relationships, be the reimbursement through formal health systems or direct consumption by the community from the provider. Our ability to meet and support patients as complex as Julie while drawing on our own embodied mastery and what she values is going to be critical. For those of us that have stepped outside the insurance system already, we know failure on our part to adapt, create and provide practical valued service each visit will lead to open spaces in our schedules and financial shortcomings the next visit because the patient quite simply won't come back. If the internet or some less expensive, possibly less qualified (sic) provider can meet the patients' needs, we are then technically irrelevant, even if we can wave the high-level evidence article about our technique generating statistically significant changes in some outcome. Creativity demands much from each of us in order to practice EBM, but then so too do our patients. Let's rehabilitate EBM while we rehabilitate rehabilitation!

How EBM Can Foster Creativity

Good rehabilitation practitioners use both individual clinical expertise and the best available external evidence matched to patient values, as none of the facets alone is enough. Without clinical expertise, practice risks becoming tyrannized by evidence, for even excellent external evidence may be inapplicable to or inappropriate for an individual patient. Without current best evidence, practice risks becoming rapidly out of date, to the detriment of patients. Great evidence paired with great practice expertise but having no value for the patient, does nothing to restore health. How then might EBM resolve Julie's dilemma about her next steps in executing a best practice for herself? Is there a way to allow the provider to fully harness the power that is possible in the rehabilitation process for both of them? Insight can be gained to these questions by combining the original intentions for EBM we reviewed above and modifying the assumptions that underlie the present day shortcomings of EBM just described.

This next section of the chapter develops those insights further in order to enhance our appreciation of how EBM and creativity do fit well together. Pairing creativity and EBM produces a robust roadmap forward into the emerging future of rehabilitation. We will address all three components in turn, beginning with the most familiar component of EBM, the research evidence.

Research Evidence

In Chapter 3 we emphasized that contrary to popular misconceptions about creativity being a call for "anything goes," creativity in rehabilitation demands an even higher level of rigor than conventional care. Being creative doesn't ignore research evidence. Instead it becomes the ultimate big box of crayons from which we choose draw from and also help point to future spectrum of additional inquiry and discovery. This section isn't just for researchers. These opportunities are available to researchers, educators and clinicians alike. So let's all enjoy that childhood memorable smell from the new box of crayons of creative research evidence.

Evidence based medicine is not restricted to randomized trials and meta-analyses. It involves tracking down the best external evidence with which to answer our clinical questions. If no randomized trial has been carried out for our patient's predicament, we must follow the trail to the next best external evidence and work from there. Each form of research inquiry has its own inherent strengths and weaknesses. Changes in technology for managing the sheer volume of qualitative and participatory research data from qualitative and action research now make those types of studies, along with mixed methods studies, much for feasible and play to the qualitative strengths of generating new understanding in complex situations.

Earlier in EBM development the research inquiry was asking how we can better know if what we are doing is the best, most efficacious practice. These inquiries were founded on the perspective of realism that there is one way reality is, and with research we can find the best way to utilize that reality to control outcomes. This perspective was the hallmark of what Sardar calls normal times. Just as our clientele are becoming more complex, so to must our ways of inquiry. Now in postnormal times, we understand that how we can come to know a best practice in complex human interactions such as rehabilitation is rarely certain. Therefore we need to expand our tools and methods (think crayons) of inquiry to capture the nuances and new possibilities that postnormal times hold for rehabilitation. Fortunately the power of technological developments gives us the ability to hold the richer complexity of these new tools and for clinicians to access the results in ways unimaginable 20 years ago. In order to create an ease of review rather than dense paragraphs, consider the following factors:

1. Research Methods: In addition to the normal time valued RCT, we need to appreciate the development of qualitative research, especially the action research methods, and the increased ease of running mixed methods studies in both data processing and reporting through the more flexible multi-media electronic formats. Each type of research answers certain questions well and others not so well, or not at all. Action research methods not only have the ability to look at complex challenges, but have an empowering political element of engagement of the participants in no longer being passive subjects, but co-researchers that ask and answer questions with the primary researchers. Such inquiries are also generally embedded in the participant's own setting and designed to yield practical results for them to use or build on going forward. This "action" orientation transforms the relationships making every party involved a creator of the new knowledge and setting up ongoing levels of inquiry/action after the study that create new possibilities in their lives. These participatory methods shift the power to the community/participants, allowing for community-based, accessible application in context specific settings. These results can also now be accessed remotely, aggregated and used to shape future best practices and further inquiry with much more context specific versatility. Coupled with quantitative measures in a mixed method, these types of research lend themselves to real-world application and clinical engagement while yielding quantifiable data for analysis. Textbooks have been written on the subject and if this is all unfamiliar, that is fine as it leads us to our next topic.

2. Reading Across Disciplines: Also known as getting out of our respective professional silos of focus. As we noted in Chapter 1, creativity itself has been trapped in a variety silos (psychology, social sciences, organizational development, etc.). Within our rehabilitation professions we need to be able to read across disciplines and have the ability to switch our lenses of perspective to understand why psychologists ask these questions, why occupational therapists focus on this, and why nurses ask additional seemingly unrelated questions. This type of reading both within and outside rehabilitation literature provides the divergent exposure to generate what later can yield unique associations in the form of convergent insights for us. The emerging pain literature is a great example where we see functional anatomists, neuroscientists, psychologists, immunologists, surgeons, clinicians and so many more now creating an eclectic chorus of input to new understanding and creative new tools

for pain management. How do we keep up with all of this information in our already overcrowded lives?

3. Learn New Information Management Techniques: Create the habit of exploring new ideas by harnessing the power of technology. Professional outlets often provide bulletins of new findings. The internet has generated sites and blogs that aggregate breaking information about areas of interests, having done the scut work of searching across resources for new findings. Joining specialty interest groups brings bullet points summaries of new discussions and findings that allow you to scan for pearls of your interest. A great habit is to once a month invest an hour reviewing what contrasting or opposing opinions are doing and saying about your area of interest. Very quickly with these creative habits, you can be exposed to so much without having to painstakingly review everything. Then of course exercise the habit of reading on regular basis some of those pearls….but see, in these postnormal times we are getting ahead of ourselves into the next section, clinical mastery, as the old normal boundaries blur.

4. Challenge All Assumptions: As a creative rehabilitation professional the most important habit is to challenge all assumptions, including this one! Paradigms are habits of mind that save us time, but also can become cages that restrict us and our creative expression. These challenges can ruffle feathers, create confusion and chaos, and also be the all-important early step in transformational learning of being a disorienting dilemma. The dilemma arises when we discover an inaccurate or incomplete assumption that then doesn't fit in our habit of mind as to how reality works. This creates an emotional response, but there we go again, we are jumping forward to the clinical mastery section. Before we head there, it's critical that we retain the discipline of knowing and examining our inquiry biases, particularly as they apply to treatment outcomes and causality.

An appropriate concern about creative interventions in the clinic is that the creator then claims causality for an intervention producing a particular outcome based on erroneous assumptions. These assumptions are problematic for both new and the traditional conventions of care, but bear listing as the zeal for some new treatment can cloud our better discernment of causality. These are known biases to review and keep in mind as we create and remember that they affect our judgment and clinical reasoning. They are listed here and we should be familiar with each if we can actually claim to have created something within EBM:

- The natural history of disease can lead to improvement in a patient;
- The regression to the mean can appear as an improvement that occurs regardless of the treatment;
- The powerful placebo effect can be the cause of the change;
- The influences on health coincident with (but independent of) the particular treatment given the many other complex factors;
- The Post Hoc, Ergo Propter Hoc effect can create a false claim of causality despite proximity to the treatment;
- Confirmation biases in general are known to generate a selective advantage, cognitive dissonance, healthcare desire and expectations, and self-fulfilling prophecies; peripheral factors can relieve perceived symptoms; and, Independent of direct, effective, therapeutic support, patients often come to feel better.

These are not trivial and as rehabilitation professionals we have an ethical responsibility to insure that such effects not be falsely credited to our creative specific treatments. How we establish this vigilance around these biases leads to our next topic.

5. Cycles of Personal Enactment and Embodiment: The blurring of these classic components of division in EBM from normal times becomes very obvious as this chapter is being constructed. Where else can we inquire as a process of our own personal research to gain insight into best practice? The dated, dry, disembodied objective pursuit of normal times has now evolved into this new, messy, intermingled, deeply subjective and embodied part of evidence review in postnormal times. Research inquiry is no longer relegated to the lab or some constrained clinical trial. The creativity of EBM now also includes that opening moment of Julie's story, where provider and participant are embodied in the present moment, each inquiring into 1.) the real-time evidence of their and the other's state; but also, 2.) all the known evidence available; AND,3.) the unknown silence of uncertainty.

These sources of evidence blur together as a combined personal inquiry as to our own and the other's state and needs in the moment (aka clinical mastery and patient needs and values).These domain practices via empathy and compassion allow us to pause and to not act from reactive patterns of habit based on something other the real time evidence of all the variables in the moment. Such a state of embodied awareness and enactment to the unique circumstances of the moment clears a space into which creativity unfolds from silence as Sanford described in Chapter 2 and was detailed in Chapter 3. Such an inquiry practice of the evidence: 1.) minimizes the risk for violating the patient's opportunity for engagement and healing behavior; 2.) also prevents the provider from missing the rich opportunity to create a new rather than the otherwise withering enactment of routine or rote behaviors; and, 3.) This reduces that threat that one or both miss their own health enhancing, creative expression. At this point we naturally blend into the classic description of an effective clinical mastery practice and confirmation of patient values and flourishing.

Clinical Mastery

"Yesterday I was clever and tried to change the world.
Today I am wise and try to change myself."
~ Rumi

The new evidence across disciplines about the complexity of rehabilitation science negates any fear rehabilitation professionals may have about top down cookbook prescriptions from EBM. These postnormal times raise the bar on what is a vibrant clinical mastery and takes the practice far further than its previous role. According to classic EBM, external clinical evidence informed, but never replaced individual clinical expertise, and this expertise was what decided whether the external evidence applied to the individual patient at all and, if so, how it should be integrated into a clinical decision. Similarly, any external guidelines were integrated with the individual's clinical expertise to decide whether and how it matched the patient's clinical state, predicament, and preferences, and thus whether it should be applied. Now when viewed from the lens of the known complexities of healing, even the most ordinary encounter in rehabilitation with students or patients leaps out in new possibilities much like a high-resolution picture of a digital television sitting next to an old analog television picture. The new evidence from research added to the ongoing practice of the conventional skills of our particular profession sets the creative stage for this bright new mastery in the following ways:

1. Exercise a disciplined practice of quieting: Reflection and introspection are parts of conventional clinical mastery. In today's always on, 24/7 hyperstimulation environment, regularly carving out such times is critical and difficult. Habit and ritual help to reinforce such a discipline.

2. Develop the skill of quieting: Once the space is made, then find a practice to become skilled at generating quieting of body, mind and breathing. Quieting is a learned behavior and as such people vary in their skill levels. Practicing one that matches personal preference is crucial. Yoga, tai chi, dance, journaling, prayer, a warm bath, sitting/walking in nature and turning one's attention inward are all popular practices.

3. Seek interprofessional embodied experiences: Exposing ourselves to fully engaged experiences of other's work will generate a wealth of new understanding and associations to draw from in the future. Even within our disciplines there are many nuances to sample beyond our routine of experience. Drop preconceptions and exercise the discipline of fully experiencing the work from an open, beginner's mind and pay attention to all the sensory and conceptual awarenesses that unfold during and after the experience.

4. Explore new communication skills: Motivational interviewing, non-violent communication, and compassionate listening can all be avenues of developing new communication. Picking up a second language, especially one that might be used clinically is known to generate new neurological patterns. The craft of writing generates new ways of ordering the patterns of thought and association while having the side benefit of enhancing friendships or business development.

5. Create a challenging mentor relationship: It is extremely beneficial to have at least one relationship with a mentor that knows us across all dimensions of our life. That mentor should be both encouraging and challenging us to move beyond our personal comfort zone of habitual behavior. The more broadly they know us the more likely they will be able to see our blind spots of imbalance and keep us healthy and in a sustainable process as described by Van Demark in chapter 7.

Practicing these five behaviors will generate a fly-wheel of development and insight to fuel our personal creative expression as professionals and within our personal lives. Part IV of this book contains many exercises and practices to further enhance clinical mastery. The fruit of these practices is the sharpening our sensitivity and insight into the final leg of EBM, patient values.

Patient Values

What began in EBM as a process for determining measurable outcomes such as magnitude of effect and level of certainty (precision), evolved into what now is considered equally as important—the balance of patient values and preferences. Our patients like Julie do want to be heard and not dismissed. But they also want to regain a sense of efficacy and a real relief of suffering that translates into unique circumstances. The normal times model acknowledged this as important, but was founded on the perspective that the provider was the expert and therapist that needed to assess those values and needs, but the therapy would come from the expert then based on their consideration of all three aspects of EBM. The post-normal times EBM has a more humble approach and acknowledges the patient as a critical peer in the creative process of healing that has their own expertise and responsibility of personal mastery to draw upon to co-create the path forward.

How do we practice this aspect of EBM? Who has time to do this even if we know what to do? Can we sense that blank canvas of not knowing mentioned in Julie's opening introduction? Can we listen to those internal voices of protest and concern? And hearing them, set them aside and listen more deeply into the not knowing? This is edge we need to find and rest in above as our mastery, but it is also the edge we must invite our patients to explore and sense if these lofty goals are to be achieved in the new patient values. This is the edge of creativity where we don't know and it's very uncomfortable at times. The pull and yearning for predictability that the normal times promised is sure to reappear, but modern science has shown us its illusory nature in most complex human interactions. So we cycle back up into our clinical mastery practices and in the acceptance of the not knowing, the potential associations of our evidence study have the possibility of coming forward in new insights and directions, while we simultaneously are able to attend to the real time state and needs of the patient. That vacuum of not knowing will be filled, our job as creative rehabilitation professionals is create the environment that makes the space, then work together with the patient to co-create their future. The authors in Part III share stories of such processes to glimpse our respective professional circumstances. The exercises in Part IV offer additional resources for generating that blank canvas of possibility for our students and patients.

CONCLUSION

In summary, despite its early origins, EBM remains a relatively young discipline and the road forward is promising with our atlas of EBM. There have been and will continue to be many contributors to include the authors in Part III to this movement. Their work has and will continue to have a profound effect on daily clinical practice. But as in any hero/heroine's journey, there remain additional obstacles to creativity on the road ahead. How do we overturn the systems limitations in our professional association and academic culture that limit creativity? What residual power imbalances in the dynamics between groups, individuals and within our culture continue to thwart creativity and how might we change those dynamics? And, how do these new creative developments emerge amidst the struggle necessary to bring them into use and once employed, can the changes be sustained? The following chapters address each of these obstacles in turn.

REFERENCES

Gray, J.A., Muir, et al. (1996). Evidence based medicine: what it is and what it isn't. *BMJ British Medical Journal, 312,* 71-72.

Greenhalgh, T., Howick, J., Maskrey, N. (2014). Evidence based medicine: a movement in crisis? *BMJ British Medical Journal,* 348-372.

Sackett, D.L. (1969). Clinical epidemiology. *American Journal of Epidemiology, 89,* 125–8.

Sackett, D.L., Rosenberg, W.M., Gray, J.A,. Haynes, R.B., Richardson, W.S. (1996) Evidence based medicine: What it is and what it isn't. *British Medical Journal, 13,* 71–2.

Sur, R.L. & Dahm (Oct-Dec 2011) History of evidence-based medicine. *Indian J of Urology, 27*(4), 487-489.

In: Fostering Creativity in Rehabilitation
Editor: Matthew J. Taylor

ISBN: 978-1-63485-118-3
© 2016 Nova Science Publishers, Inc.

Chapter 5

SYSTEMIC LIMITATIONS ON CREATIVITY IN ACADEMIA AND PROFESSIONAL ASSOCIATIONS

Staffan Elgelid, PT, PhD, GCFP

Associate Professor of Physical Therapy,
Nazareth College, Rochester, NY, US

ABSTRACT

This chapter describes the systemic limitations that interfere with creativity and innovation in academia and professional organizations. Historical, as well as present day reasons for these systemic limitations are explored. The systemic limitations in academia examined include pros and cons of the rehabilitation professions being part of the academic setting, how students and faculty are selected, how faculty advances within the academic system, who is in control of the peer review, and why we need to change "the system" to better adjust to postnormal times. The chapter closes by summarizing the interrelationships between academia and professional organizations, and how those generate additional limitations on creativity, as well as listing those that are unique to professional organizations.

INTRODUCTION

"We busted out of class had to get away from those fools. We learned more from a three minute record than we ever learned in school."
Bruce Springsteen, *No Surrender*

Does this ring true? You learn more from a "three minute record day than you ever learned in school." Is Mr. Springsteen claiming that we can learn more from practical activities than from sitting in school? Is he claiming that school is isolated from reality? Is he claiming that creativity and innovation happens while creating things? I guess we will never know and can only speculate in what one of the greatest Rock and Roll live performers ever meant by the above line. This chapter will look at if there might be limits to creativity in academia and professional organizations: Limits that might be built into the system. Limits that were built into the system on purpose and that we still have not managed to transcend, and likely will not transcend unless the system changes. First let us take a look at how the academic system was developed.

HISTORY

Academic originates from the word Akademeia, and was the name of the space where Plato held his discussions with fellow "intellectuals". The site was a space where the Goddess Athena was honored, so we can see that even in the early phases of Academia there was some involvement of sacredness (Academy, 2014; Platonic Academy, n.d.). Later on sites of higher learning in Europe and other parts of the world were usually under control of the church. Whether Christian, Muslim, Buddhist or other religions, the academies where often connected to a church or religion. This was partly due to the fact that the churches/temples was were the books were located, where people who could read were, but also by being involved with education the church could control what was taught. Many of these schools, but not all, were quite dogmatic in the teaching of the doctrine of the church (History of Early Education, 2007). While many great thinkers and scientists got their start in these academies, there were also scholars and scientists who got their works banned due to not following church doctrine or the Holy Scriptures. Innovations and creativity were to be contained within certain doctrinal boundaries in these academies, and maybe this is where we can trace the beginnings of the system that limits creativity in academia. A systemic pattern that still gives off faint, and not so faint, echoes in the halls of academia.

TODAY IN ACADEMIA

Our Universities and Colleges have produced an enormous amount of research that has benefited the world. They are also educating a larger and larger percentage of the population and are giving these students a chance to broaden their perspectives, attain better jobs and provide a living for their families. But the echoes of the history of academia are still sounding in the forms of a lack of creativity. This may be true throughout academia (Southwick, 2012), but based on personal experience the lack of creativity is very present in the education of rehabilitation professionals. Rehabilitation professionals need a good liberal arts/classical foundation, but after the required core classes the student are trained in a very specific skill and profession. It should be noted that the field of Medicine is aware of the concern about lack of creativity and has started to look at creativity in the education of MD's and in 2006 the Lancet had a full issue about creativity (Kelly, 2012; Lancet, 2006).

The echoes from the past can be heard in many aspects of academia from the selection of students, the hiring and education of faculty, promotions within the field, publishing, how practical hands-on classes are devalued compared to lecture classes, and in many other aspects. One might say that one can hear the system echoes that limit creativity in the rehabilitation professions throughout the whole educational experience. So how can we expect the future rehabilitation professionals to be creative?

How Did the Rehabilitation Professions End up in Academia?

Traditionally what was taught in the Universities in the Middle Ages were the classics. They consisted of grammar, rhetoric, dialectic, arithmetic, geometry, music and astronomy. In today's academy the traditional liberal art's consists of literature, language, art history, music history, philosophy, history, math, psychology and science (Arts 2014). Vocational schools where not part of academia. Most vocations were part of local guilds, and students were trained through apprenticeships. Healers were traditionally raised in families and the knowledge was handed down through observation and hands-on practice. In the 18th and 19th century vocational schools were established in Europe. This was in large part due to pressure from industrialization. The industries needed workers with specific skills, and training that was standardized. However the vocational schools were not considered on the same level as the universities, and the universities were still mostly for a small elite (Greinert, 2014).

Most of the rehabilitation professions did not exist at the time of the guilds and when the vocational schools were established in Europe. However a good number of medical schools were established in many countries, and many of them did not have a standardized curriculum. The medical schools in the US did not have a standard curriculum and many different models of medical schools existed. The Flexner report standardized US medical education, but also severely limited what was being taught in medical schools. Many of the alternative approaches were removed from the curriculum, and many of the schools for minorities and women were closed. (Hiatt, Stockton, 2003) No doubt making the curriculum more scientific and standardized lead to the growth of the medical profession, and research became a significant part of the workload for the medical teaching faculty. The Council of Medical Education, (CME) a branch of the AMA, was the driving force behind the Flexner report. Today organizations of many rehabilitation professions have tried to and are still trying to model their education based on the CME because the medical profession has been at the top of the rehabilitation hierarchy (See Chapter 6), and the rehabilitation professions are thereby trying to gain the same respect as the medical profession.

Today traditional rehabilitation professions such as physical therapy, occupational therapy, nursing, creative art's therapy and others are being taught in colleges and universities throughout the world. While medicine has managed to rise above the liberal arts, due to mostly having their own colleges and campuses, many of the rehabilitation professions are still being questioned in Academia since on many campuses they still are considered trainings for a vocation and not really belonging on college campuses, or there are at the very least still echoes of those thoughts on many campuses. This despite the fact that many liberal arts schools would probably not exist today if it weren't for the students studying the rehabilitation professions and other "professional/vocational" fields (Sullivan, Rosin, 2008). Getting into the academic setting has definitely benefitted the rehabilitation professions, and while the rehabilitation professions became more standardized and got increased status when they became part of the academic world, they also lost something when they became part of the academic "system."

It is ironic that the physical therapy students do not learn to move themselves, the dietitians do not track and modify their nutrition, speech and language pathologists don't enhance the vocalization, etc. The move into academia came with the risk of losing practical hands-on training, enacted practical practice and embodiment in a real world context that promotes creativity "on the spot." This move from real world practice and embodiment towards a more theoretical basis for the education might be what is hinted at in the opening lines of Bruce Springsteen's *No Surrender,* and is discussed in Chapter 4. Now that the rehabilitation professional education are firmly established within the academic system the question becomes are we changing the system towards more innovation or are we becoming part of a system that perpetuates itself instead of encouraging innovation and creativity? The answer to that question lies in how we presently select students and faculty, and how we in the future select who participates (students, faculty and staff) in the academic system, how one advances within the system, and who determines the content of the curriculum and board exam.

SELECTION OF STUDENTS AND FACULTY

To gain a better understanding if the rehabilitation professions are changing the academic system towards more creativity, we have to look at how individuals and organizations are selected to participate in academia. Since I teach Physical Therapy (PT) I am most familiar with PT students and faculty and the process that PT schools have to go through to gain and maintain accreditation. I will therefore use PT as an example. Having worked in several universities and colleges that have a number of different degrees in the rehabilitation professions, I know that most rehabilitation professions are using similar methods for selecting students and faculty and are using similar criteria for maintaining accreditation.

SELECTION OF STUDENTS

To get accepted into PT school there are a variety of selection criteria that schools might consider such as work experience, volunteer experience, letters of recommendation, interview etc., but generally what counts more than anything else is a student's cumulative and pre-requisite (science) grade point average (GPA)(APTA, 2014). Whether the school accepts student into the program as freshmen or as graduate students, the GPA is the most important factor in gaining acceptance into a program. Why is that? There are three reasons for this:

1) GPA is easy to measure and it is very easy to justify why a student got accepted or not based on the students GPA.
2) GPA gives an indication of how the student will be able to handle the course of study.
3) It appears as if pre-requisite GPA is a good predictor for passing the PT licensing board exam (Roehrig, 1988).

Also to get accepted into a graduate program most programs require the student to have certain pre-requisites. Most of these pre-requisites are science courses, often with some added psychology and statistics (APTA 2014). Does this sound like the student who will be successful with the uncertainty and unknown outcomes that will be more common in postnormal times? (Sardar, 2010) Does this sound like a creative student? The students selected are brilliant students and will function very well in the world of EBM that emphasizes the 1/3 of EBM that focuses on research (the other 2 aspects of EBM are practitioner experience/clinical mastery and patient values) (Sackett et al., 1996), but they might not be as competent at traits such as empathy, compassion, creativity and building relationships. Traits we know that are needed in the postnormal future, valued as part of clinical mastery, and valued by patients.

So why do we not select students that have more of a fine arts or liberal arts background, that show strong traits of empathy and relationship building, students that might be better at dealing with ambiguity and being creative?

Again, the limitation is in the system. For a PT program to stay accredited the program and school is being assessed on many criteria. One of the criteria is pre-requisites for students entering the program. It is suggested that the pre-requisite GPA is a good predictor for passing the PT licensing test (Roehrig, 1988). A school that decides to accept more students based on their arts and creative background might see the pass rates on the licensing exam begin to decrease. This would result in two possible outcomes. One would be from the accrediting agency inquiring about what the school is doing to strengthen the pass rate, and the other is from prospective students who might choose to attend a school with a higher first time pass rate on the board exam. Most of the prospective students and parents I see in my office will ask about the passing rate on the board exam. A low first time pass rate, no matter how creative the students are, would indicate a "bad" school to the students and parents as well as to the professional accreditation organization.

Another factor that cannot be overlooked is that students entering a rehab profession have at least 12 years, often more, of schooling behind them and they expect school to be a certain way. Here is an example of that student expectation from when I first started teaching.

> I was teaching laboratory/hands-on courses in a PT program. I wanted the students to start thinking creatively. Before the first practical exam I suggested that if the students did exactly what had been shown in class they would receive 95% on the test. To receive 100% they needed to take a chance and do something creative with the material that had been taught. Whether they managed to pull it off or not was not important, they would still get the extra % for trying to be creative. I heard some serious mumbling in the class, but thought they were OK with the way I would grade. About 30 min after the class was over I was told that I could not do that. Students had complained that they would not get a 100% on the exam even if they exactly imitated of what had been demonstrated in class. I had to back down and encourage imitation over imagination.

The students preferred the reproductive educational model (see Preface) over trying to be creative. One cannot blame the students in the above example. They have been trained since first grade or pre-school that perfect imitation is preferred and there is no bonus for being creative. Actually the student will most likely lose points for creativity, since that involves taking a chance. The message is clear, play it safe!

So the system limits the kind of students we accept into the rehab professions. I have met some, not many, faculty members who would like to have more creative students accepted into their professions, but administrators fearing a drop in passing scores on the board (and a subsequent drop in tuition paying students), accreditation agencies expecting a certain type of pre-requisites, and faculty members who have succeeded in the present system are all resisting changes to the system and their arguments usually carries the day. Some readers might be surprised that faculty members are not clamoring for more creative students, and by extension more creative practitioners? How is this possible? Let's take a look at how faculty members are trained, hired and progress in academia.

SELECTION OF FACULTY

So you want to teach in your selected rehabilitation profession? You have been in the clinic for many years, and feel like you have much to share from your hands-on, real life experience. Congratulations and welcome, but first you have a few hoops to jump through. We understand that you have done lots of clinical work, but that is not enough and most of it was probably not evidence based, i.e., backed up by research. It was only backed up by anecdotal evidence such as your patients getting better and you running a successful practice. You have not collected evidence to show that this happened so it really didn't happen. Sorry! Your PhD program will show you what works though, so welcome to 3-10 years of school to learn what works. Yeah, that is about what it sounds like when you start your academic life. So how does the system to become a faculty member encourage or discourage creativity?

To get a tenure track position in the rehabilitation professions you will need a doctoral degree. A PhD, EdD or DSci will usually do. A clinical doctorate such as the DPT will probably not. With a clinical doctorate you might get an appointment as a clinical faculty or instructor at some schools, but that comes with decreases pay compared to the people on tenure track even though the students are entering a clinical field. This salary disparity sends the message that schools do not value practical experience and hands-on work as much as theory. Theory that is usually taught by the faculty member from a textbook is valued over lab courses that can involve relationship building between faculty and students and a sharing of knowledge that goes both ways between teacher and student. Another indication of the academic value system is that one hour of lecture/theory is more highly valued than one hour of laboratory/hands-on work. The ratio is usually one hour of lecture = 2-3 hours of lab when workload is counted (US Dept of Ed, 2008). It is in the hands-on classes that we can be more creative, where we interact with the students, where we can model professional behavior, and can allow them to be creative and show what skills they already possess. It is in the laboratory that the students practice the skills that they will actually use when they are working with their patients, but it is valued less by academia than a lecture based hour. I will not comment more on that disparity, but instead focus on how the PhD student and future faculty member is shaped by the system. Again, I will give examples from physical therapy because that is the field that I am most familiar with, but there is no reason to believe that other rehabilitation professions are all that different.

Most rehabilitation professionals that decide to further their education and get their doctorate (I will use the PhD as an example, but it could be the EdD or any other terminal doctoral degree) more than likely received high grades in their entry-level degree program. That is, they were the ones who were successful in the system, and they are the professionals who will conduct research and teach the future generation of rehabilitation professionals. They may very well enter their PhD studies with great creative ideas about the research they want to perform, but once again the system may limit their creativity. Students in many, if not most, doctoral programs will have to find a professor that will agree to guide them and help them with their research. So the professor who is their main advisor must show an interest in their research, but most professors are interested in students that have research interests like theirs. A professor is less likely to take on a student who wants to do their dissertation on something that the professor has no knowledge about. Even if they take on a student with a very interesting topic, if the topic has a very poor chance of getting funded or published, the dissertation advisor will decrease his chances of getting a publication out of the student's work and thereby decreasing his chances of being promoted. Here again we see how the academic system can limit creativity.

Congratulations, you have completed your studies and just got your first tenure track job. Now you can start being creative. Right?!? Yes as a university professor you will have more freedom to be creative, but you will still bump up against reality, aka the system. Depending on what level school and what courses you are teaching that reality might still limit you, because you need tenure!

It takes approximately 5-7 years to get tenure at most higher education institutions. Your tenure will be decided by a committee of peers who will judge you by your teaching, scholarship and service to the community (but depending on the school not necessarily weighted in that order). You are ready to get rolling and have all kinds of ideas, creative ideas about teaching and research so that you can receive your tenure! Here too the system will put up limitations such as teaching to the board exam, peer review and tenure. For rehabilitation professional the biggest limitation to creativity when it comes to teaching is the board exam.

Students in most rehabilitation professions have to pass a board exam at the end of their course of study. The experts in the field write the board exams and the questions are around the established content for the educational programs in the field, the established practice of the profession and research that is accepted within the field. Not necessarily the newest research, but the research that has been included in textbooks (FSBPT, 2014a). Not necessarily the most creative research, but the research that has been included in textbooks. And who writes the board exam questions? Approximately 60% are faculty members who have the time, it is part of their job, and who are familiar with the textbooks. (Federation of State Boards, 2014b) A panel of experts will then vet the questions, before they are added to the board exam (Federation of State Boards, 2014c). The board exam might be run by the professional organization, or by an independent body that has given the power to run the exam by the professional organization. Either way these outside organizations will limit the amount of creativity that happens within academia. Even if you have been in the clinic for 20+ years and have developed all these great ideas around treatments, if they are not in the "canon" of established/approved textbooks it might not be in the students best interest to teach those methods of intervention since they will not be on the board exam. As a faculty member your creativity is limited by what will be asked on the board exam. Your job is to make sure the students will pass the board exam, or they cannot enter their chosen rehabilitation profession. You might be able to teach an elective where you have some more freedom on what to teach, but most of the time you are limited in what you spend your teaching time on. When faculty members talk about creativity it is more about how they teach. Creativity in how the material is delivered and not in what material is delivered. It is the price rehabilitation professionals pay for having a board exam that will insure a certain standardized level of competence in our profession. The above is a good example of how a system/organization is influenced by an outside system/organization. Creativity in academia is limited in itself by the academic system, but it is also influenced and limited by the systems/organizations that interacts with academia. The need for faculty members to publish is another area that is influenced by many systems interacting with each other thereby limiting creativity.

As a faculty member you will have to publish. The requirements for publications vary depending on the level of school you teach at, but there is a basic level of publishing that is determined by the accrediting organization or professional organization. (CAPTE, 2013) A research 1 school will have high demands, that you publish in high-ranking journals, and that you bring in research grants that will bring income and respect/improved rankings to the school. At a smaller school that is more focused on teaching the research requirements might not be as high, but you still need to publish peer-reviewed research to satisfy the professional organization that accredits your program. Yes peer-reviewed research. Books or articles for the general public will usually not do if you want to advance within the system. Who are the peer reviewers? They are experts within the field who are published. They will read and provide feedback and determine if your research fits into the journal and if it is high quality research. These peer reviewers will be more likely to understand and approve for publication research that is in line with the accepted norm for the field and the journal. Very creative research and research in alternative approaches generally will have less of a chance of being published (Campanario, Martin 2004; Osmond, 1983; Horbin, 1990).

In the last ten or so years there has been a proliferation of research journals and it is getting easier to find journals that will publish creative research and more alternative approaches to research and interventions. The journals might be outside of your chosen rehabilitation profession, but they are still peer reviewed and counts as scholarship when you go up for your tenure. Be aware though that the people on the tenure committee might not be as impressed by articles published in journals that they have never heard of. The tenure committee are composed of faculty members who have tenure and who have been successful in, and approved by….. (drum roll) the system!! If you don't get the approval by the tenure committee your career in academia is over. Many non-tenured faculty members therefore play it safe in order to get tenure.

They play it safe by doing research they know will get published, by doing research on topics that are only within their chosen field, by submitting for research grants on topics that are incremental improvements/changes over previously published studies, by using studies that concludes with something that is easy to measure. Nice clean studies without unpredictable, complicating factors, but with clear conclusions and outcomes. Not exactly what is needed in the postnormal times, where we acknowledge that nothing makes sense, and things are unpredictable (Sardar, 2010). In the future building relationships and empathy (See chapter 6) could be more important than the interventions we chose for our patients with chronic lifestyle disease. It is one of the limitations that the system of academia places on most faculty members though. After tenure there are similar limitations, your accrediting body want to see research related to your teaching areas and published in peer reviewed journals or presented at peer reviewed conferences. To advance in rank you must publish acceptable research in acceptable journals. The list goes on and on. We do repetitive instead of generative research and education, and we continue to perpetuate the system that is already in place and that is failing to produce creative rehab professionals.

CONCLUSION ABOUT THE SELECTION PROCESS

So we select and promote students and faculty based on tangible, predictable measures such as GPA, degrees, publications etc., even though we know that to be successful in the unpredictable future it might be more important to have empathy, learn how to build relationship, and have other "soft" skills. In addition the majority of the diseases of the 21st century tends to be chronic lifestyle disease rather than the acute disease of the 20th century. For the acute disease it was fairly easy to develop a rehabilitation program since the variables were few and the outcomes clear. For lifestyle disease the rehabilitation professional needs to understand that there are more variables and that the variables interrelate with each other. When one variable changes, the other variables change too, but in unpredictable ways. So even in the conditions we treat, we have gone from the normal to the postnormal times where we acknowledge uncertainty and that predicting future outcomes are very difficult (Sardar, 2010). However we are still selecting students and faculty based on normal times and we look for certainty and predictable outcomes. For academia to become relevant in postnormal times we must select students and faculty that can adapt to uncertainty and unpredictability. Maybe the rehabilitation professions should consider more students that are looking for a second career. That would bring in new ways of thinking into our fields. Creativity is about combining things in new and interesting ways. Today the vast majority of students are going straight through school to receive their degree, they can not combine the knowledge they gain in school with "real world' knowledge since they have spent their whole lives in school. Also they might not be as astute at differentiate between practical knowledge and "academic" knowledge. We all have heard the phrase "that is purely academic". That really translates into "that is not practical/real world." Maybe by having more students entering the field after having been out in "the real world' we can increase the amount of creativity and real world knowledge in the rehabilitation professions, but then we must also allow for a different way of accepting students into the program and as we have seen that can cause a ripple effect throughout the system when these students becomes future faculty and leaders within the educational system as well as in our professional organizations.

PROFESSIONAL ORGANIZATIONS

I hope it is clear from this chapter that the academic system can limit creativity in the people that are part of the system, but that the academic system is also influenced by other organizations that are built around their own systems. So we end up with having organizations/systems interacting with each other, and limiting each other. Two types of organizations that interact and influence/shape creativity in rehabilitation professions are professional organizations such as the American Physical Therapy Association, American Nurses Association and others, and the organizations that accredit the professional education programs. Much has been included in this chapter about how these organizations interact and limits creativity in academia. Therefore the possible limitations that these organizations might impose on rehabilitation professionals will be presented in bullet form. Please bear in mind that all of these organizations also benefit the rehabilitation professionals and they are really our voice to the outside world. In my opinion while these organizations might limit creativity, the good they do far outweighs the negative effects they might have on creativity.

Professional Organizations:

- Creating Rules and Regulations – These might interfere with creativity by specifically limit what can be practiced under a certain license as scopes of practice are delineated/defended at the state level and compromises are made to settle "turf battles" between professions that share commonalities such as the PT dry needling vs. acupuncture in 2014. This could be a problem for people with a "regulated" license such as OT, PT or Nursing in combination with a "non-regulated" field like yoga therapy.
- Approving Continuing Education – A person applying to teach a continuing education course must often gain approval by the professional organization.
- Sets standards for degree programs – Thereby limits what can be taught since the school must adhere to these standards to maintain accreditation.
- More recently as finances have tightened, associations have come to depend on corporate "sponsors" of journals, conferences and other ventures. These relationships can create pressures to limit discussion and publication especially if the vendor's product is at risk for being discredited.

Limitations by organizations that accredit schools and oversee board exams

- Requirement to cover certain topics in the curriculum – This will limit the teaching of new and "not proven" techniques that are effective in the clinic.
- Requirement that a certain amount of the faculty have PhD's or terminal degrees – Could limit the amount of clinical experts in a program, since there has to be a ratio between clinical faculty and faculty with terminal degrees.
- Board exams – Faculty has to teach content that is on the board exam
- Board exams - The latest research is seldom on the board exam since board exams are not updated yearly (FSBPT, 2014).
- Innovative Practices - Innovative practices that work in the clinic but have not been researched is not on the board exam and therefore limited time can be taken to teach these clinical approaches.

CONCLUSION

As we enter the postnormal times we are moving towards uncertainty in so many areas and professions in society, including the rehabilitation professions. We will be working with more people that have chronic lifestyle disease and the magic bullet will more than likely not be found. As rehabilitation professionals we will then have to rely more on our creativity and insight, in combination with our critical thinking, our knowledge of medicine, our colleagues and networks, and everything we learned during our entry-level and post graduate level trainings. To develop our creativity some of the limitations that are built into our formal education must be loosened up. Our basic rehabilitation training is phenomenal but we are still training for normal times. The challenge is for the institutions and continuing education providers to add training for rehabilitation professionals who will be able to thrive in these postnormal times.

Undoubtedly to make space for this type of training some of what is in the trainings now must be removed or less emphasis must be placed on the quest for certainty in predictable outcomes and measures. We must be careful not to lose what is good with the system, but still prune some of the information that is not useful for today's and future's rehabilitation professionals. I have no doubt that books like this and the work that the contributors to this book and very many likeminded rehabilitation professionals are doing right now, will make us succeed in providing professionals that will be ready for postnormal times. While the echoes will still be there, they will grow fainter over time, and the halls of academia will be filled with a vision of the embodied and enacted creative future instead of the echoes of the past. I am excited about the future and wish you well in making your own creative mark in rehabilitation. Remember, *No Surrender*!

REFERENCES

Academy. (2014). Encyclopedia Britannica. Retrieved August 3, 2014, from http://0-www.britannica.com.libra.naz.edu/EBchecked/topic/2615/Academy

APTA. (2014) Physical Therapist (PT) Admissions process. Retrieved August 4, 2014, from http://www.apta.org/ProspectiveStudents/Admissions/PTProcess/

Campanario, J.M., Martin, B. (2004). Challenging dominant physics paradigms. *Journal of Scientific Exploration, 18(3)*, 412-438.

Commission on Accreditation in Physical Therapy Education (CAPTE). (2013). Position papers. Retrieved August 5, 2014, from http://www.capteonline.org/uploadedFiles /CAPTEorg/About_CAPTE/Resources/Accreditation_Handbook/PositionPapers.pdf

Federation of State Boards of Physical Therapy. (2014). Ensuring validity. Retrieved August 3, 2014, from https://www.fsbpt.org/FreeResources/NPTEDevelopment/Ensuring Validity.aspx

Federation of State Boards of Physical Therapy. (2014). NPTE & PRT item writers. Retrieved August 3, 2014, from https://www.fsbpt.org/Volunteers/Volunteer Opportunities /NPTEPRTWriters.aspx

Federation of State Boards of Physical Therapy. (2014). General information. Retrieved August 3, 2014, from https://www.fsbpt.org/FreeResources/NPTECandidateHandbook /GeneralInformation.aspx

Greinert, W.D. (2004). European vocational training "systems" – Some thoughts on the theoretical context of their theoretical development. *Journal of Vocational Training (32)*, 18-25.

Hiatt, M.D., Stockton, C.G. (2003). The impact of the Flexner Report on the fate of medical schools in North America after 1909. *Journal of American Physicians and Surgeons. 8(2)*, 37-40. Retrieved August 5, 2014, from http://www.jpands.org/vol8no2/hiatt.pdf

History of Early Education (2007). International world history project. Retrieved August 3, 2014, from http://history-world.org/history_of_education.htm

Horbin, D.F. (1990) The philosophical basis of peer review and the suppression of innovation. *Journal of American Medical Association. 263*(10), 1438-1441.

Kelly, N. (2012). What are you doing creatively these days? *Academic Medicine* 87(11),1476. Retrieved August 4, 2014, from http://journals.lww.com/academicmedicine/Fulltext/2012 /11000/What_Are_You_Doing_Creatively_These_Days_.20.aspx

Lancet. (2006). *368,* 2-67.

Liberal Arts. (2014). Encyclopedia Britannica. Retrieved August 3, 2014, from http://global.britannica.com/EBchecked/topic/339020/liberal-arts

Osmond, D.H., (1983). Malice's wonderland: Research funding and peer review. *Journal Of Neurobiology. 14*(2), 95-112.

Platonic Academy (n.d.). In *Wikipedia.* Retrieved August 5, 2014 from http://en.wikipedia.org/wiki/Platonic_Academy

Roehrig, S.M.. (1988). Prediction of licensing examination score in physical therapy graduates. *Physical* Therapy. 68, 694-698.

Sackett D.L., Rosenberg W.M., Gray J.A., Haynes R.B., Richardson W.S. (1996) Evidence based medicine: What it is and what it isn't. *BMJ, 13,* 71–2.

Sardar, Z. (2010). Welcome To postnormal times. *Futures. 42(5),* 435-444. Retrieved August 4, 2014, from http://ziauddinsardar.com/2011/03/welcome-to-postnormal-times/

Southwick, F. (2012). Academia suppresses creativity: By discouraging change, universities are stunting scientific innovation, leadership and growth. *The Scientist.*

Sullivan W.M., Rosin M.S. (2008). *A new agenda for higher education: Shaping a life of the mind for practice.* San Francisco, CA: Jossey-Bass.

US Department of Education. (2008). Structure of US education system: Credit systems. Retrieved August 3, 2014, from www2.ed.gov/about/offices/list/ous/international/usnei /us/credits.doc

In: Fostering Creativity in Rehabilitation
Editor: Matthew J. Taylor

ISBN: 978-1-63485-118-3
© 2016 Nova Science Publishers, Inc.

Chapter 6

THE ROLE OF RELATIONSHIP AND CREATIVITY

Ginger Garner, PT, ATC

Director, Professional Yoga Therapy Studies, Emerald Isle, NC, US

ABSTRACT

This chapter draws from both personal experience and studies in the role of relationship as it applies to creative expression. It will explore the effect of "power-over" based relationships in health care, which include interprofessional collaboration, gender context, provider-patient interaction, and cultural competence, all of which have direct effects on the delivery of health care. The collective shift to a healthier relationship model is critical for the creative process in rehabilitation in situations that range from research and innovation to patient care and adherence. That process involves moving from personal internal experience to the larger role of interprofessional collaboration and interfacing with our communities in creating health.

INTRODUCTION

- Relationship in Health care
- Historical Hindrances
- Relationship Continuum
- Cultural Competence
- Relationship Layers
- Domination Pedagogies
- Relationship in Mindful Leadership
- Sustainable Partnership for the Future of Rehabilitation

RELATIONSHIP IN HEALTH CARE

A very specific type of relationship, not just relationship in general, is critical for fostering creativity in rehabilitation. We have all had experiences where we felt belittled, marginalized, or outright ignored in the health care system. As rehabilitation professionals, these stories may sound familiar:

Scenario 1:

A patient, "Deborah," had this experience during a consult with a surgeon, "Dr. D." from a well-known, elite teaching hospital. The interaction with Dr. D that left her feeling powerless and humiliated.

Dr. D came into the examination room where Deborah was waiting with her husband. The doctor did not introduce himself when he entered the room. After a casual exam, which she knew to be inadequate to diagnose a serious shoulder injury, Deborah tried to discuss her symptoms. Dr. D interrupted her and dismissed her inquiry as irrelevant. Dr. D did acknowledge Deborah's presence, but when it came time to respond he turned to her husband to make eye contact with, and speak to him. Deborah's final attempt to ask a question about evidence-based alternative treatments for pain management in order to avoid unnecessary prescription drugs received the following response: Dr. D. literally rolled his eyes, turned to her husband, gave him a "knowing" sarcastic smirk and condescendingly remarked, "No, that (alternative treatments) will not work."

Scenario 2:

"Emily," confided that treatment she received from her ob/gyn practice was horrendously humiliating, as she was regularly belittled by her caregivers at the practice and her concerns marginalized. She felt it was because early in the doctor-patient relationship she questioned the evidence-base behind recommended "standard" procedures. She made it clear that she desired a natural pregnancy and birth if at all possible(i.e., asking why some of the testing, an ultrasound and repeated Doppler, was needed and also asking why less invasive forms of monitoring baby couldn't be used.) The physician turned to Emily and her husband and, peeking out the door in mock-fashion as if to "look" outside said, "What? Did you ride in here on a horse and buggy?" Despite repeated requests to consider her birth plan, Emily went on to have two births with the same large ob/gyn practice. Both ended in "emergency" C-sections, which put her in dire straits as an uninsured, self-employed, new mother.

Deborah and Emily are real people with real stories. The relationship with their health care providers stunted their input and ignored their personal concerns. It labeled them as medical conditions first and people second, and left lasting scars of humiliation and dehumanization which they will associate with the health care system for years to come. Their stories are the unfortunate norm in not only orthopaedic and maternal care, but in health care today. But let's also consider these relational scenarios that implicate patient care as well as policy. How might they impact creative potential through relationship?

- "My association says that we cannot discuss alternative therapies such as yoga with patients because they are not considered skilled therapeutic exercise."
- "My doctor says therapy will not help for my back pain and that injections or surgery are the best route; but when I question him he cannot tell me why."
- "My PT says he will only allow me to sit in this position so my disc does not bulge."
- "Hospital policy mandates that external fetal monitoring must be carried out on all laboring mothers every hour, regardless of their pregnancy risk or health status."
- "Organizational policy cannot consider integrating coursework from, or completing research, outside of our own department for completion of your allied health degree."

All of these real life cases describe a single type of relationship. A relationship in which patients are disempowered by health care providers and where health care providers or students are disenfranchised by the health care system or its academic body. Everyone's potential is radically diminished in this type of hierarchical relationship. Health care providers and patients alike are stuck in the antiquated cogs of a "my way or the highway" sick care system.

In the cases above, three observations can be made. The first is that relationship which is not well developed negatively impacts patients self-efficacy, stifles outcomes, suppresses leadership potential, and limits creativity. The second is that if the patient does not feel their story or experiences are heard or respected, they will be far less likely to engage the provider, participate in, or follow through with their health care plan. In a real way, patient outcomes are dependent upon the quality of relationship with the provider. The third is that collaboration with a patient should not kill evidence-based medicine. Rather, consideration of a patient's input should expand the definition of evidence-based medicine, which would foster creativity via considering all possibilities for best care. In other words, evidence-based medicine and provider-patient collaboration are not mutually exclusive.

Given these three points, then the very nature of relationship must change in our current health care system. Fostering creativity in evidence-based rehabilitation, though, must be pursued in the name of sustainable innovation and equitable research that will establish trust, improve patient care, and reinforce caring relationship in the patient and public.

HISTORICAL HINDRANCES

Relationship is often discussed as being an essential part of health care delivery, but what is its role in creative rehabilitation culture? In today's biomedical paradigm, two distinct variables have prevented development of relationships that foster creativity and sustainable innovation. Those variables are ingrained socialization and cultural conditioning, which will be explored through the remainder of this chapter.

Ingrained socialization and cultural conditioning are perhaps most apparent in the "powerful and pervasive myth in biomedical health care systems that the domain of medicine belongs solely to physicians" (Eisler & Potter, 2014; position 522). This has perpetuated two myths. One is that patients should blindly follow "doctor's orders" without question. This issue could be theorized as more of a generational gap issue, since younger generations are beginning to question the "power of the white coat." The second is the myth that pits men over women. Traits stereotypically assigned as feminine, including compassion, nurturing, and empathy, have historically been devalued and viewed as "soft or weak," with their development particularly stigmatized, discouraged, and even overtly scorned. Masculine traits like competition, aggression, and assertiveness, however, have historically been lauded, considered stronger, and given more value. These cultural attitudes have impacted gender equity, which fundamentally stunts creativity for both men and women.

These patterns of social ingraining negatively impact relationship and effectively make relationship not only an individual, but a social phenomenon (Eisler & Montuori, 2007). Further, cultural conditioning related to gender inequity has created a "discourse on creativity which has been almost exclusively by and about one gender: the male." (pg. 479). If relationship is part of a larger social phenomenon, then it is that relationship, more than individual effort alone, which will ultimately determine the creative potential in rehabilitation. Only when both men and women are respected for what they can contribute can we recognize our full potential in the field of rehabilitation.

For creativity to thrive in the rehabilitative field, two things are needed. The first is an ungendered definition of creativity (Eisler & Montuori, 2007). The second is an evolution of health care culture toward a new relationship paradigm free from the trappings of inequity and domination of one gender (literal and the traits associated with) over another. This paradigm shift would affect all levels of relationship, from physicians and health care providers to providers and patients. But first, we must deconstruct the continuum of relationship that defines creativity as a holistic pursuit that affects the larger social collective.

RELATIONSHIP CONTINUUM

Cultural transformation theory (Eisler, 1987) posits that human relationships fall along a continuum from domination to partnership. While no society purely operates from one of the models, the degree to which society a supports the development and vibrancy of all its members, not just the few at the top, depends on its alignment with partnership (Eisler, 2002; Eisler, 2007). Deconstruction of these relationships reveals two observations: 1) the dominator model limits creativity and, 2) the partnership model fosters creativity.

The dominator model is based on a hierarchy of rigid top-down rankings that is maintained through physical, psychological, and economic control. The dominator model, also viewed as a "power-over" relationship (Eisler, 1987; 2000), maintains its rigid hierarchy by historically favoring only one gender: male (Eisler, 1987). The shadow that the dominator model has long cast over health care has not been fully considered until recently (Eisler & Potter, 2014).

The biomedical model has traditionally been organized under a dominator relationship, historically pitting one profession over another and one gender over another. However each field or profession in health care brings its own medicine to support patient healing and wellness (Eisler & Potter, 2014). Eisler (2007) identifies four distinct characteristics about the dominator model. The dominator model favors:

1) institutionalization of hierarchies that rank men over women,
2) an authoritarian and inequitable social and financial structure,

3) a high level of institutionalized social violence, from violence against women and children to violence in war, and

4) beliefs and stories that justify and idealize domination and violence.

The Partnership System

Democratic and economically equitable structure

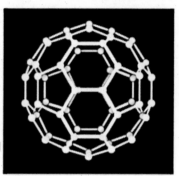

Mutual respect and trust with low degree of violence

Equal valuing of males and females and high regard for stereotypical feminine values

Beliefs and stories that give high value to empathic and caring relations

The Domination System

Authoritarian and inequitable social and economic structure

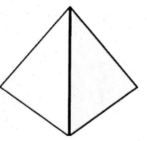

High degree of abuse and violence

Subordination of women and "feminity" to men and "masculinity"

Beliefs and stories that justify and idealize domination and violence

Figure 1. Dominator/Partnership Model.

In contrast, the partnership model is based on a democratic and economically equitable "power-with" structure that:

1) equally values both stereotypically male and female traits and work contributions,

2) has low levels of violence and functions in an atmosphere of mutual respect and trust,

3) demonstrates democratic and economically equitable structure, and

4) invests in beliefs that give high value to empathetic and caring relations (Eisler 2007).

CULTURAL COMPETENCY

Our current definition of creativity is biased. Socialization practices designate creativity as an individual creator or "lone genius" treating the world as objects to be used in service of a creative vision rather than viewing creativity as an open-ended and evolving conversation between subjects with their own internal integrity and vision. The historical definition of creativity then, is skewed by dominator model socialization that perpetuates cultural beliefs and practices that devalue historically stigmatized "feminine" characteristics such as nurturing or compassion, thereby valuing masculine traits as more desirable or beneficial than feminine traits.

The patriarchy that institutionalized this definition of creativity is damaging for both men and women, since it limits relationship and creative expression with one another by only recognizing the contributions of half of humanity's potential. Men and women alike are socialized to negate femininity in all areas of social construct, from "not running like a girl" in sports to "being more aggressive in the boardroom" in order to compete in the workplace. Even our everyday language perpetuates the dominator model with common phrases and clichés like "That's above my pay grade." or "My doctor said he will only allow me to _____." continue to erode the partnership potential of our health care system.

The current domination model in health care creates barriers to receipt of health care services by identifying physicians as "gatekeepers," with all other health care professionals ranked as subordinates. Their determining what services all other disciplines provide is a short-sighted approach. No checks and balances exist to ensure patients are getting services they need or that the decisions physicians make are based on best plan of care rather than what's convenient or financially best for the physician or their employer. Communication is also stunted because the physician hands down directives rather than using a team approach that creates accountability for a patient's best care. What results is disjointed continuity of care, which erects barriers to receipt of necessary rehabilitation services and erodes creative potential by not considering the input of rehabilitation professionals.

Insurance companies also have a "power-over" relationship with rehabilitation professionals. Use of the dominator model reduces utilization of needed non-invasive services by providing a distinct barrier: requiring orders from a physician who may know little or nothing about the highly specialized fields of rehabilitation. The ideals of capitalism are exploited by bringing gross financial profits at the expense of the society that needs health care. The cost of health care in the United States is the most expensive in the world, spending more of its GDP (17.7%) than any other developed nation; and yet performs the poorest, ranking last of 11 other wealthy nations studied (Davis et al., 2014), especially on measures of access, efficiency, and equity. Worse, the US has ranked last in previous reports as well, including 2010, 2007, 2006, and 2004 (Davis et al., 2010; Davis et al., 2007; Davis et al., 2006 & Davis et al., 2004).

Without an advocate experienced in negotiating the current dominator system of health care, a patient does not know what services are needed, what services to ask for, or that they even have a right or option for rehabilitative or preventive services. The patient is left feeling like they have very few options, very little voice, and therefore oftentimes feel their real problems are left unaddressed. This scenario works against society's best health, quality of life, and economic prosperity, further illustrating why rehab needs rehabbing.

The patient has been left feeling dominated, marginalized, belittled, dismissed, or outright ignored as a patient. But how does the dominator model affect us, the providers? In "Transforming Healthcare Culture: Unlocking the Foundational Barrier to Improved Patient Safety, Quality, and Experience," a workshop offered through the Center for Partnership Studies, Julie Kennedy-Oehlert posits that the dominator model can create:

- Lack of validation in (health care) roles
- Patient and employee "policies and procedures" that are steeped in domination theory (urban legend-like outdated policies)
- Punitive-based policy
- Lack of common language and a name to call out things/relationships where they are on the continuum (domination/partnership)
- Culture that doesn't allow for partnership and interprofessional collaboration

Additionally, perpetuation of the dominator model in rehabilitation can take the form of:

- lack of health literacy in both health care professionals and patients that perpetuates the dominator view of MD at the top,"
- lack of direct access to rehabilitation services and providers in all states, and
- lack of public health policy and social policy to support individuals and families who care for the young or old.

Ultimately everyone loses in the domination model. Physicians lose because they cannot possibly supervise and carry a sufficient knowledge of all rehabilitation practitioners, nor do they have intimate knowledge of the skills and services each profession is able to provide. Rehabilitation professionals lose because another profession controls their expertise and contributions to patient healing. Most importantly, the patient doubly loses because they feel neglected and dehumanized by the system and their needs go unmet.

Partnership-based health care would maximize the healing potential of all therapies and forward creative problem solving in rehabilitation through several means. Use of a partnership model in health care:

1) views the patient as the leader in his or her health care, wherein the individual's feelings and stories are listened to and considered in mutually arriving at a best plan of care,
2) fully engages the patient and family members as active participants in their own health and well-being, and
3) empowers the patient to take responsibility for her or his own health.

Use of partnership-based model is also a more sustainable means for a solvent health care economy because it increases the likelihood of patient adherence through patient engagement and focus on relationship thus leading to better overall long-term all-health outcomes and a lower burden of cost for the individual and the system. Ideally, partnership should see a relationship where clinical doctors and health care professionals practice "shoulder-to-shoulder" with one another. This approach was described at the First Physical Therapy Summit on Global Health as a horizontal, than the historical vertical, approach (Dean et al., 2011) to clinical practice, which is congruent with the definition of a partnership relationship between health care providers.

The partnership model is also based on the egalitarian principle that both male and female are capable of creativity and leadership, and that one gender or person does not need to be considered superior to another. Creativity then, must be redefined to include "both the female and male halves of humanity to be more congruent with research" (Eisler & Montuori, 2007 pg. 480). This egalitarian definition of creativity depends on shifting from the domination model to the partnership model. In other words, we do not have to disembody compassionate, nurturing, and the caring state of being from the self. We are both.

The Domination/Partnership Continuum

   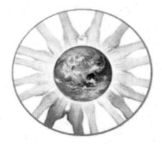

Hierarchies of Control   Hierarchies of Actualization
Superior/Inferior relations   Relations of mutual respect
Dominate or be dominated   Shared focus on nurturing
                                            and sustaining life

Figure 2. Domination_partnership continuum.

Partnership-base health care depends on harnessing the power of "feminine" values, including empathy, compassion, and nurturing within a biomedical system that is largely driven by "masculine" values. Partnership also allows health care professionals to apply the same feminine values to relationships with patients, their coworkers, families, and ultimately, themselves (Eisler & Potter, 2014). Strengths on the feminine part of the continuum (again, seen in both women and men) include (Turner, 2012):

- Building relationships and establishing community in the workplace
- Structuring teams and groups in non-hierarchical, egalitarian networks that encourage involvement
- Collaborating (as well as competing)
- Making decisions by paying attention to process, gathering input and synthesizing perspectives (vs. driving to a goal)
- Influencing by persuading (vs. commanding)
- Sharing information, credit and power

Where on the relationship continuum does your organization or workplace fall? The remainder of this chapter will help identify where organizations may fall on the relational continuum through elaboration on the deeper layers of relationship, patterns of domination in health care culture, how relationship affects leadership, and how cultural competency affects the paradigm shift toward sustainable partnership in rehabilitation and health promotion.

RELATIONSHIP LAYERS

When a patient goes in for a health care visit, how many layers of relationship are visible to the clinician? How many layers does the provider recognize e.g. self and patient, patient and family, patient and community, etc.? How do those layers of relationship, and their quality, affect the patient's prognosis or potential for well-being?

In Deborah and Emily's cases, how did their relationship with health care providers factor into their overall health outcomes? With their self-efficacy? With future relationships with health care providers? And how did the stunted relationship affect the caregiver's creative potential in determining the best plan of care? Did either Deborah or Emily's provider even consider their unique and creative abilities could contribute to the healing process?

What about interprofessional or educational interaction? How many layers of relationship are visible between a physician and therapist? Or between a therapist and student therapist? Instructor and student?

At the most basic level, there are two types of relationship in which the individual participates: 1) intrapersonal and 2) interpersonal. Intrapersonal relationship describes the depth and health of the relationship you have with yourself. Interpersonal relationship describes the way you relate to, and communicate with, others. As described in Chapter 3, healthy interpersonal relationships depend on an accurate sense of self-communication, or intrapersonal relationship.

But both types are equally important to the health of both the patient and the provider. Eisler's cultural transformation theory challenges health care providers to rethink all of their relationships including relationship with self, patients/ clients, colleagues, other professionals, and communities (Eisler & Potter, 2014, position 1051-1052). The layers of relationship should then be considered at the following levels:

- patient and provider,
- patient and clinic staff,
- provider with the self and environment (staff, family, community, and society)
- individual with the self and environment

These intersecting relationships must also be considered within the virtual plane of interaction via digital culture. Digital citizenship and engagement have drastically influenced how we receive and interpret information, permanently changing the collective social landscape and creative potential in healthcare. Whether a digital native or digital immigrant, digital citizenship - the idea that a person can be a multi-cultural member of society from their desktop - is a powerful method of communication that has given birth to vast creativity.

Seven dimensions of transcultural citizenship have been identified that can further affect creative potential via digital relationship, which include (Pathak-Shelat, 2014) an individual's:

1) Identities/Affinities
2) Values
3) Knowledge/Information
4) Connection/Communities/Networks
5) Expression/Voice
6) Dialogue/Deliberation
7) Action (which also describes the sense of one's efficacy)

Online or distance education is another forum through which the creative muse can be lost or found, and which affect all seven dimensions of transcultural citizenship. Both forums, digital citizenship and digital education, encourage us to develop a more critical outlook on relationship, perhaps viewing citizenship or belonging as something that happens with human beings, rather than occurring only in the context of one government or organization.

Relationship also happens on a larger scale at all seven dimensions, because citizenship includes not only relationships with people, but with the environment as well. In the partnership model, being in relationship appeals to an obligation to "respond to others with hospitality and the feminist theory of ethics of care" (Pathak-Shelat, 2014, pg. 62).

Even more complex is the degree of culture competence and sensitivity that exist in relationship. At a basic level, there is the quality and quantity of relationship that exists between rehabilitation professions and between those same professions and other health care providers, including medical doctors and nurses. For example, the struggle for autonomy and so-called "turf" wars has led to many battles between medicine and rehabilitation professions, as well as between rehabilitation professions ourselves. One discipline fights to have exclusive rights and privileges over another profession without considering how both professions can work together to dually provide aspects of service in order to increase access to, and efficacy of, care.

These layers of relationship must be considered, as well as their context, because of the complex template they provide to negotiate the creative path in rehabilitation. In addition to lack of literacy, access, and policy, there are also barriers to creation of health care literacy, direct access to rehabilitation services, and caring public health and social policies. In order to earn the trust of patients and public, those in health care fields would "likely need to develop radical new means of thinking and acting collaboratively" (IOM 2013 pg. 1-1). Statements like this reaffirm the need for adopting a partnership model in rehabilitation, in hopes that the shift to an egalitarian model would eliminate some of these age-old barriers.

DOMINATION PEDAGOGIES

Another relational realm in rehabilitation culture that can affect creative potential is the way we teach and learn. The growing body on interprofessionality points toward a pedagogical model aligned with partnership. Transdisciplinary professionalism, "an approach to creating and carrying out a shared social contract that ensures multiple health disciplines, working in concert, is worthy of the trust of patients and the public" (ABMS, 2013).

The way a teacher views and instructs a student is a reflection of the pedagogical relationship model the teacher has knowingly or unknowingly adopted. Use of a dominator model pedagogy, may take on the following characteristics:

- the "expert" teacher resides over the student and views the student as a blank sheet of paper waiting to be "filled" with the teacher's knowledge, while
- the "underling" students operate only under the knowledge given to them by the "expert" teacher, excluding their own experiences and prior knowledge.

Teaching in this way limits and often disqualifies a student's own experience, inherent knowledge, or inborn talent and genius, thereby limiting teacher-student interaction, the student's ability to be creative, and as a result, subsequent innovation in the classroom. Dominator interaction during a student's medical education, can exact negative consequences, such as an instructor belittling the student in front of colleagues, or creating an atmosphere of fear in a clinical residency or rotation where the students avoid asking questions for fear of being ridiculed. These negative experiences can affect the self-esteem of students across professions (Eisler & Potter, 2014). If students in medical training "cannot trust their own observations, how will they become full partners in health care if their self-esteem is weak?" (Eisler & Potter, 2014, position 2637). Overall, any system where rigid hierarchies reign supreme do so at the expense of proactive collaboration and true innovation, because they are built on competition and control or "power-over," rather than on establishing relationship based on mutual respect, trust, and authenticity, or what Eisler & Montuori (2001) describe as "power-with".

By contrast, a partnership model in health care exists within a framework that validates authentic experiences and unlocks people's potential, says Sara Saltee of the Center for Partnership Studies. Frenk et al. (2010) calls for major education reform in health care in The Lancet, citing that breaking down professional silos through interprofessional education should occur alongside increasing "collaborative and non-hierarchical relationships in effective teams" (Frenk et al., 2010 p. 1924), which is congruent with the definition of the partnership model.

The Institute of Medicine (IOM) reports that transdisciplinary professionalism would facilitate improved interprofessional teamwork and may even synthesize and extend discipline-specific expertise to create new ways of thinking and acting" (IOM, 2013 pg. 1-1). The IOM (2010) also states that physicians should be educated with other health care professionals both as students and throughout their careers (and vice-versa) in lifelong learning opportunities, an approach well supported by the World Health Organization (WHO), the Centre for the Advancement of Interprofessional Education (CAIPE) in the United Kingdom, and the Canadian Interprofessional Health Collaborative (CIHC), to name a few (WHO, 2010; WHO, 1978).

Developing innovative thinkers in rehabilitation must consider cultivation of collaborative skills, behaviors, and values to students in health care programs, as well as developing leadership that can facilitate "ongoing research and innovation for transformative change" (IOM, pg. 1-1). This movement toward interprofessional education and collaborative practice (IPECP), in existence for decades, is finally receiving increased attention. Especially in the face of the health care crisis in the United States today, there should exist an increased sense of urgency and deliberate effort to work together in partnership.

"Health systems research, which aims to capture such complexities, by necessity, needs to be multi-disciplinary and multi-method" (Swanson et al., 2012, pg. 58.; Mills, 2012).

RELATIONSHIP IN MINDFUL LEADERSHIP

The new creativity discussion in rehabilitation recognizes the crumbling silos and tension between professional identity and integral understanding. But to shift the paradigm of practice in health care from a dominator to partnership model, effective leadership must also be addressed.

Leaders become so because of the quality of their relationship and interaction with others. If we learn who we are from others, then we become who we are because of the quality of interaction with others, says Daniel Siegel, clinical professor of psychiatry at the UCLA School of Medicine and Co-Director of the Mindful Awareness Research Center. Relationship, then, is the context for creativity, including creating our own sense of self and health.

Partnership-based health care in the community would look flatter and less rigid than the hierarchal organizations we are accustomed to seeing (Eisler & Montuori, 2001). Chapter 4 on evidence-based practice underscores that research and community-based inquiry are both affordable and efficacious. In evidence-based practice, hierarchies often rank quantitative evidence over qualitative (Potter & Eisler, 2014), placing randomized controlled trials (RCT's) above all other types of research. "RCTs in isolation are inadequate to address complex challenges inherent in the context of health systems" (Swanson et al., 2012, pg.58, Mabry et al., 2010). Evidence-based medicine should not be ranked above the experience of the patient or practitioner.

International commentary on strengthening health care systems identify three themes as being most prominent or critical to systems-thinking approaches:

1) collaboration across disciplines, sectors, and organizations,
2) ongoing, iterative learning, and
3) transformational leadership (Swanson et al., 2012).

A global, partnership-based conversation is necessary as advocacy groups and global health leaders address the epidemic non-communicable disease rates, combined with achieving universal health care coverage and strengthening weak health care systems. The conversation shift, and success of achieving global health initiatives, depends on leaders' "ability to collaborate with other key stakeholders around a shared vision…through creation of "learning organizations" that bridge across communities, sectors, and disciplines, continuously working together toward a common future" (Swanson et al., 2012).

Twentieth century medicine and rehabilitation were built around the necessity of dealing with acute disease and injury; however, 21st century health care must respond to the overarching social and behavioral determinants of health, chiefly chronic diseases caused by lifestyle choices. Since medical intervention affects a person's lifelong health by an overall estimated 11%, while lifestyle and personal choices dictate 62% of a person's health (Kaufman, 2012; Kaufman & Pomeroy, 2012), health care of the future must focus on setting "common goals and targets with patients and relevant stakeholders, ensuring that each person is properly informed and engaged" (Swanson et al., 2012). This means that transformational leadership is not defined in terms of the traditional, patriarchally-defined hierarchy. Instead, transformational leaders will exist at all levels of an organization and will serve to challenge old ways of thinking and practice. Leadership representation will be found through the organization and will be built around a "shared vision of equity and efficiency...encouraging collaboration across disciplines...to break down traditional professional and disciplinary silos" (Swanson et al., 2012, pg. 58). Moving away from a dominator-style leadership in education would not require elimination of hierarchies, but instead encourage the development of leaders at all levels of an organization.

Leadership in health policy has also been linear and short-sighted in application. In the past, "Policy makers too often approach health systems from a mechanistic perspective, assuming that implementing a particular policy will lead to a predictable change in the behavior of local actors (such as providers, professionals and citizens), thereby ignoring the interactions between them. This line of thinking leads increasingly to detailed incentives and regulations from the top down, a so-called 'command and control' approach to policy" (Rouse, 2007). This approach leads to a loss of locus of control, self-efficacy, and dependence, which ultimately undermines leadership thinking at all levels by defaulting to punitive strategies and reward-type incentives. This type of approach also fails to consider that there are many determinants of health and a wide variety of efficacious interventions available.

From a neuroscience perspective, leadership must be considered according to brain-based thinking. The prefrontal cortex is "responsible for many competencies of good leaders," and is ironically dubbed the executive center (Siegel, 2014). Effective, mindful leaders must create an organization not through the old dominator mentality, but through helping those in the organization become their best self, described as helping the "latent self" in others to emerge (Siegel, 2014). Meaning, the potential for greatness lies in the individual already and a good leader will help the individual recognize the unrealized self. A truly visionary leader communicates in ways that motivate, instead of through old dominator patterns which would use intimidation, threats, or ultimatums.

SUSTAINABLE PARTNERSHIP IN REHABILITATION AND HEALTH PROMOTION

"Much of what is happening today (in health care) is the conflict between the shift to partnership systems countered by domination/hierarchical resistance" (Eisler & Montuori, 2001). The organizational development and cultural transformation field is moving toward an overarching partnership model. For example, the University of Arizona's vision for academic medicine embraces partnership theory by focusing on unifying culture via (Kennedy-Oehlert, 2014):

- Service/patient experience
- Faculty and staff experience
- Diversity and inclusion
- Multi-dimensional communications
- Joint planning
- Interprofessional practice

Hospitals, clinics, and human resource departments in organizations and private practices can focus on partnership by addressing vestiges of dominator-relationship in (adapted in part from Kennedy-Oehlert, 2014):

- Patient policies (e.g. strict limitations on visitation/attendance at appointments that prevent patient inclusion and family engagement),
- Employee policies (e.g. staff bullying and interprofessional relationship; rigid work schedules that do not consider flextime, job-sharing, etc.)
- Procedures, Research, & Development (e.g. encouraging interprofessional collaboration and research through creating accountability policies that require interaction between professions and departments)
- Leadership development (e.g. Do leaders carry interprofessional goals and share responsibility? Are leaders responsible for engagement and who is included as a leader? Is there a team approach used? Is there lateral violence, high turnover, or discrimination in recruitment policies?)
- Patient-Provider Interaction (e.g. See the sample letter/conversational template that promotes collaborative person-provider interaction*)
- Provider-Provider Interaction (e.g. Establishing healthy dialogue between providers at all levels of an organization or between practices)

*Consider this sample letter used to encourage collaborative person-provider interaction encased in a partnership model:

It was a privilege to meet and work with you today. Thank you for sharing your story, your birth experience, and your fears and hopes with me today. I am glad you felt an environment of trust and respect to do that. This is how medicine should be and it is why I operate outside of the typical/conventional mode of practice. Healing is affected by our environment, the attitude and outlook of our health care providers, and as a result, I try to provide a welcoming, nurturing environment to each individual that becomes a patient. Your health care is very important and should warrant a team approach in every instance. That means your health care providers should always work together to provide a holistic, biopsychosocial plan of care. I am glad to hear that you have/are doing...Please see the attached program for your IHP (individualized home program).

Grace and Peace,
Ginger Garner PT, ATC

CONCLUSION

We are staged to use partnership in American health care, but we are not using it. Creativity in rehabilitation requires leadership that moves past the rhetoric of political and social conditioning and gender discrimination. Leadership development includes a balance of both feminine and masculine traits, encased in a partnership model. When both genders thrive, a country's economic system is stronger, which is a boon for potential health care, not to mention economic, reform. "Abandoning preoccupation with material wealth and profits and elevating ourselves to a more empathic worldview will require embracing feminine characteristics that foster peaceful communities and sustainable economies" (Perkins, 2011). A nation's quality of life is inextricably connected to the status and power of women. When their status is threatened, an entire nation's quality of life suffers (Eisler, 2007).

From boardroom to bedside and beyond, the partnership model can allow rehabilitation professions to pursue their vision more effectively, sustainably, and certainly, more creatively. We must press on toward cultural transformation in health care that fosters health literacy and collaborative education to truly see active partnership thrive and forward the creative agenda in rehabilitation.

REFERENCES

ABMS (American Board of Medical Specialities). (2013). ABMS professionalism definition. Retrieved July 23, 2014. http://www.abms.org/News_and_Events/Media_Newsroom /features/feature_ABMS_Professionalism_Definition_LongForm_abms.org_040413. aspx)

Davis K., Schoen C. & Stremikis S.C. (2010). *Mirror mirror on the wall: An international update on the comparative performance of American health.* New York: The Commonwealth Fund.

Davis, K. Schoen, C., Schoenbaum S.C., Audet A.-M. J, Doty MM, & Tenney K. January (2004). *Mirror mirror on the wall: An international update on the comparative performance of American health care through the patient's lens.* New York: The Commonwealth Fund.

Davis, K., Schoen, C., Schoenbaum S,C., Doty, M.M., Holmgren, A.L., Kriss, J.L., & Shea, K,K.May (2007). *Mirror mirror on the wall: An international update on the comparative performance of American health care.* New York: The Commonwealth Fund.

Davis, K., Schoen, C., Schoenbaum, S.C., Audet A.M., Doty, M.M., Holmgren, A.L., & Kriss, J.L. April (2006). *Mirror mirror on the wall: An international update on the comparative performance of American health care through the patient's lens.* New York: The Commonwealth Fund.

Davis, K., Stremikis, K., Squires, D., & Schoen C. (2014) *Mirror, mirror on the wall. how the performance of the US health care system compares internationally.* New York: The Commonwealth Fund.

Dean, E., Al-Obaidi, S., De Andrade, A.D., Gosselink, R., Umerah, G., Al-Abdelwahab, S., Anthony, J., Bhise, A.R., Bruno, S., Butcher, S., Fagevik-Olsen, M., Frownfelter, D., Gappmaier, E., Gylfadottir, S., Habibi, M., Hanekom, S., Hasson, S., Jones, A., Lapier,

T., Lomi, C., Mackay, L., Mathur, S., O'donoghue, G., Playford, K., Ravindra, S., Sangroula, K., Scherer, S., Skinner, M. & Wong, W.P. (2011). The first physical therapy summit on global health: implications and recommendations for the 21st century. *Physiotherapy theory and practice, 27*(8), 531-547.

Eisler, R.T. & Montuori A. (2001). The partnership organization: A systems approach. *OD Practitioner, Vol. 33*, No 2.

Eisler, R.T. (1987). *The chalice and the blade: Our history, our future.* San Francisco, CA: Harper & Row.

Eisler, R.T. (2000). *Tomorrow's children: A blueprint for partnership education in the 21ˢᵗ century.* Colorado,CO: Westview Press.

Eisler, R.T. & Montuori, A. (2007). Creativity, society, and the hidden subtext of gender: Toward a new contextualized approach. *World Futures, 63:*7, 479 – 499.

Eisler, R.T. (2002). *The power of partnership: Seven relationships that will change your life.* Novato, CA: New World Library.

Eisler, R.T. (2007). *The real wealth of nations creating a caring economics.* San Francisco, CA: Berrett-Koehler Publishers.

Eisler, R.T., Potter, T.M. (2014). *Transforming interprofessional partnerships: A new framework for nursing and partnership-based health care.* Sigma Theta Tau International.

Frenk, J., Chen, L., Bhutta, Z. A., Cohen, J., Crisp, N., Evans, T. & Zurayk, H. November, (2010). Health professionals for a new century: Transforming education to strengthen health systems in an interdependent world. *The Lancet, 376*(9756), 1923-1958.

Institute of Medicine (IOM). (2010). *The future of nursing: Leading change, advancing health.* (Report brief). Washington, DC: National Academies.

Institute of Medicine (IOM). (2013). *Establishing transdisciplinary professionalism for improving health outcomes: Workshop summary.* Global Forum on Innovation in Health Professional Education. Washington, DC: The National Academies Press.

Kaufman A. & Pomeroy C. (2012). *Social determinants of health.* The New York Academy of Sciences.

Kaufman A. (2012). *Linking university health resources to social determinants in the community: Prioritizing health disparities in medical education to improve care.* New York, Academy of Sciences.

Kennedy-Oehlert, J. (2014) *Transforming healthcare culture.* Session 4: Operationalizing a partnership culture. April 28, 2014.

Mabry, P.L., Marcus, S.E., Clark, P.I., Leischow, S.J. & Mendez, D., (2010). Systems science: a revolution in public health policy research. *American journal of Public Health, 100*(7), 1161-1163.

Mills, A. (2012). Health policy and systems research: defining the terrain; identifying the methods. *Health Policy and Planning, 27:*1-7.

Pathak-Shelat, M. (2014). *Global civic engagement on online platforms: Women as transcultural citizens.* Unpublished dissertation for PhD in mass communications. University of Wisconsin-Madison.

Perkins, J. (2011). *Hoodwinked: An economic hit man reveals why the global economy IMPLODED -- and how to fix it.* New York: Crown Business.

Rouse, W.B. (2007). Health care as a complex adaptive system: implications for design and management. *Organization Science, 38*: 17.

Sackett, D. L., Rosenberg, W. M., Gray, J. A., Haynes, B., & Richardson, W. S. (1996). Evidence based medicine: What it is and what it isn't: It's about integrating individual clinical expertise and the best external evidence. *BMJ: British Medical Journal, 312*(7023), 71-72.

Siegel, D. (2014) *Discussing the Leader's Mind.* Podcast 59. From leadership: A master class. Interviewed by Daniel Goleman. More than sound. Retrieved July 1, 2014. http://morethansound.net/2012/11/15/discussing-the-leaders-mind-with-daniel-siegel/?utm_source=BenchmarkEmail&utm_campaign=leader's%20mind&utm_medium=email#.U7LM817o0dt

Siegel, D. (2014). *Discussing the leader's mind.* Podcast 117. (part 2) From Leadership: A master class. Interviewed by Daniel Goleman. More than sound. http://morethansound.net/2014/04/15/ep-117-discussing-leaders-mind-daniel-siegel-part-2/?utm_source=BenchmarkEmail&utm_campaign=leader's%20mind&utm_medium=email#.U7LOvF7o0du

Swanson, R.C., Cattaneo, A., Bradley, E., Chunharas, S., Atun, R., Abbas, K.M., Katsaliaki, K., Mustafee, N., Mason Meier, B. & Best, A., (2012). Rethinking health systems strengthening: Key systems thinking tools and strategies for transformational change. *Health Policy And Planning, 27* Suppl 4, Iv54-61.

Turner, C. October (2012). *Difference works: Improving retention, productivity, and profitability through inclusion.* Retrieved July 24, 2014. http://www.forbes.com/sites/womensmedia/2012/10/24/can-feminine-women-make-it-to-the-top/

World Health Organization (WHO). (1978). *Primary health care. Report of the international conference on primary health care.* Alma-Ata, USSR. Geneva: World Health Organization.

World Health Organization (WHO). (2010). *Framework for action on interprofessional education and collaborative practice.* WHO Department of Human Resources for Health. Geneva, Switzerland: WHO Press.

In: Fostering Creativity in Rehabilitation
Editor: Matthew J. Taylor

ISBN: 978-1-63485-118-3
© 2016 Nova Science Publishers, Inc.

Chapter 7

CREATIVITY, STRUGGLE AND SUSTAINABILITY

Cheryl Van Demark, PT, MA
Director, Health In Motion, Chino Valley, AZ, US

ABSTRACT

Fostering creativity is a process that continues to unfold across time and while enjoying a romantic notion in our day, very often involves significant resistance. The earlier chapters thoroughly documented some of the biggest barriers to creative emergence in rehabilitation. This chapter bridges those issues with a look at the personal requirements to undertake this process. It also prepares for the next chapter on implementation of our creativity both personally and within organizations. Once implemented, the new creation must also be sustained. This sustainability requires a much larger lens of focus beyond the walls of our local experience, yet the ability to stay focused and have the systems in place to be fully incorporated.

INTRODUCTION

"Creativity is about liberating human energy"
Howard Gardner.

In the moment when you become inspired to create and then empowered to sustain the creative process without struggle, what could be rehabilitated about rehabilitation? It is my intention to guide you in liberating your creative energy. It is my hope to inspire you to contribute your voice and your will to engage others in the necessary revolution that is to follow the devolution of our present form of rehabilitation. Through the ages, Mother Earth continually re-balances herself with demonstrations of her natural power in the form of earthquakes, hurricanes, tornados, floods, droughts, volcanos, fires, plagues and blights that all have profound effects on humanity. Our present health systems are being overcome by a tsunami of populations with chronic illnesses that are lifestyle and stress-mediated. This tsunami represents a global health challenge that affects the whole human continuum; those whose illness is related to excessive consumption of resources on one end of the continuum and those whose illness evolves from lack of consumption of resources at the other end of the continuum. Make no mistake; we have collectively created this tsunami. Einstein counseled us long ago to recognize the power of thought in creating our reality: "We cannot solve the problems with the same thinking that created them." How can we begin to reflectively disrupt *our thoughts* to collectively co-create a system of health and healing for ourselves and our patients to rehabilitate rehabilitation? The fact that you have opened this book speaks to your readiness to engage in this creative journey.

As I write this chapter, I am enjoying my thirty-first year as a physical therapist and navigating the "empty nest" stage of parenthood. I am well practiced in fostering creative states that are facilitated by tolerating ambiguity, learning to face fears, inviting a curious state of mind and growing my knowledge base. The tap to my creative flow re-opened considerably when I returned to contemplative practices over the past decade. Creative ways to rehabilitate continue to unfold in rich relationship with others as I move through the world flavoring my physical therapy with my life experiences as a yoga student, teacher, yoga therapist, teacher of yoga therapy and entrepreneur.

Creative energy is liberated by invoking the power of story, metaphor, imagination and visualization. To that end, I have invoked a Rehab Muse for our creativity in this chapter. Consider how the qualities of muses relate to creativity. Muses are imaginative, mischievous, light and agile. When they appear, muses disrupt our version of reality; shifting our perspective on what we believe to be true and possible. Muses have kind and playful hearts that guide them effortlessly into ingenious solutions. Muses are also capable of focusing their powers for significant magical acts. Lastly, muses tend to appear when you need them the most: "Necessity is the mother of invention." Given that you are reading this book, I presume you agree that it is a necessity for us to foster creativity in rehabilitation. I invite you to pour a steaming cup of tea and take a comfortable seat near a window with natural light. Prepare to liberate your creative energy.

CREATIVITY

Inspiration is both a foundation for creativity and the oil for our internal fire, as a metaphor for struggle and sustainability. We all know inspiration is part of the creative process, but what is it? Being a modern girl, I perused Google and chose this definition from dictionary.com: "a divine influence directly exerted upon the mind or soul." Within the construct of your belief system, allow "divine" to take on whatever form you can most comfortably invite as catalyst for the flow of creativity that exists within. Our Rehab Muse, as with the ancient Greeks, will represent our creative inspiration. Picasso apparently knew this feeling well, as he authored the phrase: "I do not seek, I find". To help you find your inspiration, your Rehab Muse, I highly recommend a self -imposed "retreat" to invite the energy of the creative process to percolate into your conscious mind. Begin with just a few minutes of ritual retreat or refuge each day. You may find the experience so pleasurable that you decide to expand your retreat/refuge into a few hours, a day, and then eventually a weekend and beyond! It is especially helpful to set intention to invite inspiration to be revealed. (See Part IV: Action Steps to Creativity for exercises addressing the following qualities of inspiration.).

IMAGINATION

Inspiring moments occur primarily when you feel relaxed and the mind is freed to explore and imagine. Imagination is a crucial element of creativity and must have no bounds. "What could be?" is a fundamental creative question. Invoking imagination is another reason for the choice of a Rehab Muse. Freedom of the mind to imagine often accompanies freedom from our routines and especially from our habits. When is the last time you were freed? When we step outside of the familiar, our five senses are refreshed. We can best refresh our senses when our environment soothes them. Recall your last experience outdoors in a beautiful setting and note your ability to recall the sights, sounds, smells tastes and feels. Our minds flow more freely when we relax our bodies, or use them in familiar rhythmic movement patterns. Have you noticed that habitual thought and habitual postures are often interrelated? Habitual behaviors perpetuate functioning on autopilot. Autopilot perpetuates the status quo. When we engage in new physical experiences, or enter a playful state, we facilitate the imagination. Our attention is stimulated by new sights, sounds and experiences. *"Originality is simply a pair of fresh eyes." Woodrow Wilson.* In a novel playground of cleansed senses, the mind becomes more mobile. A mobile mind generates novel thoughts. A non-distracted, attentive mind notices them. Where is your attention in this moment? Is it with you as you read this book or is it divided? If it is divided, what is dividing it? Anticipating the next text, e-mail, phone call plan etc. or rehashing something? Attract your own attention so that you can get into the pilot seat. Recall that creativity requires liberation of your energy. Energy follows attention.

ATTENTION

As a future change-maker in developing a new model of rehabilitation, consider the profound implications of this statement about attention by Otto Scharmer, a leading corporate change expert affiliated with MIT, *"…the success of our actions as change-makers does not depend on what we do and how we do it, but on the inner place from which we operate….The essence of our view concerns the power of attention: We cannot transform the behavior of systems unless we transform the quality of attention that people apply to their actions within those systems, both individually and collectively."* (Scharmer, C. O., 2007). Creating new approaches to rehabilitation will require us to start with attracting our own attention and learning to redirect it inward. Self-inquiry as a key component of clinical mastery builds the skills for bringing our attention back out into our world with sharper focus and the capacity to attend to broader views of ourselves, others and the systems we have the potential to co-create to serve society. Practicing mindfulness is a very effective way to train attention.

AWARENESS

Paying attention to our attention cultivates self-awareness. Self-awareness is pre-requisite for something far more important to creativity: Awareness. It is our Awareness that recognizes the arrival of inspiration. To engage Awareness, we must learn "presencing" or pre-sensing, which involves a combination of present moment awareness and a sensing of future possibility. Awareness or connection to Source is a "blind spot (it is our nature, but what is *its* nature?)" (Scharmer, C. O., 2007) There is a helpful metaphor for understanding this concept. It depicts a lame man who can "see" (Source/ Soul/Awareness) being carried through the world by a blind man who can move (human body/self). Making this self-awareness to higher Awareness connection, is "a necessary reintegration of mind and matter" (Scharmer, C. O. & Kaufer, K., 2013) that allows us to understand where our actions originate and how our collective intentions create thoughts, words and deeds that shape our social and environmental reality. Contemplative practices cultivate presencing, which allows us to learn "see" with our blind spot.

CONSCIOUSNESS

Aware change-makers collectively co-create from the inspiration they attune to and, through their will, the emerging future can unfold. An alternative term for this Awareness is Consciousness. This viewpoint on accessing our creativity from our blind spot is one in which form follows consciousness; sometimes referred to as downward causation. There are numerous descriptions of consciousness on various levels. "Personal consciousness is awareness—how an individual perceives and interprets his or her environment, including beliefs, intentions, attitude, emotions, and all aspects of his or her subjective experience. Collective consciousness is how a group (an institution, a society, a species) perceives and translates the world around them. In its largest sense, consciousness has been referred to as a "milieu of potential," a shared ground of being from which all experiences and phenomena arise and eventually return." (Scharmer, C. O., 2007) To foster creativity in rehabilitation, we can raise our self-awareness to a higher Awareness, learn presencing and access our blind spot. We can invite Consciousness to drop in via inspiration so we become vehicles for change-making. As rehabilitation professionals, it is likely we have all experienced those times in the clinic where we have a breakthrough in how to work with a patient in a novel way to help them succeed in achieving their goal.

COMPASSION

Awareness opens your head oriented thinking mind to receive inspiration through the heart-felt insights that arise through imagination and attention training. Heart-felt insights are rooted in compassion, which the Dali Lama describes as a feeling of closeness to others combined with a sense of responsibility for their welfare. Compassion for self and others opens the heart for inner guidance to direct the action that I will represent as "hands." A heart-head-hand connection can then be sustained. Working in the rehabilitation professions requires great compassion for others, but how often do we extend a similar degree of compassion to ourselves, our colleagues and even to those who are cogs unaware/asleep at the wheel in the current health system? Compassion does not lead to economic systems that treat health, human beings, the earth and money as commodities. The compassionate heart remembers its nature as "unstruck, as capable of presencing the common experiences and needs of the human race through the eyes of love (Scharmer, C. O., 2007)." Most traditions speak to love of self as the basis for being able to love others, and having compassion for the self as a starting point for learning to love. If we truly embrace our innate nature as Awareness, then what is not to love about ourselves? If this same Awareness is the innate nature in all living beings, then what is not to love about others? Strong heart-head-hand connections create awareness-based collective actions (Scharmer, C. O., & Kaufer, K., 2013) that align push and pull. Push refers to awareness that keeps pace with continual external changes. Pull refers to our mindful awareness of our inner domain as Awareness. Aligning push and pull as we engage others in the co-creative process of rehabilitating rehabilitation gives us the capacity to sense common intention and to act from an Awareness of the whole. The words healing health and holy all share the same root word: hal - to make whole (Cragie, F., 2010).

ACTION

Attention, mindfulness, compassion and cultivation of awareness are about far more than personal liberation of creative energy. It starts there, but then attracts like energy. The whole point is to come together and use our collective awareness as a conduit for the transformation of rehabilitation. Creative change-makers shift their awareness from "ego-systems (focus is on me) to eco-systems (focus is on we)." (Scharmer, C. O., 2007) Beyond attention, it is this quality of awareness of those creating the system that will determine the quality of results we see from the system in action. It is time roll up our sleeves and gets our hands dirty by tossing out what does not work in the old models to make space for the new. Start prototyping and motivate colleagues to do the same. Circles of conversation grow into forums for co-creating based on the lessons we all have learned from our prototypes. In order for any system to change, the change-makers must engage self-awareness to listen with empathy and "see themselves and the system through a multiplicity of views (Scharmer, C. O., 2007)." Change makers need to try "presencing" with each other so something new and wonderful will emerge. A right view will evolve a future for rehabilitation that embraces a "profit" (originally defined as learning) that yields a triple bottom line; a profit for people, the systems they are a part of and our environment. (Scharmer, C. O., 2007) Applying an ecosystem (focus on we) mentality in rehabilitation would expand our outlook far beyond individual functional outcomes to include ecological, social, intellectual and spiritual outcomes. Are you ready to make this shift?

SUMMARY

Intend to foster creativity by taking retreat or refuge, preferably out in nature, to invite inspiration. Practice mindfulness to train your attention to pay attention, thus cultivating self-awareness. Use self-awareness to learn presencing. Presencing allows self-awareness to be released into Awareness of a divine influence being directly exerted upon the mind or soul through the pathway of a compassionate heart. Limitations of what might be possible are in our heads. Strong heart-head-hand connections enable us to become a gateway for the co-creative process which Consciousness is trying to emerge. Moving through the world inter-connected in heart-head-hand prepares us to cope with struggle and find sustainable solutions. After all, Rehab Muses only appear to those who are inspired to imagine and see with fresh eyes!

STRUGGLE

Struggle is the result of disintegration of our heart-head-hand connection or lack of compassion for ourselves along the way in our creative process. Cynicism is said to result from disconnection to the heart; Depression from a disconnection to the will and denial from a disconnection to the mind. At this writing, I am in my fourth year of a creative journey integrating mindful movement arts into rehabilitation. A personal story of inspiration from my Rehab Muse is offered in Part III of this book. I have come to know struggle on an intimate basis as a change-maker engaging in awareness-based collective creativity, which I presume led to my friend and mentor, Matt Taylor's invitation to write this chapter! Moving creative inspiration into form and function through countless prototypes requires courage and resilience to navigate the many challenges that arise. (I was raised a Lutheran, so believe me, I have a strong work ethic fed by many a casserole.) Again, the value of contemplative practice cannot be overemphasized in maintaining a heart-head-hand connection to endure the growing pains that come with the mantra of "fail early to learn quickly." Letting go into trusting Awareness as the inner compass for navigation is a work in progress and the foundation of clinical mastery. Ego will always think it knows better than surrendering to the softer Awareness!

Habits of thoughts and subconscious core beliefs are a common source of struggle. The beliefs generate the habits of thought that take on various voices in the head. Fear, judgment and cynicism are common voices that generate struggle. The stronger our self – awareness, the more we can practice observing the sources for our struggle. For example, my first response to Matt asking me to write this chapter was deep gratitude for being invited to the table for this wonderful book. My fearful habits of thought "I don't know enough yet" led to more fearful mental chatter such as "Oh no, what if he wants me to share my creative process as an example of what not to do!" Hello struggle. A helpful practice when we notice such destructive habits of thought, is to ask ourselves "Is this true?" (Hanson, R., & Mendius, R., 2009)

The experience of struggle may also depend upon your perspective on obstacles. Obstacles are likely to arise. Surprise! Don't take them personally. If we keep the focus of our creative endeavor on the greater good, then we can avoid the 'I", "Me", "Mine" thinking that feeds into taking things personally, whether they go wrong or right. If we trust in Awareness as our inner compass, obstacles may be strategically placed in our path for our protection. Consider treating them with curiosity. Look for a lesson. These recommendations are not as simple as they may appear. Practice with them. An important last word about struggle is to look closely at whether your upbringing and conditioning have led to a core belief that struggle is necessary! That life is hard! All good things will require sacrifice, etc. Again, "Is this true?" is a helpful question. If you expect struggle, you will likely encounter it!

SUFFERING

Struggle builds character for some and leads to suffering for others. The ever-widening socioeconomic divide has invited many struggles. Growing numbers of people around the globe are facing hunger, poverty, inequality, loss of political voice and violation of basic human rights. Only 1 in 5 has access to clean water. Many people are being overcome by the magnitude and diversity of struggles that surround them and suffer through life. An alarming number of children in this country are presently growing up below the poverty line. The health status, educational and societal impacts of this is monumental. Suffering is an uncomfortable topic. If you think suffering is a strong word to associate with struggle, consider these statistics: "In the past 45 years, suicide rates have increased by 60% worldwide. In the year 2000, the WHO reported more than twice as many people died from suicide as died in wars. Suicide is the second leading cause of death among American high school and college students (after accidents) and is in the top 3 causes of death on a global scale for those aged 15-45."(Source Theory U) Depression is the leading cause of disability in our country for this same age group. I find these statistics tragic. Healing has been defined as "the transcendence of suffering." How will we address suffering in a new model of medicine and rehabilitation?

Picture our Rehab muse might carry a bow and arrow, which is relevant to discussing suffering. In the Yoga tradition the bow and arrow is used as metaphor wherein the body is the bow, the postures are the arrow and the target is the soul. Yoga is said to have been offered to humanity as a means of coping with suffering as an inevitable part of the human experience. In fact one definition of Yoga is "the union of the disunion with suffering" (Feuerstein, G. 2000) Influenced by yoga, the Buddhist tradition also uses the metaphor of the bow and arrow to address suffering. In this metaphor, suffering is not about being struck by the first arrow; getting injured, having a disease or struggling with whatever obstacles arise in your life. Suffering is described as being struck by a second arrow, which is self-inflicted. The second arrow represents the stories we construct, and then narrate on a continuous mental feedback loop, around getting stricken by the first arrow. The Christian narrative around the cross and pierced heart of Jesus is transformed through the apostle's new story on Easter Sunday. We run these stories in our central nervous system like a simulator (Hanson, R., & Mendius, R., 2009) such that they create our perception of reality based on *the simulation*. This continuous running of our simulator creates neuroplastic changes in the brain (neurons that fire together wire together) that get bigger, stronger and faster at generating the stories from this simulator until suffering becomes our only narrative. Chronic pain can be well explained in this way. The Therapeutic Neuroscience Education approach emphasizes our capacity to change our story of pain, resulting in immediate change demonstrable on functional MRI.

SELF-DIRECTED NEUROPLASTICITY

To reframe suffering, we can tap into our capacity for self-directed neuroplasticity. We can unlearn the story of that second arrow, and create a new narrative. What are your personal sources of suffering around the current model of rehabilitation? You can probably generate a pretty big list: workload, time constraints, paperwork, reimbursement, communication, technology, etc. Here is the kicker. As rehabilitation professionals, we personally have to learn to transcend suffering so that we can act as guide for our patients in this new model of rehabilitation we create. How do we access self-directed neuroplasticity to re-write our personal narratives?

Contemplative practices that employ mindfulness are at the heart of self-directed neuroplasticity. Mindful movement is one of the mindfulness tenants. Mindfulness stands out in the literature as our present best medicine for reducing stress and stress mediated chronic illnesses. Yoga, a science of the mind that uses our embodiment as our laboratory, is the platform for modern mindfulness based stress reduction and cognitive behavioral therapies. The myriad physical practices in the Yoga tradition are used primarily to train attention, generate mindfulness and prepare the body-mind for meditation. These practices represent a treasure trove for mindful movement that could be useful for priming for rehabilitating rehabilitation. Is yoga sustainable? Well, it has been practiced by humans around the world for at least five thousand years or more....What are your thoughts for other sources to prime us for what we need to recognize our innate wholeness and capacity for healing as we create new narratives about rehabilitation?

SUSTAINABILITY

Mindfully self-aware, inspired, compassionately connected in heart-head-hand, engaged in awareness-based collective action and empowered to transcend suffering, we can now address the sustainability of a co-created vision for rehabilitating rehabilitation. That is where the metaphor of fire comes in. I have fire in my belly. So do you and your colleagues - otherwise we would not be in the rehabilitation professions. Borrowing again from the Yoga tradition, the energy of fire has many qualities. It relates to digestive processes (everything coming into your 5 senses), to clear vision for discernment of the meaning of the 5 sense inputs and to higher intelligence (recall the burning bush metaphor in the Bible). Fire energy purifies, sharpens and hones our will, and its heat fires the belly to endure. Fire transforms form. In collective creativity, you will need to manage fire qualities to see your vision of rehabilitating rehabilitation through to its full becoming. And, it helps not to set each other on fire!

Using the discernment quality of fire, sustainability calls for the ecosystem and triple bottom line viewpoints that arise from operating from our blind spot, as previously discussed. Transformative qualities of fire will recreate a responsive sustainable model for rehabilitation that considers access to care for all populations who need it. Think of all the facets of "access"; location, centralized services, adult/child care, hours of operation that working people can make, language, affordability. I am just starting the list. Once access is unconstrained and everyone can come to the table, how do we use fire to feed them education? How do we light a fire in their bellies to improve health status if difficult lifestyle changes are involved? How do we sustain interest to rehabilitate "the whole house"? How do we facilitate more ownership in the value vs cost of the services? Most importantly how to we entice the client into co-creation of rehabilitation? Dean Ornish suggested our focus in heart disease has been misdirected for all these years. Cardiac medicine focused on fear of dying instead of joy of living. Have we missed the mark in similar ways in rehabilitation?

How do we sustain? How do we keep from burning out our fire, our passion as rehabilitation professionals? What gives you will-power/motivation? What do you truly value or hold sacred in your life? Do you align your time/your actions with what has most meaning-based on your core values? At the end of the day, we all want to feel that our life has meaning. We must see our connection and contribution to a greater good. Our behavior needs to be driven by passion and purpose. We ultimately spend our "free" time doing what has meaning to us. How does this look for you? Perhaps the results of this exercise are not sitting well with you because you don't feel in charge of your time. You actually are in charge, so look again with compassion at your habits of thought, routines and beliefs. Find your inspiration. As we personally learn to do this, we can get better at looking for opportunities to help our patients move through the same process. To help them connect meaning, passion and purpose in their rehabilitation process to what they value (i.e., EBM), to what is vital and sacred for them.

Align your vision with your core values and a mission/creative endeavor for rehabilitating rehabilitation will emerge for which you will have no problem keeping the fire in your belly burning. You will have the appetite to sustain your vision when you love what you do and do what you love. Finding what you love in your inner domain, not seeking it externally, takes us full circle back into a recommendation for bringing contemplative practices in some form into your life. Embracing a triple bottom line (people, systems, and planet) in the vision, so that it is aligned with the greatest good will ultimately determine if your creative contribution is sustainable.

If there is no stillness, there is not silence. If there is no silence, there is no insight. If there is no insight, there is no clarity. Tenzen PriYadarshi
May you be inspired to adopt a contemplative practice.

CONCLUSION

Where to go from here? What might you do with your inspiration to rehabilitate rehabilitation? Start talking about your ideas with others. Read the inspiring stories of others that have walked this path ahead of you in Part III and then dive deep into exercises of Part IV. Share this book! By giving creative ideas voice, you will invite other voices to speak. Listen deeply! You will feel and hear where the creative ideas are weak and where they are strong. Get your hands dirty by diving into to prototyping so your ideas take form. Form is tangible and therefore easier than abstract ideas as a means to collaboratively co-create.

As you engage in awareness-based collective actions, remember, what people ultimately remember is how you make them feel- what experience was created. As we co-emerge a process to rehabilitate rehabilitation, I hope we facilitate healing. Recall that healing is ultimately about learning to transcend suffering and the root of the suffering is separation. Separation from our innate wholeness, from our creative freedom, from our inspiration "a divine influence directly exerted upon the mind or soul." We sense ourselves as being separate people, separate systems/institutions and separate from our planet. Separation is deepened when we focus on our differences (race, religion, socioeconomic status, genders, political views, etc.) instead of our similarities as one human race. When we emerge our future from our blind spot (Awareness), we all look the same! When we as rehabilitation professionals feel separate, we suffer in a system we feel too small to change. We all have a Rehab Muse waiting to inspire and empower us, to liberate our energy. What could be if we did not regard ourselves as limited or separate?

References

Craigie, F. (2010) Positive spirituality in health care. Minn, MN. Mill City Press.

Feuerstein, G. (2000). *Shambhala encyclopedia of yoga.* Boston: Shambhala.

Hanson, R., Mendius, R. (2009). *Buddha's brain: The practical neuroscience of happiness, love, and wisdom.* Oakland, CA: New Harbinger Publications.

Scharmer, C. O. (2007). *Theory U: Leading from the emerging future as it emerges. The social technology of presencing.* Cambridge, MA: SoL Press.

Scharmer, C. O., Kaufer, K. (2013). Leading from the emerging future: From ego-system to eco-system economies. San Francisco, CA: Berrett-Koehler Publishers.

In: Fostering Creativity in Rehabilitation
Editor: Matthew J. Taylor

ISBN: 978-1-63485-118-3
© 2016 Nova Science Publishers, Inc.

Chapter 8

THE IMPLEMENTATION OF CREATIVITY

Matthew J. Taylor, PT, PhD

Director, Matthew J. Taylor Institute, Scottsdale, AZ, US

ABSTRACT

The two sides of innovation are the idea and the execution of the idea into reality. This chapter proposes a functional model to utilize when addressing the execution of an idea into your environment. That action might be as an individual or as part of a bigger institutional system. Execution requires different skill sets, resources, and management than idea generation. Building a system for yourself or assembling one in an organization involves discipline, perseverance and a rapid learning cycle. Managing the ongoing responsibilities of rehabilitation service while bringing in new delivery models or techniques is not just an art, but a management science.

Inspired that we can express our creativity in both ordinary and sometimes even extraordinary ways, now what? Julie still sits with us. Or the troubled, disillusioned student/colleague sits with us. Or our friend, neighbor, or the stranger on the train. Most of all, we still sit with ourselves, teaming with inspiration, new insights and deep compassion. But what now? There's so much to do or that could be done that we never imagined. Too often this bright flame is followed shortly after by the dampening "reality" of how truly hard meaningful, lasting change is to affect... Julie returns from what you both saw as a breakthrough session only to report relapse or exacerbation... You snap at your child after faithfully performing your practices in Part IV for months...what gives? Welcome to the illusion of creativity as an event or an endpoint. Our creating is in the end an ongoing emergent process of Life unfolding, ever changing in an ever shifting context. There is no destination to arrive at. Only the ongoing process to re-commit and begin anew again. We will do well to remember the old Buddhist saying, "After enlightenment, time to chop wood and carry water." Well, it's time for Julie, and for us, to chop and carry. The good news is that others have gone before us and with the application of their experiences we can sharpen our axe and make the carry feel just a bit more downhill.

INTRODUCTION

This chapter addresses what Govindarajan and Trimble in "Beyond the Idea" (2013) describe as the "mountain climb" of innovation: executing new ideas into reality. They describe the generation of a novel idea as half of innovation and contend it is the relatively easy ascent to the top. Creating systems to then bring the ideas into reality is the other half. That second half is a treacherous, grueling process of descent where accidents and all manner of misadventure can occur through the fatigue of implementation. Gone is the fresh enthusiasm for the start of the climb of creativity, but we aren't home yet as we attempt to see the idea into enaction. In Chapter 7, Van Demark provided excellent insight into the aspects of sustainability and struggle that accompany this "chopping and carrying" half of the climb. From that context of self-care, watching for the illusion of separateness, and her broader philosophical perspectives, we will now craft a working metaphor based in part on Govindarajan and Trimble's "Beyond the Idea" (2013) and in large part on my lived experiences of birthing and rehabbing rehabilitation and other organizations.

AFTER THE IDEA

The generation of novel ideas will occur as you undertake the practices outlined in earlier chapters and Part IV of this book. Chances are that at some point in your career you already have had a few that you tried to implement without success, or just haven't quite gotten around to starting. Those have been your second half the climb of innovation. Either way, the insights and ideas will really emerge in abundance if you engage the domain practices in the days ahead. In this chapter we are presuming you have the idea, now what?

Unless you are blessed with financial independence, unlimited time and personnel resources you have a problem. The problem is you will almost certainly have to tackle two tasks at once: sustaining what already exists and trying to implement this new idea. The problem is compounded by the fact that the two tasks have almost nothing to do with each other. In fact, Govindarajan and Trimble (2013) state the tasks are very distinct and are inevitably in literally in conflict with one another. On the one hand you have to take care of today's customers and competitors, operate efficiently, be accountable to management and payers, be punctual, deliver a best practice level of care, and be profitable. But to implement involves risks, unknowns, additional expenses with scarce resources and uncertainty regarding long term success of the new idea. Bear in mind, any creative project that is new to you or your organization has an uncertain outcome. That uncertainty is real, it is an accurate reflection of postnormal times and will require all 3 axes of noncreative practices to navigate down the mountain.

For example, let's say you have a new treatment program you developed, but work full-time with patients in a very busy clinic schedule. How and where are you going to put this program? Work overtime? Cutback office hours and current revenue? Work on the weekends or evenings? Who will market it and pay for the development of the supportive materials? How will you keep upgrading the current operations and delivering the same high level of care there? …Can you feel it? Have you been there before? That's the rub of implementation and why there are so many great ideas out there, but why so few ever get implemented.

And yet, some new ideas do get started and eventually fully implemented, don't they? Of course! So what's the secret?

As you will read in Part III, our colleagues learned that while they were very good at the clinical skills of maintaining an ongoing clinic or classroom, no one had ever trained them in this other task of implementing something new. Over and over you will read how they had to gain new skills, find new support and develop new relationships. Lifelong learning personified and across a wide variety of domains! The good news is that having once done it, they no longer fear striking out into new territory, and each one looks forward to doing so again. Most achieved their goal by persistence and happenstance. The purpose of the remainder of this book to sharpen your axe and make the carry a bit lighter by applying the systems of implementation that follow.

WHERE IS OUR SUPER HERO(-INE)?

The former understanding of how things got implemented generally involved some tale of a creative superhero (almost always male) that saved the day. Chapter 1 dug deep into how this came about, but the notion still permeates our culture. Govindarajan and Trimble call this fictitious character of normal times, Innovation Man (2013). Innovation Man not only brings the bold new ideas, but lifts mountains of obstacles, inspires legions of followers and miraculously finds resources to bring the project to a successful implementation before flying onto the next adventure (think Steve Jobs mythology). Their research, and that of many others, dispels the legend of Innovation Man. Turns out it is almost always a context-sensitive situation with multiple factors coming together while participants incorporated certain skill sets and behaviors. So look in the mirror because that is where you are going to find Innovation Person.

OK Innovation Person, ready to go? Regardless of whether you just want to deliver a bit better care for your clients or save the world, let's get you properly outfitted. We need to get you some tools for implementation for your superhero belt, some systems to sustain you when your powers begin to wane, and a cape of perspective to assume the necessary heights to save the day. Of course entire departments in bookstores are devoted to this topic. In this chapter we will limit our outfitting to just two broad resources that would have saved me and the other contributors considerable struggle or mis-directed use of our superpowers. First there will be a review of resource that I have found to be the single most influential factor when answering the question of "How do you get so much done?" Then we will summarize the Govindarajan and Trimble's work as it can apply in not only corporations, but as individuals.

THE MAKING OF AN INNOVATION PERSON

For the first thirteen years of my career I was a replicator. Both a CEU and self-help book junky, I consumed and then replicated the directions and techniques of as many successful people as I could muster. The ultimate normal times rehabilitation professional.

This a common theme in the chapters ahead of our colleagues as well. Then one day after small incremental changes and shifting circumstances, I was doing things that hadn't been done and having fun. The first glimpses of "superpowers" I suppose. In a town of 3500 I went from an employee of a tiny physical therapy (PT) department with a part-time aide to now business owner, boss, payroll dispenser and eventually found myself as director of a fully integrated medical gym and PT department with 17 employees in the mid-1990's. Whoa, how did that happen? Well, while that was all well and good, I had an unstable lumbar spine that was increasingly debilitating... so much for superpowers by the expert backcare guy.

Long story short, I hear at a national fitness conference that this yoga stuff is suppose to be the next hot thing, so I find the only yoga teacher in our remote rural area and begin to attend class once a week. Little did I realize, I was beginning to dive deep into the noncreative domain practices of attention, affect, insight and embodiment. I had had the intention axis to improve and serve others, and I engaged those self-help behaviors regularly as the remaining axis. In 1997 the non-linear dynamics of complex being ignite an intense four year period where I was afraid to ask a question at a CEU course began to teach my own. From their invitations to write articles, collaborate on projects, chair organizations, etc. came fast and furious. As fun as it was, there also was a sense of overwhelm between opportunities, a very dedicated marriage and family life as well as community participation. So I decided to get a distance-learning PhD too! As "luck" would have it, one of my classmates was an expert in time management teach internationally. He introduced me to a resource that I continue to use to this day.

I had tried a variety of time management systems, but they always seemed to create more, not less work and bother. What he shared was "Getting Things Done" by David Allen (2002) that is now classic system of implementation. In hindsight I can see that what separates this system from the others, and I believes further fuels creative emergence, it that is embodied and enactive. Rather than the conceptual/mental axis focus of most systems, this one begins with context: where are you and what actions can you perform now? This embodiment orientation is artfully tied back into a system of insight, attention, intention (re-committing to what he calls commitments of action) and setting up systems to capture new ideas and to enact the ideas into practice. The system uses modern day tools of electronic calendars, email management, etc., as well as old fashion manilla folders and paper planners for the luddites.

These systems capture, process and track all those loose ends that otherwise overload our nervous systems and suppress creative emergence via allostatic overload. Finally, a way to be in my embodied state, satisfy my intellectual pursuits, keep balance on life priorities and most importantly, see my passion enacted. The mechanics of the system once set up, facilitates the creation of space and ensuing silence that will be explored in Chapter 24. Again priming additional creative emergence via the positive systems feedback loops of complex being. It isn't necessary to fully use the system, but reading the book and pulling just one idea out will give you another, if not many, "superpowers" of implementation while protecting your health via the embodied axis of awareness.

Lest this begin to devolve into what might feel like a late night infomercial of the rich and famous, did I mention elsewhere that destruction is the first step in creativity? Well, it is.

OH-OH, DIDN'T SEE THAT COMING

Fast forward to Fall of 2003. Cruising through the academic portion of my doctorate, lining up my dissertation subjects, eldest two children away at out-of-state college, spouse in a full time master's degree program 2 hours out of town, president of the local Rotary group etc,, etc… context shifts. The new administrator at the hospital where we have had our contract for 14 years doesn't have the partnership mindset of the former administrator. Short version: we live in different worlds, the board hired him and by systems effect must back him since they chose him, and we are effectively pushed out of our contract. (That destruction part I mentioned.)

The summer of 2003 finds us in Scottsdale, AZ trying to build a new clinic where there is one on almost every corner. Living on a new grad's social work salary and retirement funds, and not knowing anyone to recruit for that literal thing called a dissertation study on chronic back pain. Let's not romanticize this period. It was not fun to understate. But the destruction has cleared space in my life for something new to emerge…literally the Phoenix archetype. Personally it was my Julie moment from a personal narrative. What now? Well that earlier that Spring I'd seen what the new clinic would be as I lay metaphorically dying in my yoga corpse pose. Where it came from is open to interpretation, but the fact is via my noncreative embodied practice of yoga and inviting silence there it was, a new way to deliver integral physical therapy. Somehow I convinced my banker back in the Midwest that I could take a clinic with no standard PT equipment, only yoga blankets and blocks, and no experience billing (the hospital had done that in the past) and make it work financially while presently unemployed and not knowing a single referral source. At this point, a grateful nod to Sister Toban, my high school creative writing teacher! So I had the idea, the money to build and open, now the implementation half of the mountain climb. Needin' some serious superpowers here.

LIVING "BEYOND THE IDEA"

This is as good as any point to introduce my understanding of the term "sacrifice", or to "make sacred." In our Julie moments of darkness or Sanford's lying in bed paralyzed as a 13 year old boy, there are moments of choice. We can bag it, quit and withdraw from life or we can do that uniquely human thing of taking from the crucible of fire and transforming our life circumstance to have new meaning and purpose. At these moments we aren't talking about minor shifts in perspective or direction, but full speed, gut wrenching turns that often burn old bridges of being. I realize now that I was enacting our bones of domain practices at this point in my life with a complete sense of "not knowing" how it would all turn out. And this is no creative genius tale either, the sacrifices that my wife and children made during this period were significant. We never do it alone…never.

The happy "ending" …and there is no end in creating, is that this morning as I type things have worked out. By holding true to our family intentions of supporting one another and trying to ease suffering in the world, the kids are grown, successful in their own right, my wife and I are enjoying the new life of empty-nesthood, and my practice is a too busy, insurance-free cash-based business with a waiting list coming out of the worst economic period in our country's history. There were so many times when we had to re-engage the "making sacred" what mattered most to us. There was no vision-board construction and magically creating this life. And this life still has plenty of serious challenges, and that is even before turning on the news. The humility of practicing these domains for priming creative emergence is a deepening insight into the uncertainty of reality and with that insight, a deep appreciation for interconnectedness of causality that pecks away at the small ego's grasp for claiming credit of any kind for outcomes. All of this echoes back to Halifax's (2012) model of compassion and the creation of space for compassion to emerge not in some timid, weak fashion, but with the creative force of life that transforms and makes sacred our ordinariness in every moment.

My Phoenix experience has left me with two pearls to share that I see as key to our individual and collective health while sitting in the *silence* of life . These two pearls inform who I am, what I hope for our children and our world, and I believe will empower us as colleagues to more effectively rehab rehabilitation.

TWO PEARLS

It is important to repeat from Chapter 3, "A New Understanding of Creativity" that innovation and creativity are not the same things. A person can innovate a better, more effective showerhead at Auschwitz or a new weapon for killing humans but not damaging property. Creativity as we are using it in this new understanding of the complexity of being, first and foremost should be grounded in an ethic enhancing life's flourishing, diversity and sustainability. Without those hallmarks, it becomes mere innovation. This distinction is crucial and is the foundation for the two pearls I have discovered.

The first pearl is that implementation is worth little without compassion. A deep, reflective understanding of the intention behind the implementation and the results of its enactment should be sought prior to the first act of implementing. The discernment of insight from a place of affective attunement around the motivations behind the implementation fosters such an understanding. As Halifax writes so eloquently, this compassion begins first with self-compassion which in turn allows for deeper empathy for others. If the implementation is driven by the wrong or misdirected motivation, there is then a good chance that the outcome might generate rather than relieve suffering.

My insight around this pearl of compassion rooted in self-compassion occurred over years. At first my motivation was pure survival to care for my family. During this time there were plenty of doses of "should haves/could haves" and other berating of my self about the circumstances around the changes that led to our move to Arizona. At other times it was influenced by "showing them" or grasping to be secure or safe. Those impulses still arise of course, but with practicing the domains of Chapters 24 and 25, they become less frequent, I notice them sooner and can attune back to a greater perspective of equanimity. As a result, my intention sharpens to both care for myself AND relieve the suffering of those that seek my services. When I am able to do so, the quality of my life and theirs is enhanced and creativity emerges. The shift can be from a unique insight to redirect a treatment, the expansion of the sense of time when needing to cover a great deal or the serendipitous event that surprises us in a session (a Ganesha-type experience such as the Julie story).

I have some ideas about how this might happen, to include suspecting the neuroanatomical and physiological effects of the domain practices, but that is the stuff of future books. For now, gain the experiential knowledge of the practices, conducting your own individual case study on yourself. As I tell every patient on their first visit, "You've been told a great number of stories. I am telling you another. Don't believe me. But, try the story and if it seems to serve you, use it." So there it is, the first pearl. Develop and adapt a practice of self-compassion that fosters greater compassion for yourself and others. Upon this first pearl, take the second pearl of implementation and create greater human flourishing.

The second pearl is the unfolding realization that our incredible power to enact change is both terrifying and exhilarating. When implementation is not rooted in self-compassion it can lead to horrific results from drug studies gone bad to patients seeing only the backs of their care providers as the provider engages the electronic record. Implementation can be exhilarating when we transform the ordinary of our experience from profane "being processed through a system like a factory" to having a sacred, moment to moment, however imperfect, sense of being cared for and being heard. If the implementation is not anchored in our hearts before being executed by our intellect and enaction, violence ensues and all this talk of implementation destroys rather than rehabilitates. This heart talk is important but it must also be paired insight, attention and effective engagement. Plenty of good intentions for the flourishment of humanity are not doing a single thing in reality to actually serve others! So there is a grain of sand that irritates to create this second pearl of implementation. That irritant is the knowing that there will always be the conflict between your/your organization's ongoing operations and bringing something new into existence. Always.

If you forget this irritant of essential tension between ongoing and innovation, it will disrupt your attention, generate affective upset, and mental projections of blame or self-pity. All of which lead to the numbing of your embodied experience and then misdirected enactment as a result of the imbalances on these axes. These recursive loops of complex relationship are either going to generate virtuous loops of effective implementation or just as powerfully, vicious loops of degrading relationships thwarting implementation and causing further suffering. The creative rehabilitation professional then needs to be developing their domain practices across all axes. However, they also need some new, non-clinical skills based on this grain of sand. First some a couple of examples of how I came to discover this second implementation pearl the hard way through the past 10 years before we describe the skills.

My doctoral program emphasized practical application as an essential aspect of our scholarly development. I have been fortunate to have numerous "experiments" in implementation from my new clinic, to being board president of the International Association of Yoga Therapists (IAYT), a two year research study in Minnesota at a full scale research center, and this collaborative textbook process. In my experiences on the IAYT board I saw first hand how much resistance there could be to trying things that hadn't been done before; how important learning quickly by measuring results and revenues is to implementation of our international research conference and electronic library especially during the recession; and, how recruiting a capable board and committee team members ultimately determines if implementation actually occurred. We had some home runs and some pretty grand failures! The process was honing my skills and by the time Matthew Sanford and I approached the Courage Center in Golden Valley, MN the learning curve was paying dividends. I had learned how to tell a better story from the consumer's perspective, how to explain systemic benefits, and most of all to listen more than talk. We were able to garner two years of statistically significant organizational change and only stopped when the 2009 downturn dried up their research funding. Chapter 27 has more of the results of that process.

This book represents the third experiment. Could I pitch a story to a publisher, then 18 contributors, convincing them to write about a topic that hasn't been addressed before in rehabilitation? Even if I could, would they follow through (hint: there's no money in it for them), would their work be quality, and would it have practical value to the eventual reader? And would the publisher allow a slightly different format that blends didactic instruction and theory, autobiographical narratives and practical exercises for the reader to employ? If you reading this, the answer is "yes". Without my prior "experiments" and the development of the various interpersonal and technological skills, this book could never have been executed in less than seven months and on time. So thank you for reading this and let's now layout some more detail about the second pearl of implementation skills: holding the reality of the conflict between keeping the current operations running and initiating something new.

In retrospect, had I had this pearl of knowing the conflict was both normal and inevitable, I would have been a great deal easier on myself (self compassion) and others. Not only would it have been more pleasant emotionally, it would have been much more productive as I would have altered course sooner or acquired different resources for implementing the changes knowing it was normal and not personal. So even if you have initiated implementations for decades, scan the following summary of the science of managing this conflict as I suspect we can all find one more smidge of superpower, if not an entire new tool kit.

Being Comfortable in Conflict

Much of what we do is on a small scale and often private, the ordinary creativity. Sometimes though we will have a creative endeavor that involves anywhere from a few to an international reach. Chapter 26 addresses specific practices for the smaller projects while Chapter 27 discusses pertinent issues to taking things really big. It doesn't matter if you are just committed to smiling at your grumpy co-worker as they complain at lunch or establishing an international children's rehabilitation referral system, the conflict will be waiting for you.

My suggestion for dancing rather than wrestling with this conflict is to first just buy and read both "Beyond the Idea" (2013) and "Getting Things Done" (2002). They are both extremely readable and will flesh out the details to this summary for you. Allen's (2002) book sets up a simple system for you to regularly recommit to your dance, generating the ongoing intention to see the implementation through or modify the course. This pause/reflect/act is of course the heart of clinical mastery. Unfortunately in our very full days without a system, we don't and it's in not attending to this part of the intentional domain, that the dramas of the conflict gradually generate affective dysregulation, misdirected attention with ill-appropriated engagement. Let's look at the commitment to smile at your grumpy co-worker project to illustrate this principle.

You did great the first week and after much self-congratulating, started to slip when the receptionist called in sick throwing the office into chaos for two days, accompanied by another glitch in the EMR system. By that second Wednesday you caught yourself clenching your jaw as she was going on and on about the idiots that bought that system (you were on the selection committee by the way). Had you done your brief weekly review of commitments over the weekend, you might have had the ability to note the embodied response to the affective dysregulation she had provoked in you. That may have allowed you insight into the fact that it was occurring and the subsequent creative, equanimous of a compassionate response recognizing her comments as a reflection of her suffering, not an attack on you. Without that "space" of insight, the affective dysregulation may have prompted an angry reaction to include a comment about her really needing to take basic computer course to enter the 21st century...and all the fun that would have followed that not so creative slip of the tongue!

While this ordinary example of trying to institute a creative response may seem silly, it holds the important principles both of these resources detail in order to manage the conflict inherent in implementing change. You need a system that regularly re-assesses your experiment in starting something new, recognizing it will take additional resources and may require outside support as well. Allen's book (2002) gives you specific systems to set up and "Beyond the Idea" (2013) offers the following broader rules for management based on management science. Understanding these rules and employing the technique allow the dance with conflict while still awkward, considerably more comfortable.

We will use the corporation metaphor from here on out, so whether it is your ordinary implementation within your personal "corpus" on a small scale such as the above example or that multi-national project involving many, the conflict is the same. Implementation takes both a metaphoric and literal team. You will want to design a very specific structure to succeed and it will require a team. The team structure is a partnership between a "dedicated team" and a 'shared staff'. The action steps to manage the conflict between maintaining the ongoing and starting the new are:

Define the mission: As in any goal-setting exercise, the greater clarity you can articulate on the intention and final outcome of the mission, the better your chances of constructing a system to manage the conflict.

Specify the work: Gather as much detail around the work to be done as possible beforehand. Any unanticipated work will later need to be negotiated and could become a source of additional conflict.

Design the team: Now that you know what needs to be done, "who" is going to do it. Be very clear about what "hats" will be needed to complete every part of the work.

Divide and quantify the work and assign roles for the shared and dedicated teams: Govindarajan and Trimble (2013) differentiate between dedicated or shared resources. Dedicated are resources that are solely used to work on the new mission. In big systems, maybe a new IT specialist or research assistant that is only going to do the work of the mission. For the individual, it might be more metaphoric, e.g., I'm going to dedicate for the next 3 months instead of shopping on Sunday afternoons I am going to block that time to work on this mission only. You are dedicating some part of your non-ongoing operation resources to the mission. For the shared work, you squeeze extra work from those already part of the ongoing operation. Maybe you identify John in HR to work a budget for the new program personnel costs. As an individual, possibly you decide to devote that last 15 minutes at lunch for drafting the new program instead of chit-chatting in the breakroom. That is, you are sharing some resource out of what you were already doing by squeezing it out of the bit of inefficiency or waste in your current habits of ongoing operations. This section is key to anticipate adequate resources and clarity of roles. Failure to do so will generate either your own personal internal conflict (I didn't realize Sunday shopping was my way of relaxing and now I'm exhausted by midweek) or John will run screaming to his upline because PT just asked him to do some additional project for them. Whether your personal corporation or the bigger corporation, give this section much time and detail.

How much training required? Will you or some team members need new training as part of the overall project? If so, who and how much? Who will pay for it?

Prove it works: Lastly, Govindarajan and Trimble (2013) use the experiment analogy for setting up a rapid learning cycle of forming a hypothesis of what will happen, making measurable predictions, executing and measuring results, changing course based on frequent meetings (by yourself if personal or as a team), and being brutally honest in what is working and what isn't. It is at this point where we see the crossing over of these practices with the domain practices of Chapter 25. Inability to sustain attention, monitor and adjust affective response, sustain intention through embodied reflection will all influence the quality of insight gained and resultant actions of future engagement. Fail fast and fix fast requires this embodied set of practices as we have all witnessed the painful slow death of new innovations when the leaders can't pull the plug and the effort limps along well past the obvious failure point. The experiment mindset is systematic way to reconcile behaviors to results by asking are our predictions getting more accurate and is it resulting in either lower costs or better outcomes or both? They suggest formalizing the experiment by developing a custom plan with custom metrics that assess the outcomes AND costs. Then schedule a separate space on calendars to review plans, results and lessons learned.

Questions to ask during these sessions are: Is the planning process being done seriously? Is there a clear hypothesis? Is it understood and the implications clear throughout the process? Are the unknowns (especially most critical) clear to you? Are revisions based on identified lesson? Is there quick reaction to new information? Are all of you facing the facts? Are predictions improving? Their mantra is "Try to spend a little, learn a lot."

While this is only a short review of processes, hopefully there are components that as you read them, they brought to mind either current conflicts or those from past implementation efforts. The adoption of these noncreative systems will set the stage for reduced conflict of the second half of the mountain climb while enhancing the emergence AND implementation of your creativity in rehabilitation and your life in general.

CONCLUSION

It has often been said that the first step to creativity is destruction. Something old has to give way to something new. The Phoenix arises from the ashes, the artist makes the first brush mark on the blank canvas, or your Sunday shopping is eliminated. So too for your creative emergences and having the space to employ these techniques and this model of implementation. We can't keep filling an already overflowing cup. First we have to pour something out to make room for more. What are you willing to destroy or eliminate in order to make new room? How much will you will sacrifice to create? Before beginning, please learn and explore with our colleagues in Part III about how they birthed something new into rehabilitation and what they are presently creating. Afterward, with their inspiration, you can pick up your axe and water bucket as you head into Part IV, "The Action Steps that Foster Creativity," to make more of your unique contributions.

REFERENCES

Allen, D. (2002). *Getting things done: The art of stress-free productivity.* New York: Penguin Press.

Govindarajan, V., Trimble, C. (2013). *Beyond the idea.* New York: St. Martin's Press.

Halifax, J. (2012). A heuristic model of enactive compassion. *Curr. Opin. Support Palliat. Care* Vol 6 2: 228-235.

PART III: CASE REPORTS FROM CREATORS IN REHABILITATION

In: Fostering Creativity in Rehabilitation
Editor: Matthew J. Taylor

ISBN: 978-1-63485-118-3
© 2016 Nova Science Publishers, Inc.

Chapter 9

OCCUPATIONAL THERAPY

Arlene Schmid, PhD, OTR
Associate Professor of Occupational Therapy
Colorado State University, Fort Collins, CO, US

WHAT CHALLENGES AND OPPORTUNITIES ARE SPECIFIC TO YOUR PROFESSION?

As with all of health care, there are many challenges and opportunities. In general, all of rehabilitation is threatened with numerous challenges, including but not limited to high 'productivity standards', making quick gains that may or may not be relevant to the client, less time to foster a client's independence after an injury or event, and insurance/payers often controlling rehabilitation outcomes and goals. There are a few very concerning challenges specific to occupational therapy (OT) at this time. For example, there is a concern that other professions/professionals are trying to be everything in rehabilitation and are not valuing the unique role of OT. OTs have a long history of meaningful or purposeful and functional activities, often including creative activities. Much of this has been lost as we moved forward with a medical model and an increased focused on bio-mechanical aspects of the person. Additionally, in some rehabilitation venues there appears to be a reduction of collaboration among therapists and this is somewhat related to payment systems. I think it is a true loss to the client when therapists are not able, or not interested, in working with each other for the best of the client via interprofessional collaboration. This may also be attributed to some health care professionals not valuing the role of OT. An important need for OTs, as stated in our strategic goals, is to be able to demonstrate and articulate our value to others.

OT will be celebrating its 100th anniversary in 2017 and this is a wonderful opportunity for our profession. It is very validating to be part of a profession that has a long and solid history of clinicians and researchers supporting the idea that how we occupy our time is important and essential to the rehabilitation and living process. OT was founded on the ideas of treating the whole person - mind, body, and spirit (not just a body part) with a holistic approach. This allows us to weave the idea of focusing on a chosen way to occupy one's time; OT is therefore very client-centered and addresses the whole person and that person's goals and occupations (activities). There is great opportunity here as much of (western) society is quickly moving to the idea of treating the whole person. OT often is and should be at the forefront of these changes in health care. This shift to whole person care provides great opportunity for OT as it is incredibly intuitive for us to think this way about our clients and treatments.

An exciting aspect of OT is that we truly wish to focus on improving life for people, we frequently state that a priority of OT is helping individuals 'live life to its fullest'. In relation to fostering creativity in rehabilitation, I think many OTs are intuitively creative and want to bring this to the rehabilitation table, a huge opportunity for us as a field. I am happy that I found OT and that I have been dedicated my career to help people, and help students help people, to add life to years, not just years to the life….

WHAT DID/ARE YOU DO/DOING?

I have been an OT for nearly 20 years. The opportunity to create is one of the reasons I found and chose OT; I think this is true of many of today's OT students. After I graduated from OT school in Buffalo, NY I moved to Hawaii and worked in multiple clinical settings. I gradated in 1997 when the prospective payment system changed rehabilitation as we knew it and it was a challenging time to get a job or keep a job. Creativity was of key importance to companies and hospitals who managed to work through the new payment system. While I was able to maintain a position as an OT, after just five years of clinical practice, I felt as though I was no longer challenged as a clinician. My last clinical position was as a hand therapist, a very prescriptive type of OT to say the least! Maybe my lack of feeling challenged was actually the acknowledgement that I was not able to be creative as a clinician? Regardless, I then decided to pursue my doctorate and received a PhD in rehabilitation sciences, an interdisciplinary degree.

While I had been in the clinic, I had personally found yoga and it had a tremendous impact on my life. Yoga helped me to feel better physically but also really helped me to feel more grounded and more comfortable in my own skin. I then began to use yoga with my clients, in an adolescent mental health facility and then in outpatient rehabilitation. I found this led to great results, both better and faster than with traditional exercise. It was at this time that I had decided it was best to pursue a doctorate to be able to study the benefits of integrating yoga into rehabilitation. Since I completed my doctorate I have developed and studied yoga interventions as an aspect of rehabilitation. It is very rewarding, but I think my desire to be able to change practice and integrate yoga into therapy and health care may still be very far away.

WHAT SUPPORTED YOUR PROCESS?

The most important support in my academic and research position has been my mentors. My mentors helped me to establish myself and reviewed my work as I wrote manuscripts and grants. They truly supported me as a stroke rehabilitation researcher, and were happy to go along for the ride as I delved into my yoga specific work. A lot of people thought it was not very smart for a research scientist to study yoga, but my mentors who really cared about me and my happiness were supportive of this idea.

WHAT INHIBITED IT?

Sadly, trying to earn tenure in the university setting greatly restricts creativity. At the end of the day, to receive tenure, one needs to write and receive grants and publish heavily. Ideas that are funded and published may be not your true passion, stifling creativity. Therefore I find myself torn between trying to fund research about yoga and being on grants that may or may not allow me to fully be passionate about the topics.

DO YOU HAVE ANY PERSONAL PRACTICES THAT YOU THINK SUPPORT YOUR CREATIVITY OR WORLD VIEWS?

I try hard to be outside at least a little bit every day. I now live in Colorado and there is great opportunity for this. I know I feel better and work better, and am more grounded when I am able to be outside and play. Of course keeping up with some yoga is a personal practice and I always feel better when I am more consistent with my yoga practice. I think achieving a high level of education and being able to travel and meet people from around the world has greatly changed my views. I try to remember we all come from different places…

HOW HAS THE EXPERIENCE INFLUENCED YOUR CURRENT CREATIVITY?

I think this depends on the day! Being an academic, every day is different for me. I have a lot of autonomy that I really cherish and enjoy. The days that I truly enjoy are when I am creating something from nothing…whether this is creating new lectures, teachings students new concepts, or writing a new manuscript. I find that I can be really focused on these types of activities. I love teaching, and in OT we teach students to be critical thinkers. Critical thinking is an opportunity for being creative, however students frequently want the black and white answer, and this most often does not belong or exist in OT. It is wonderful to help them acknowledge their creative self and help them to move forward. All of that said, there are many days when creativity is not a real option.

DESCRIBE YOUR EXPERIENCE WITH CREATING ...IS IT A STEADY PROCESS? EPISODIC? MANIC? DROUGHT? DOES IT FEEL LIKE IT COMES FROM "YOU" OR ELSEWHERE?

This is an interesting question. I think it somewhat depends on the task at hand, so episodic. While I love starting a new project, I do sometimes get stuck and have trouble actually beginning it, but once I start I tend to get almost obsessed with it and I think about it and talk about it and work on it until it is done! Maybe that is a bit manic….For sure, this comes from me. I'm often surprised when others don't feel this….

HOW DO YOU NURTURE OR NURSE FLEDGLING IDEAS?

I have a colleague who is also a best friend, and I feel like I can really talk about any ideas with her. We can nurture such ideas together, or importantly she can help me put some ideas to rest. I think this is equally important as we only have so much time in the day and it is important to wisely choose which ideas to nurture. Once I have decided to pursue an idea, I begin reading about and start writing about it, and probably talking to others about the ideas and where those ideas may lead. I also spend a lot of time in my office with the door shut, writing and thinking.

WHAT ROLES DOES/DID YOUR COMMUNITY/COLLEAGUES PLAY IN YOUR CREATIVE EXPERIENCE?

My mentors were incredibly helpful in progressing my academic career. However, I think most important is building relationships with people where you can go and sit and chat with colleagues and throw ideas around, always feeling comfortable. I think just being open to thinking outside of the box, and finding others who are too, is a key step in maintaining a creative mind.

WHAT WOULD YOU DO DIFFERENTLY?

I would consider an academic position in an integrative medicine research center, not only rehabilitation.

WHAT'S NEXT?

I really want to help take new possibilities into the classroom and the clinic. I do not think that large randomized clinical trials are what will change or better rehabilitation. I think we have to be open to the possibilities of looking at research and therapy with a different lens. I think it is essential that we move to trials where we can truly tailor the OT intervention, as it is highly unlikely that the exact same intervention will work for every person with a stroke or every person with an amputation. It is time to make rehabilitation research more clinically relevant. It is time to really engage the clinicians and clients as we move forward with trials and decision making.

WORDS OF WISDOM/INSPIRATION?

Embrace occupation and the abstractness of occupation and OT! OTs by background are creative, embrace this too! It is what makes us unique in healthcare and we should be proud of it.

In: Fostering Creativity in Rehabilitation
Editor: Matthew J. Taylor

ISBN: 978-1-63485-118-3
© 2016 Nova Science Publishers, Inc.

Chapter 10

PHYSICAL THERAPY

Mary Lou Galantino, PT, PhD, MS, MSCE

Professor, Physical Therapy
Richard Stockton College of New Jersey, Galloway, NJ, US

WHAT CHALLENGES AND OPPORTUNITIES ARE SPECIFIC TO YOUR PROFESSION?

The challenges in our profession are the ever demanding paperwork and healthcare systemic issues that may lead to burnout. When I completed my post doctoral fellowship and research on stress in healthcare professionals, I was struck by the initial passion as everyone endorsed the work, but that passion was soon lost over time. Clearly, strategies need to be in place for creativity and self-care, and this includes the training of our rehabilitation graduate students across the nation. My *Wellness Coaching* for DPT students is one example of a way to incorporate strategies throughout the curriculum which may be applied in patient care. Practicing what one preaches is key to authentic delivery of care. Self care is an important component of clinical mastery and essential in replenishing the art of creativity.

WHAT DID/ARE YOU DO/DOING?

Take the road less traveled, find new areas to open doors for others and explore how one could serve locally and globally. What ignites a passion inside is translated into a natural extension of what we do in the world. We are blessed by the inner voice which guides us and I am grateful to have listened along the way. Why are we inclined to serve others and not ourselves? Where have we given into the demands of the system to overtake our perspective of a profession turned into the drudgery of work?

Reinventing myself in the context of what I love is key to my facilitation of others in my role as a family member, friend, wife, mother, professor, researcher and clinician. Having a variety of venues in which I serve fosters the colorful palate of the legacy I wish to impart. While I enjoy my work in the northeast region of the U.S., every opportunity to travel, whether it is to China to oversee our acupuncture training, Haiti to treat patients where disability is not accommodated for, or to South Africa, where I visit the HIV townships to conduct population based research, I embrace the challenge of meeting new people and immersing myself in learning about the culture of healing and open my eyes to the fact that we are all interconnected, finding our way to wholeness and wonderment of life.

WHERE DID YOUR IDEAS/DESIRE COME FROM?

My desire to engage in the fullness and variety of life started in during my hospice care as a new graduate in the early 1980's. I was fascinated by the end of life process and the inherent human spirit trying to survive amidst impending death. The curious nature of navigating ambiguity and jumping into the unknown was a creative force that emerged moment by moment, as I deeply connected to each person and family member. In that restlessness of being unaware of the timing and ending of a precious life, I learned much about interfacing the inevitable. This fostered a deep resonance of spontaneous creativity and compassion in my role as a health care professional as I had no previous training in hospice care. I then embarked on the art of self-compassion when I realized I could not prevent the death of so many in the end stage of the disease process.

I was 23 when I started my profession and during my training at MD Anderson Cancer Center in Houston, TX I was touched by so many people of all ages grappling with the side effects of cancer treatment, eyes begging for a cure, another opportunity for optimal health and family members feeling helpless, yet willing to support from all levels. Even the caregiver of loved ones requires special nurturing so the intervention expands to support the entire family. I am constantly curious about the *art of resilience* and the courage one has in facing adversity. Living in third world countries has also added to the definition of resilience beyond measure and I continue to be inspired by the human spirit.

This inspiration breathes intuition which is not an intellectual or emotional process but rather being present to the "gentle essence" which is effortless and confirming. It formulates clarity amidst chaos or decision making in the moment because this intuitive and creative connection transcends cognitive interruption or emotional takeover. It is a guiding force which has fluidity and grace.

WHAT SUPPORTED YOUR PROCESS?

The internal drive to serve patients who were dying in the early 1980's provided the foundation to spring forth creative interventions in young patients my age (at the time). Their exploration to uncover every opportunity to live was remarkable in so many ways, knowing their fate was death since we did not have a cure for an unnamed disease. My process was supported by my work with people living with AIDS in drug (AZT) trials alongside the first clinical research I conducted in the use of exercise and quality of life (QOL) even at the end stage of the disease. Indeed, the groundbreaking research showed enhancement in strength, endurance and improvement in quality of life even when the outcome would be death.

What supported me during those fragile years was the realization that these men deserved optimal care despite the stigma and prejudice imparted by the media and surrounding communities. I was motivated to foster holistic rehabilitation within the framework of living to the fullest, everyday. Therefore, when the first HIV hospital in the nation closed (*Institute for Immunological Disorders*), I opened a private practice - *L.I.F.E. Physical Therapy (Living in Full Expression)* and carried the banner to serve those with chronic diseases. I never required a marketing strategy, for the entire community supported my efforts. Given the fact these patients would lose insurance, I started writing federal grants to supplement our care. I further developed wellness programs for people with HIV disease throughout the city of Houston and surrounding areas and now for the Garden State Infectious Disease Clinic in New Jersey. Since the 1980's, I continue to write grants to further the art of integrative therapies for individuals with HIV and cancer diagnoses.

Knowing the success rate of NIH grant funding (only 8%) need not be a barrier but a call to be *even more creative* in the next submission. While we may feel overwhelmed by the minutia of detail, we can be equally open to the playfulness of constructing the "art" of a grant. It is a deeper invitation for our own creative growth and willingness to connect with another source to manifest a vision or goal.

WHAT INHIBITED IT?

I am not sure I would say it was ever "inhibited" but I was certainly looked askance at the work I was doing with people living with HIV/AIDS. The stigma attached to this patient population was extended to me and I did have a difficult time hiring rehabilitation specialists at the first HIV/AIDS hospital in the nation in 1985, the Institute for Immunological Disorders. "*Consignment TENS units need not be returned*" was a common response when I called equipment companies after families returned the unit for pain management of their deceased loved one. Even discussions about purchasing a life insurance policy in my line of work because I was a "high risk" healthcare professional further fueled my desire to forge ahead and continue to serve. Men I dated were worried I would contract this horrible disease but there was never a moment when I thought my life was in danger. The sense of trusting in the process of caring for the disenfranchised of society was ignited by the deep and abiding connection with individuals in the final phase of life. There were times I wondered *who was the patient* and *who was the therapist* as this reciprocal connection of humanity in the most fragile of moments has momentum of its own. It is the co-creativity in those experiences that time itself was elusive.

DO YOU HAVE ANY PERSONAL PRACTICES THAT YOU THINK SUPPORT YOUR CREATIVITY OR WORLD VIEWS?

Yes, an inquisitive mind, an open heart and a drive to "right" what is wrong when discrimination is present. I appreciate that human dignity is the intrinsic value of life which each person is deserving of moral protection and reverence. I suspect attraction to these populations has always been part of my upbringing as an extension of outreach in our community. Therefore, person-centered compassionate care with special attention to vulnerable populations through interrelatedness should be characterized by justice. My personal practice is an abiding presence, a commitment to truly listen and know that the person I encounter in the healing process unlocks the answer to his/her reclamation of return to health or a peace filled and serene death.

My personal practice to cultivate my creativity includes morning yoga and meditation, being in nature and jogging through various cities to discover the nuances unnoticed by car or train. I start each day with a loving kindness meditation and set forth to be mindful with each encounter. I enjoy journaling and wonder if my children will be reading my journals as we see in the opening of the *"Bridges of Madison County."*

HOW HAS THE EXPERIENCE INFLUENCED YOUR CURRENT CREATIVITY?

My engagement with individuals in the HIV epidemic has inspired me to answer questions posed, find the evidence in mind-body medicine and translate it into everyday compassionate living and practice. Since I sat at the bedside of hundreds of patients dying in the 1980's, I held on to the hope for medical advances to find a way to prolong life of patients with HIV disease. My Master's and PhD research focused on exercise interventions for this population and the definitive outcome was always positive in the realm of physical activity whether it was traditional exercise, or tai chi. Because we recently received funding from the Oncology Section of the APTA for a small clinical trial, we are exploring the feasibility of yoga for the side effects of the antiretroviral treatment and impact of painful distal sensory neuropathy. However, I have conducted many clinical trials on the impact of yoga for various chronic diseases (osteoarthritis, low back pain, cancer, fall prevention in seniors). So for over three decades, there are consistently new areas to explore, novel research projects to complete and brilliant colleagues and incredible people to connect in profound ways.

DESCRIBE YOUR EXPERIENCE WITH CREATING ...IS IT A STEADY PROCESS? EPISODIC? MANIC? DROUGHT? DOES IT FEEL LIKE IT COMES FROM "YOU" OR ELSEWHERE?

I admit, while I do find myself to be "driven", I must say it is a force beyond me that fosters my creativity. I enjoy the challenges presented to me and just when I think I am on the brink of not solving an issue, a breakthrough occurs, a new idea emerges and I am guided to the next project, idea and focused journey with humanity.

There is a somatic and visceral experience that occurs in the creative process. It is blocked by taking a stance or attempting to "control" the process or event. Tension arises and I feel an urgency that is perceived as a pushing rather than gentle prodding or *presence* in the moment. This is the moment where self-compassion peeks through the incessant self-imposed demands of myself, the healthcare system and others wanting more of me, in the moments I am depleted. Giving myself permission to relinquish my humanness and revitalize in silence, permits an opening that is unknown through this process. This episodic dark and light opens to various mergers and intensity of colors and opportunity. Permitting ideas to take me on a circuitous route provides a freedom to manifest in creative ways. My practice of yoga and mindfulness is essential for the creative flow in any aspect of my day. My breath is the key to tuning in at any given moment, for I return to my body for sparks of creativity and intuition.

HOW DO YOU NURTURE OR NURSE FLEDGLING IDEAS?

My passion for integrative therapies emerged from working with patients in end stage of life as they tried EVERYTHING under the sun (moon and stars) to try to garner one more day to live. Thus, meditation, yoga, tai chi, homeopathy, nutritional dimensions and so much more were explored alongside my role as their PT. Even as I was the lone person aiming for rehabilitation in a tenuous situation, I was assured that it made a difference in their lives and this nurtured me to continue with the vision for people living with chronic pain and various diseases. Feedback from patients and family members assisted in the design of a variety of creative rehabilitation approaches within the framework of traditional medical care. Colleagues noted the value of rehabilitation in maximizing function and offering possibilities in the face of death.

This inspired me to do more research in this area alongside integrative therapies. My post-doctoral work on the use of meditation for stress in healthcare professionals revealed the incredible amount of burnout and loss of empathy with the lack of self-care, and I yearned to intervene and mitigate this disenchantment experienced by my colleagues. This was not the way these individuals entered the healthcare arena and I have been inspired to foster wellness in our doctoral students in order to have our new graduates appreciate their wellbeing as they approach each individual they partner with in PT.

This "noticing" of my students' stress levels gave me pause years ago as we advanced our profession to the DPT. *Were we implementing the "seeds" of burnout by not providing coping strategies while meeting the demands of an intensive curriculum?* I embarked on a wellness coaching training through the American College of Sports Medicine and initiated a 7 week coaching experience for our first year students. Since I view every opportunity to collect and analyze data through a mixed methods approach, we found the implementation of such techniques to enhance graduate students' stress management techniques and greater self-awareness. Because I took the time to "notice" and do the research in the area of integrative mindful practices for these students, we published our findings and have been asked several times to present our strategies at APTA National Student Conclave Meetings. Another example of sustaining the "spark of creativity", for if we teach self-care in health care professional training, we can better serve patients in the long trajectory of health care delivery.

WHAT ROLES DOES/DID YOUR COMMUNITY/COLLEAGUES PLAY IN YOUR CREATIVE EXPERIENCE?

Mentors are a gift in life and I have been fortunate to have several key people who guide me in my journey as a clinician, academician, and researcher. I count on my colleagues to share ideas, brainstorm strategies and quite frankly keep me up to date with all the computerized needs in the clinic when it comes to health electronic records. Despite the increasing demands in healthcare, the patient-practitioner/ student-professor interaction is always the key aspect of each day.

Prioritizing where I desire to spend my time and energy is essential. Learning the art of "no" for "knowing" if I can or am unable to fulfill a commitment is key to balancing my personal and professional life. Knowing how and when to engage with the outside demands within my profession, meeting the needs of students, patients, colleagues and friends and family is the creative art of balancing each and every day. I find that conversations in vulnerable moments in someone's life however tend to provide meaning and purpose to the spontaneous connection of even a stranger on the street. Touching the lives of my colleagues through humor, sharing creative strategies and being present to the vicissitudes of life is the joy of everyday!

WHAT WOULD YOU DO DIFFERENTLY?

I would do nothing differently, as I have learned from my tumbles and triumphs. Even in the face of becoming a patient in my own healthcare system as a breast cancer survivor in 2003 gave me a unique perspective - *"on the other side of the table"*. It fostered a kaleidoscope view when my husband was diagnosed with head and neck cancer and we are grateful to be able to tell the story. When I was asked to present a Ted Talk regarding my experiences as a cancer survivor last October, it opened a platform to interrogate what it means to be a "survivor". Can one survive "survivorship"? http://m.youtube.com/watch?v =mJ-kSrZ2z5E&desktop_uri=%2Fwatch%3Fv%3DmJ-kSrZ2z5E

What is it like to simply witness oneself in the experiences of the unknown? How can we resource centeredness and mindfulness in the art of ambiguity? Can we unleash resilience in the face of adversity and healing?

This talk culminated in sharing my journey as a survivor and co-survivor and fully embracing my vulnerability as a patient and caregiver. No amount of intellectual or emotional maturity could prepare me for a diagnosis that could lead to our potential death. The experience was a rather surreal introspection on the very nature of my career and although I thought I understood my patients, *did I really? Did they think the same thoughts as I had?* This would be the real test of integrative medicine. I received chemotherapy for months while I did meditation and yoga practice, recovered from five surgeries, obtained acupuncture treatments for severe neuropathy pain (and I thought I appreciated the nature of this type of pain in patients...). I permitted myself to cry in despair and be vulnerable in front of my colleagues and deepened my resilience which provided insight I did not have prior to my diagnosis. Interrogating the question of my two children ages one and three - who would raise them if I were to die and then answering their question "Will Daddy die too" took me to the core of my being as I answered "I don't know". Witnessing and seeing life through the different lenses has opened me to various dimensions beyond measure.

WHAT'S NEXT?

I just returned from a Fulbright experience in South Africa as I envisioned working globally in the area of chronic disease. This closed the loop for my work in HIV rehabilitation and has spawned new population based studies. Furthermore, it sparked rich creative endeavors with a new culture and wonderful colleagues at the University of Witswatersrand in Johannesburg. I wish to continue my work with teenagers and adults, teaching mindfulness in the classroom and inspire my own children to carry the torch of service locally and globally and to be fully present through the journey.

WORDS OF WISDOM/INSPIRATION?

THRIVE and SURVIVE:

*T*hink in the now - be mindful
*H*armony of mind and body
*R*evitalize the soul
*I*nspiration through self-reflection
*V*alue positive affirmations
*E*vaporate thoughts of uncertainty

*S*implicity in the sacred
*U*nconditional acceptance
*R*ecognition of beauty
*V*itality in the present moment
*I*ntuitive and insightful openings
*V*ision for the future
*E*mpathy for our humanness

*C*larity of thought
*R*eflection of the day
*E*ager to take the road less travelled
*A*bundance in health
*T*rust in oneself
*I*nnovation fosters creation
*V*itality fuels momentum
*E*volve with each lesson in life

During my time in South Africa, I experienced Ubuntu which translates: *"I am what I am because of who we all are"* Archbishop Desmond Tutu offered a definition in his 1999 book: *A person with Ubuntu is open and available to others, affirming of others, does not feel threatened that others are able and good, based from a proper self-assurance that comes from knowing that he or she belongs in a greater whole and is diminished when others are humiliated or diminished, when others are tortured or oppressed.* May your creativity unfold in thriving and surviving the very essence of each day. May your vulnerability and resilience be part of each experience, and may all humans feel the freedom to be affirming and creative in all realms of life. *Ubuntu, Be well....*

RESOURCES

Articles

Galantino, M.L., Baime, M., Maguire, M., Szapary, P., Farrar, J.T. (2005) Comparison of psychological and physiological measures of stress in health care professionals during an eight-week mindfulness meditation program: Mindfulness in practice. *Stress and Health 21*, 255-261.

Spence, D.W., Galantino, M.L., Mossberg, K.A., Zimmerman, S.O. (1990). Progressive resistance exercise: Effect on muscle function and anthropometry of a select AIDS population. *Arch Phys Med Rehabil. Aug; 71* (9), 644-8.

Zweir, A., Galantino, M.L., Frank, M. (2011) Longitudinal impact of wellness coaching for graduate students in a doctorate of physical therapy program. *Journal of Physical Therapy Research.* Spring Issue.

Books

Galantino, M.L. (ed). (1992). Clinical assessment and treatment of HIV disease: Rehabilitation of a chronic illness. Thorofare, NJ: SLACK, Inc.

Galantino, M.L. (ed). Complementary medicine in orthopaedic physical therapy. (2000). Orthopaedic Physical Therapy Clinics of North America, 9:3.

Standish, L., Calabrese, C., Galantino, M.L. (eds). (2002). AIDS and alternative medicine: Current state of the science. Churchill Livingstone.

In: Fostering Creativity in Rehabilitation
Editor: Matthew J. Taylor

ISBN: 978-1-63485-118-3
© 2016 Nova Science Publishers, Inc.

Chapter 11

A FRACTURED PATH

Sara M. Meeks, PT, MS, GCS

Director, Sara Meeks Seminars, Gainesville, FL, US

WHERE AND WHO I "AM" IN MY JOURNEY

With my diploma in hand and a few months later my license to practice, I have been a Physical Therapist (PT) since 1962. I am also a Kripalu-Certified Yoga Teacher (KYT) since 1984 and an American Physical Therapy Association (APTA) Certified Geriatric Clinical Specialist (GCS) since 1994. In addition, I received my Masters in Physical Therapy (MS) at the age of 60 and am so very glad I went back to school to learn more. I've been focusing on the management of the patient with osteoporosis and/or osteopenia since 1984 when I saw my first patient with known osteoporosis and an acute compression fracture. I now have a telephone and on-site private consultation and treatment practice and also travel internationally to teach seminars on the physical therapy management of patients with low bone mass to medical and exercise professionals.

Throughout this long career there have been times when I thought I knew something. However, as time goes on, I become more aware of how little I know, how much there is to know and what little time I have to do it in. This awareness keeps me focused on my path of bringing safe and therapeutic movement and exercise into the lives of those who seek my help. It also keeps me open to new information that comes my way, whether through the research literature, the next patient I see, a conversation with a colleague or a participant in one of my seminars who asks a question that I can't quite answer and which leads me onto the path to find out more.

When I am preparing to see someone for the first time, I have a plan based on principles of movement that I've honed over the years but, until that person actually appears before me, I have only a vague idea of what I am going to do and how it is going to turn out. So much depends upon the life history of the person and how that person has adapted or compensated to what has happened to him or her during that lifetime. And so I've learned to have few pre-conceived ideas until I am in the presence of that person.

When someone comes to see me, I make initial eye and handshake contact even before the initial assessment. I begin to watch how a person moves from the first moment and continue to do so as we go through assessment, positioning, and exercise. In this way, I've learned to be very much in the moment in order to observe subtle reactions to what I'm asking them to do. In this way, I can alter my "plan" according to what I see, hear, touch, feel and, somehow, sense. From the onset it is a reciprocal relationship as we exchange information and decide together what will happen next.

Even when I do venture into an area of body restriction or weakness with which I'm not familiar, I do follow certain principles of movement. I call the process a Return to Optimal Alignment in all positions. With an underlying principle of safety to minimize the risk of the next fracture, the intent is to build stronger bones and lead this person into better function in daily life.

And, underpinning all of that is the physical and mental capacity as well as the personality of the patient as we work together to figure out the best program. Firm but gentle touch, eye contact, response to questions and close listening help engender a feeling of trust that this visit to physical therapy is going to be different. Many have told me of their relief that, at last, they have a sense of arriving at the right place for help.

I believe this process that I teach in my seminars and have been following for at least 30 years, to be in alignment with the most recent APTA vision statement adopted in 2013: "Transforming society by optimizing movement to improve the human experience." I believe I do this, one person at a time. My vision is that optimal movement experience will then be taken out into larger and larger realms until The Meeks Method becomes an integral part of the whole of physical therapy practice.

This journey of mine is nowhere near finished. I learn every day from my own body, the bodies of others, the research literature, and the students who come to my on-site seminars.

My current "plan" is based on a recent encounter with an 86 year old sculptor who wants to keep on doing what she is doing until some higher power decides she can no longer do it. This is my plan—to continue as long as I can to help people live life the way they want to live it, with some modifications, as safely and as independently as possible.

And so, now that I've told you where I "am", let's take a look at how I got here.

THE FIRST STEP

The phone call that was to profoundly change my path in physical therapy came in 1984, 22 years after graduating from college. A physician called me with a request to see a 65 year old woman with known osteoporosis who he had just admitted to the hospital with a vertebral compression fracture at the T9 level. He further said "Sara....you're the expert in this area; I'm going to turn the care of this patient over to you." Little did I realize then the impact that this request would make on how I would practice physical therapy in the future.

I knew that osteoporosis existed as a condition primarily in ageing populations, but this was the first patient I would see with known osteoporosis and an acute compression fracture. I was excited and also honored at this opportunity.

With no clinical pathway or research evidence to dictate my treatment plan, I set out with my usual intent to help her return to her former lifestyle as safely and independently as possible.

I first reviewed her X-rays for some needed guidance. What I was later to learn was called an anterior wedge fracture was clearly visible on the X-ray. My next step was to consult my trusty Gray's Anatomy text book that I still had from physical therapy school. After reviewing vertebral column anatomy and biomechanics and knowing that the first step in fracture management is to reduce the fracture, I reasoned that to reduce a compression fracture I needed to de-compress or unload the fracture site. I needed to, somehow, preserve optimal vertebral column alignment as much as possible. And so, my first order was to have the patient positioned supine with the bed flat, a small pillow under her head and a bolster under her knees. With this, I began to design a program which is still the foundation of what I do today. During her 10-day hospitalization, my assistant and I saw her 2-3 times daily for pain-relief, back extensor isometric strengthening exercise and instruction in body mechanics. Post-discharge she was seen for follow-up as an out-patient.

At approximately 6 months after the initial injury, I had the chance to review her recent X-ray and could see the increase in vertebral body height at the fracture site. This was a successful healing of the fracture! She had also returned to her previous busy life as a part-time bookkeeper, grandmother, wife and homemaker, and volunteer to many civic groups in town.

Somehow realizing I was "on" to something new in my career, I began to look closely at how I was practicing as a physical therapist. Noting that I had gravitated towards focusing on the geriatric populations and presuming many of my patients already had osteoporosis although undiagnosed and unrecognized, I changed my focus from primarily muscle and joint issues to how the positions and exercises were affecting the bones. That shift changed my practice profoundly. My patients with other challenges such as back pain and post-surgery and even neurological conditions began to respond positively to this new approach.

And so, now I knew that I was on a unique and unmarked path. Little did I know what was to come or how it would affect me on such deep professional and personal levels.

THE FORMATIVE ANTECEDENT YEARS

As I thought about writing this "case study" of myself as a physical therapist, the initial step was an easy one to describe. However, as I wrote, I began to think about the path my life had taken to arrive at the time when I could "step outside of the box" of what I thought I knew and begin to create a meaningful, effective and successful intervention, based on anatomical and biomechanical principles for this patient.

Briefly, I was born in 1940, grew up in small-town America, decided I wanted to pursue a career in Physical Therapy when I was a senior in high school, applied to one school – Ithaca College – and was accepted. I graduated with a BS Cum Laude in Physical Therapy and, basically, have "never looked back" nor questioned my decision.

As I looked back at that time, I realized that early in life I had learned to care for people and to think of others rather than always of myself. My mother's sister, Mary Helen Kelly, was born in 1898 with cerebral palsy. Not expected to live long, maybe a day or week certainly not to adulthood, she outsmarted everyone and left this earthly life 2 months shy of her 80th birthday. A "sunny" soul, always an inquisitive person, she studied library science and became one of the most beloved faculty members at the local high school.

As I grew up, Aunt Helen had many surgeries and I was the one chosen to help her with her exercises as she stayed in our house during her recovery. I believe that this experience somehow laid the groundwork to what I was to become.

Although my career as a Physical Therapist has taken many turns, I have always been happy in my chosen work and never wanted to do anything else. I never stayed in one job long enough to earn any tenure; rather I began in rehabilitation, moved on into hospital outpatient, then to several years in research followed by home care, back into hospital outpatient, and then, 12 years after seeing my initial patient with osteoporosis in 1984, into an outpatient clinic where every patient I saw was diagnosed with osteoporosis and/or osteopenia by bone density scan. I honed my approach in that clinic for fourteen months and then opened my private practice. I also began teaching seminars on what has become known as The Meeks Method of the physical therapy management of the patient with low bone mass and/or compression fracture. To say that this has been a simple, smooth journey would be disingenuous of me as my path has been winding and curving, sometimes beset by detractors and, through it all, I have had but one simple goal—the well-being and safety of the people who come to me for help.

THE PROFESSIONAL YEARS

My ability to rise to the occasion of managing this initial patient rests not only with my early life as I was growing up, but also in the firm foundation I acquired in the profession both in physical therapy school and immediately after.

One of my professors in my senior year was Arthur S. Abramson, MD, one of the founders of Rehabilitation Medicine. A trail-blazer, hit by a sniper's bullet in World War II rendering him paraplegic, he changed his chosen field of medical practice from surgery to rehabilitation and became a leader in this new field of medicine. From him and his dedicated staff, I became grounded in principles of perfection, innovation, persistence and adaptation in the face of personal adversity and this experience helped shape me into the therapist I am today.

After graduation, my first job was as a staff physical therapist at the Institute for Physical Medicine and Rehabilitation (IPM&R) (Rusk Institute) in New York City. This institute was founded by Howard A. Rusk, MD who was another innovator and trail-blazer in the field of Rehabilitation Medicine. Through personal association with Dr. Rusk and his staff, I developed a solid foundation as a treating therapist.

I was mentored by senior therapists and learned the strength and importance of a team approach to patient care. Although the work was sometimes very physically exhausting, it was always mentally challenging as I learned to help with the rehabilitation of patients with many conditions. It was there that I learned a valuable lesson from one of my patients. A woman was admitted to the institute about a year post-CVA with left hemiparesis. She was ambulating with a cane but had no function of her left upper extremity. Her goal was to return to her role as an independent homemaker. I remember many of my colleagues wondered why she would want to come back into a hospital to do that. My own perspective was that this patient exhibited what I thought was at the real heart of rehabilitation medicine. Her goal was to learn how to cook, clean and do general housework despite no use of one arm and limited use of one leg. I marveled as she achieved that goal with her indomitable spirit and the interdisciplinary approach to rehabilitation present at the institute.

After her discharge, she invited me and the occupational therapist to her house for dinner. She had cleaned her house, prepared the meal and set the table for this celebratory occasion of her independence entirely by herself. She was so proud and I was delighted to be a part of her joy. I have often remembered this woman and this lesson as I continue to strive to assist people to safely live the life they want to live even in the face of devastating physical challenges.

Osteoporosis is one of these challenges. It does not affect people equally, occurs in all populations (from birth to death), with intrauterine antecedents, and does not necessarily occur as a lone diagnosis. It can be concurrent with every condition we physical therapists see in our practices. One of the challenges faced by a physical therapist is the management of patients with osteoporosis and how to design an exercise and movement program that will take into account not only the forces on the bones but also the co-morbidities of the patient, some of which have conflicting approaches (e.g., spinal stenosis).

My professional and personal life changed very profoundly and in ways I never expected when I began bringing the forces on the bones into the equation of exercise prescription. As time passed from that initial patient with osteoporosis, I refined my approach based on clinical experience and a definite trend towards looking more at the whole patient. I began to wonder why:

- People with back pain would come in for treatment, feel better but then return weeks or months later with a recurrence of similar but more severe symptoms,
- People on my program would feel better with their initial symptoms but as treatment progressed, would come in with different ones at a later date. For example, people with back pain would get relief from back pain and then begin complaining of knee pain.

I sensed that I was missing some critical link to peoples' over-all well-being and began to look more closely at the "whole patient", taking a more exhaustive history, checking out other parts of the body as well as assessing the symptomatic area.

I was also becoming more aware of the research surrounding back pain and even, osteoporosis itself. During these years, Robin McKenzie came on the scene with his new and controversial ideas on back pain management. I took a course from Moshe Feldenkrais and I also discovered Kripalu Yoga. I also took continuing education courses with John Barnes. All of this new information was woven into my thought process and practice in patient care.

As I prepared to specialize I took more continuing education specifically for geriatrics, assuming that all my patients would be elderly, Caucasian, thin-boned, asymptomatic women. In front of 300 colleagues I asked one prominent geriatric physical therapist what she thought of my working in such a clinic with only this population and she did not think it was a good idea, commenting, "I wouldn't touch that with a 10 foot pole." Maybe it was just this stubborn streak I've always had, but tell me I can't do something and I see that as a challenge. This interaction, while troubling, really only spurred me on in my quest to help people and I began the work anyway.

By the time I began work in this specialty clinic for patients with osteoporosis (in 1996), I was an entirely different therapist from the one I was in 1984. The changes that had occurred however turned out to be nothing compared to what was ahead.

My "Dream Job"

I had been working as a home care therapist since 1990 when, one day in 1996, I noticed a small ad in the newspaper. The ad stated that a locally-owned physical therapy clinic was looking for a physical therapist to work in the specialty practice of osteoporosis management. My "Dream Job" was about to become reality.

I interviewed, was offered the position and began full-time within a physician's office complex where I was to be the sole therapist working with patients all of whom had been diagnosed with osteoporosis and/or osteopenia by bone density scan. Before beginning work, I took continuing education courses and had two weeks to set up my program. I was ready…or so I thought!

The patients weren't what I had imagined. I quickly found out that although they were mostly women, I saw people of all ethnicities, all body types, ages 23-92 (I've since seen younger and older), and they were mostly far from asymptomatic. As I worked with this population, I often had to "think on my feet" especially when the first patient with both osteoporosis and spinal stenosis stood before me. I had to quickly devise a program that would focus on safety for this individual with these conflicting diagnoses regarding spinal movement.

I had many "Eureka" and "aha" moments and surprises along the way. Not only did my patients have known low bone mass but they also came in with just about every other physical therapy diagnosis one can imagine: COPD, neurological conditions such as CVA and multiple sclerosis, hip and other fractures, joint replacements and many back pathologies. Many had not just one, but several co-morbidities. To focus on the bones and take into consideration other conditions plus the personality and goals of the patients was a challenge and one that caused me to become even more focused and aware with exercise prescription. It was during this time that I identified what I have termed The Patterns of Postural Change©, postural changes that appear to happen as, but not necessarily because, people age. I began to realize that good body alignment is important for better muscle contraction and weight-bearing forces on the bones.

As a result of these 14 months of experience, I decided that I was going to treat every patient as if they have low bone mass unless they could prove to me they don't. In this way, I could be more assured that I was creating safety in movement with my assessment and exercise prescription.

As people experienced pain relief, gained body height, and returned to former more active lifestyles with this program, I began to realize that I was working on something that had greater ramifications and with its focus on body alignment, would prove useful for patients with many other diagnoses as well.

Unfortunately, all of this happened during a time of great change in the health care system. Small practices, including the one in which I was working, were being sold to larger corporations and I was increasingly being asked to see more patients in less time with little or no help. Thinking that I would have to compromise my professional ethics, I realized I could no longer work in this environment. This was a practice filled with mostly geriatric patients with several co-morbidities and who had not received help elsewhere. Even though I was known as the "osteoporosis therapist" and was receiving referrals from an increasing number of physicians, I found I was not able to give the care I wanted to and that not only was I being stressed, but my patients could not get the help they needed. So I resigned and returned to work in home care. As I worked in home care, I began to realize that, as my patients progressed, I had no place to send them for further therapy. This led to my opening a cash-based Private Practice and, at a colleague's suggestion, the beginning of traveling and teaching seminars to health and exercise professionals on the management of the patient with low bone mass.

And so, I turned the proverbial lemons into lemonade.

ON MY OWN

Quite frankly I never thought I would have my own private practice. Yet, here I was, a therapist with 35 years of experience, opening my own clinic, forging a new path in not only a specialty private practice but a cash-based one at that. I was very soon busier than I thought I would be, juggling two careers-one in patient care and one traveling and teaching seminars. In this practice, I was now unbound by time and reimbursement restraints, could see patients at their own and my best times, and could spend plenty of time exploring movement in their bodies and, in the process, unraveling the tapestry of their lives.

Although I would never say that I have many answers to the condition of bone loss, the "answers" to some of the questions about recurring and "new" symptoms that I had in the past, began to emerge. As patients' alignment improved, old injuries and surgeries would re-emerge and patients would re-visit old symptoms. Usually, with one or two sessions of very site-specific work, these problems would be resolved and the alignment work would continue.

During this time, the evidence-based movement became a strong force in therapy practice. I began to peruse the research literature with great enthusiasm and energy, discovering that all of the ideas I had for the management of osteoporosis were well-supported in the research literature.

Even though my specific program has not yet been subjected to the rigors of a scientific study, the principles of what I do and teach were then, and are now, well substantiated in the literature. Even so, I've been faced and am still being faced with nay-sayers and detractors along the way. There are people who say:

- I don't need to be as conservative as I am in exercise prescription.
- There is no such thing as silent fractures, even though the research literature and the statements of large, reputable organizations continue to report silent fracture rates as high as 70-80% of all fractures,
- It's ok to flex, side bend and rotate the spine in osteoporotic patients because it "feels good," it's necessary for function and they're going to do it anyway,
- My program is not evidence-based.

Simultaneously, I've developed a large network of therapists who have taken my work and used it with great success, melding it with other physical therapy and movement approaches. There are now over 6,000 medical and exercise professionals who have taken my trainings, which now include three levels of instruction. Knowing that my candle will someday burn out, I have developed a program of certification in The Meeks Method and there are therapists who are preparing to teach my Level 1 course. I continue to learn new things everyday – no two patients are alike; no two seminars are alike—and I stay open for that next moment of insight into this epidemic and growing problem of osteoporosis with its severe quality of life and financial impact on peoples' lives.

WHAT DOES THE FUTURE HOLD FOR ME?

No-one can predict the weather very accurately, much less the future. However, my intent is to continue seeing my greatest teachers, the people who come to me with devastating fracture cascades and all sorts of surgeries who "have been everywhere and done everything" all to little or no avail. Whether through telephone or on-site consults, I intend to continue to help people find ways to live their lives the way they want, with safety and freedom from the fear of falls and fractures. I also plan to include continuous exploration of my own body movement and to develop and be open to new ways of moving to improve and maintain optimal alignment for better, more independent function. And, with new research indicating an intrauterine component to future risk of osteoporosis and fracture, my plan also includes reaching out to more therapists to assist me on this path.

At the age of 65, I received the diagnosis of osteoporosis and went through stages of denial, grief, anger, bargaining and frustration until I finally came into acceptance. That was when a whole new world of movement possibility really opened up to me.

As Dr. Alfonso Montuori has stated in the preface to this book, some of the problems in rehabilitation are related to the "sheer volume of information, increased productivity and documentation demands, technology changes, dwindling reimbursement and high rates of professional burnout." Add to this, the admonition from professional organizations "to practice only what has high-level research evidence to support the practice" and one can easily see that original thought and creativity can easily be stifled. My current idea is to take what I have created and hone it down to a system which will be more "do-able" by practitioners who are faced with these demands while at the same time maintaining the heart and extremely personal approach of The Meeks Method.

When I was 4 years old, I stood in front of my home in Alexandria Bay, NY and decided I wanted to live to be 99 years old. I thought, then, that 100 would be pushing it. Now, with the advances in medical care in the U.S., I've decided that 109 would be more like it. My idea is to be as sound of mind and as sound of body as possible for as long as possible.

I now have 35 years to achieve my dream of safety and therapeutic result for all persons who enter into a movement and/or exercise environment. I invite all of you to join me in this endeavor.

FINAL THOUGHTS AND WORDS OF "WISDOM"

I am fairly certain no one could, or might *want* to, duplicate my path. I've had opportunities to work with patients up to 3 hours at a time or until either their or my endurance wears thin. I've also had a myriad of influencers and experience in various specialty areas of physical therapy that make my practice somewhat unique. Nevertheless, I believe there are certain threads that run through my life and work that you might find helpful. Here are some of my ideas.

- *Listen to your patients and they will be more likely to listen to you.* If you are paying attention, they will *tell* you what to do. The trick is to give them as close to what they want and, at the same time, let them know that they may have to modify certain lifestyles if they want to live as independently as possible into a fulfilling old age. To do this in less time with little help, you need to listen closely.
- *Open all your senses, and your heart, to the next patient who comes to you.* This may make you feel more vulnerable. But, if you do this, on a very human level, knowing that you need each other, you will grow in many more ways than you can imagine. You have the education and the skills….now be your own self in the process.
- *If you have an idea, capture it before it flies away.* Write it down. Mull it over. Give it space. Stay away from initial nay-sayers. Who knows, those ideas may lead you, as mine have led me, into product development, book writing, a career that has taken me to parts of the world I never thought I'd be and a knowledge of the human body that I might never otherwise have had.
- *Go back to the basics.* Review your anatomy, kinesiology, physics, and biomechanics many times over. It's amazing how I, with anatomy as a favorite subject and with all I've studied, continue to learn more.
- *If you are drawn to a specific specialty area in practice, follow it.* Ask your supervisor to send more patients with that diagnosis your way. Take better notes. Do a more complete assessment. Keep all your senses on alert to pick up the nuances that can occur in patient-therapist interaction. And notice how, even with the same diagnosis, each patient is unique. Rather than relying only on ideas from a book or a research study, use your clinical expertise and experience to design your programs to meet your patients' specific needs.
- *As soon as you think you know something, watch out!* Something or someone will come along to make you think otherwise.
- *And remember, in the end, that you are just one of a team who may see this patient.* You don't have all the answers and you may end up with more questions than answers. Learn to live in the question and be open to what comes.

You chose this wonderful profession of physical therapy for certain reasons, some of which you know and some of which you have still to find out. Stick with your idea of making this a better life for one person at a time. That will spread out into society and around the world. You may not see all the fruits of your labor in your lifetime, but do it anyway!

And so, I have come to the end of the story of my life thus far. My dream continues and I'm hoping that you who are reading this will join me in that dream. If we are to "transform society by optimizing movement to improve the human experience" then we need to definitely bring the bones and our own heart into the exercise equation. When you do that, your practice will change and in ways you might never expect.

Be prepared for a roller-coaster ride and have fun along the way.

Sincerely Yours in Good Bone Health,
Sara Meeks

In: Fostering Creativity in Rehabilitation
Editor: Matthew J. Taylor

ISBN: 978-1-63485-118-3
© 2016 Nova Science Publishers, Inc.

Chapter 12

SPEECH AND LANGUAGE PATHOLOGY

Michelle Garcia Winner, SLP, MA-CCC
Founder of Social Thinking®, San Jose, CA, US

I am a speech language pathologist (SLP) who has been working as a clinician since the mid -1980's when I received my Master's degree.

My profession fosters creative treatment planning. SLPs are taught about speech, language, auditory processing, cognition and learning strategies in a developmental manner. We problem solve the needs of each individual client and then create a unique set of treatment plans and goals based on how the individual presents through face to face interactions and testing. We are to consider the best evidence available, communicate with the client, consider their families' values and wishes, and utilize the knowledge of experienced clinicians in order to determine what we consider to be the best treatment pathway. We also have to consider the very real limitations our different delivery systems present (school schedules, in-patient needs, etc.).

To do our job well, we also need to consult with other professions that are working with our same students/clients.

We also have flexibility in our career paths. SLPs work across all the age groups from birth through geriatrics, communication challenges across many diagnostic labels, and we work across a large range of service delivery systems (schools, hospitals, private practice, etc.).

The fact that our profession highly values developmental and cognitively based information across the lifespan through the lens of evidence-based information afforded me a large range of treatment experiences through the early years of my career. I was able to work in grant funded autism research treatment programs; Head Start; and on medical teams associated with hospitals in acute, sub-acute, and home based treatments; school systems; and finally private practice. In each treatment placement I was able to assess the value of communication and related learning concepts as they were influenced by culture, client's age, presenting demands for use of concepts, insights of other professionals and, of course, family concerns. When working in Head Start I had to learn how to be really sensitive to the needs of immigrant families, many who were highly educated but now presented with little time to attend to their children's learning because they were holding down so many menial labor jobs and had subtly different cultural communication styles. In medical treatment programs I learned about integrating the view point of medical, psychological, and occupational needs as all of this influenced what would be meaningful to teach clients to help them re-establish functional use of their communication systems. In the schools I learned how the core factors that contribute to our communicative success also help us to interpret and respond to different aspects of our curriculum, work well in group learning environments, as well as make and keep friends. Hence, being an SLP has provided a very large palate of experience and has encouraged constant new learning, flexibility and personal/professional growth.

One of the challenges our profession presents is that our work is often done in the quiet confines of a treatment room, with the client experiencing few distractions, yet this same client is expected to incorporate and apply these lessons in a large range of vastly complex and confusing situations. We are constantly faced with the question of how we can help our clients utilize the information they are learning across a range of environments and situations.

Another challenge is that while our national professional organization, the American Speech-Language-Hearing Association (ASHA), reports that they embrace an evidence-based model that encourages all therapists to be creative and use their best information available combined with clinical judgment, they appear to be moving us in a different direction; they are conflicted. While they know that our clients need creative treatment strategies, ASHA is heeding the political call for all clinical practices to only utilize treatments that have been proven through research studies. This is truly problematic as the studies are often limited in scope and fail to account for complex variables that surround my client, which begs the question: if we are to only utilize proven treatments, then how does the field foster innovation? Don't we need to develop innovative treatment philosophies and related strategies *before* a group can prioritize what merits deeper research? While I embrace utilizing the published research (not all of which is clinical) to foster my own clinical creativity, I find this call to limit our practice to proven research studies means that I am depending on the history of the researchers to not only have faced every one of my client's challenges but also had the ability to turn it into a research project that they then have time to write up and share with the public (preferably in a journal). This is obviously an unrealistic call to action that shuts down our ability to meet our clients' individual needs. Take for example the age-old recognition that good treatment is the result of applying both the art and science. Ironically, while we can document through the science of research core lessons we should teach on any given topic, our teaching of this information is often ineffective without a teacher or clinician being "artful" in how they present this information to their students/clients. The art of teaching values how the core information to be taught relates to our students and sustains their motivation on the worst of days – not their best of days. The research struggles to find a strongly scientific method for measuring something as creative as the "art" in much the same way that researchers have found it difficult to measure our "soft skills" or our interpersonal skills, which happens to be my area of fascination and wonder.

WHAT DID/ARE YOU DO/DOING?

I developed Social Thinking®, a framework and related strategies to help make the implicit expectations of the social world more explicit. This information based on our social cognition applies not only to how we teach students social skills but also relates to lessons we use to guide our students to more efficiently interpret socially based information carried through the curriculum (e.g. reading comprehension of literature), be more active onlookers in our communities (social detectives) or respond to information provided through the media.

My passion has always been in the study and treatment of people who have difficulties with developing functional communication and, more specifically, their social communication skills. This led me into the field of autism in the late 1970's before autism was a condition mentioned in the media on a regular basis. I began my work with adolescent students with autism who also had intellectual impairments and had little to no access to formal communication skills. There were no standardized tests available to understand their learning challenges, so the only way to understand their needs was to move with them across difficult situations and observe how they processed and responded to changes in environments. I was lucky enough to have a terrific mentor who encouraged us to be creative and give us time to think deeply to create innovative treatments. I was part of a cutting edge program, housed in a university that strongly encouraged interdisciplinary engagement between the professionals so that our clients were receiving consistent lessons across treatment providers. Consistency in teaching was the name of the game. As a young professional in my early 20's, I had no idea that this was the only time in my professional life that I would get to experience working on a team dedicated to developing creative treatments, supported 24 hours a day by a range of professionals and assistants. This early lesson of professionals truly working together on a team to help an individual significantly impacted my lens as a teacher/therapist from that point on.

In the late 1980's and early 1990's, I chose to switch my focus by taking jobs working in hospitals and sub-acute rehabilitation teams. Now I had clients who had strong intellectual skills but their brain injuries had robbed them of immediate access to those skills. I learned a lot about problems associated with more subtle but significant learning challenges related to poor executive functioning, etc.

In 1995, I took the job as an SLP in our local high school district, so I could be on the same holiday schedule as my 2 daughters who had just entered public elementary school.

In 1994, unbeknownst to me at that time the groundwork was laid for autism to expand into what is now known as ASD or Autism Spectrum Disorder, through the introduction of Asperger's Syndrome into the DSM IV. I also had no idea that the last 12 years of working with "lower functioning" students to working with those who had brain injuries provided me with tools I needed to address the emerging needs of a brand new population of students who were flooding into school districts en masse. Research had not yet been done on clinical treatment of this higher functioning group of students, but I had a lot of students who needed treatment plans developed now! I also noticed that this new diagnostic label of Asperger's Syndrome overlapped with other diagnostic labels such as ADHD, social anxiety, social phobia, gifted learners, Tourette's, etc. Those who work in the schools know that each teacher is supposed to be a specialist in any diagnostic label known to man! Armed with my years of previous clinical experience, as I evaluated my students I saw strong similarities across different diagnostic labels; I also saw significant differences in how my clients processed and responded to social information within the same treatment label! Given that school based services require SLPs to provide instruction in clinical groups, I was noticing that when I paired my clients by their similar learning traits and communicative needs, three different students could come into the group with their own diagnostic label (e.g. one had ADHD, one had Asperger's Syndrome and another had autism) yet they had similar learning needs. I found that if I grouped them simply by their diagnostic label, (e.g. a group of students who all had Asperger's Syndrome) the manner in which they processed and responded to social information was so discrepant, I struggled to run a treatment group that was relevant to all their needs. At the same time, I had students who were quite offensive, telling me they didn't care how they made anyone feel. Furthermore, I noticed that the academic issues they were experiencing in their classroom seemed to relate to their social communication limitations. I was very willing to explore these students' needs in the context of the greater school day. I spent a lot of time talking to their teachers and looking at their curriculum based expectations. Psychologists and teachers started referring even more students who were struggling in class to relate to others and within their coursework; some had no clear diagnostic label. It felt like I was in the wild west of learning about a newly identified group of students (e.g. those who had relatively strong language and learning skills as measured by tests, but who were limited in their social communication skills), for which we knew relatively little in terms of treatment.

I began reading all types of research, articles, books to better understand core concepts related to social learning while also investigating how reading comprehension and written expression, two areas many of my students showed struggles, related back to the social communication process.

At the same time, I began evolving treatment frameworks and related strategies to help teach social communication concepts to those we consider "high functioning." I also began to get the attention of other treatment providers in the school system. Parents and professionals were interested in learning more, and mainstream teachers began to talk to me about their students.

I began to describe what I was teaching, as helping our students to become better "social thinkers" and I stressed that this treatment philosophy and related strategies was exclusively for individuals with social communication/social learning challenges who had a verbal IQ of at least 70 to as high as gifted and normal to strong expressive language skills. Now, 19 years later we have treatment strategies based on the evidence that helps students/clients from age 4 through adulthood.

The core of what I teach through Social Thinking is that social skills do not start with a social behavior (the social skill itself). Instead, it starts within our brains to think socially about the situation and the people in the situation (including ourselves) to help us interpret each others' thoughts, emotions, motives, beliefs, etc. to try and understand what is happening around us. We use our social thinking not only to interpret and respond to people we are talking to, but we also use this core social thinking to make meaning out of TV shows/movies we watch, information we read, etc. When involved in social interaction, we then use this social thinking information in split second timing to adapt effectively with our own social skills to the people and situation we are immersed in so that those around us can interpret and respond to us in the manner we want them to think and feel about us. Others emotionally interpret our social behavior, and how they feel about us can impact how they treat us, impacting how we feel about them and ourselves.

Social Thinking is a paradigm shift, moving many treatment professionals, across a range of fields, away from a vastly over-simplified idea of how to teach social skills to understanding the more dynamic, synergistic processes the social brain interprets and responds to for those who are expected to blend into a crowd, maintain friendships, hold a job in the community, share space in a classroom effectively, etc.

While I am trained as an SLP, my work is now being utilized across all types of mental health and educational professions and across a range of diagnostic labels. Social Thinking's more sophisticated concepts are also being used with business professionals and with persons working with adjudicated youth, etc.

WHERE DID YOUR IDEAS/DESIRE COME FROM?

When I realized that the way I was taught to teach social skills to "lower functioning" individuals did not transfer well to my more argumentative, fully verbal teens in my high school program, I decided to re-think what I had learned based on what my clients were currently experiencing. It led me to many discoveries, some of which are reviewed below, that have now become the groundwork for my creativity in developing social thinking:

- People with solid to strong language skills and learning skills need a dedicated program that utilizes their language learning abilities to help them understand the complexities of social communication. This is different from teaching students social skills by asking them to memorize social behavior.
- We need to avoid making assumptions about our students' functional abilities based on their IQ and language skills.
- We need to see how social cognition provides the groundwork for accessing academic curriculum related to reading comprehension of literature, written language, working as part of a group, making inferences, taking perspective, etc.
- Across professions (psychiatry, psychology, SLP's, educators, counselors, OT's, behaviorists) there is a consistent lack of training in our formal education programs. This means that the core concepts involved in teaching Social Thinking and related social skills is new learning for even the most seasoned professional.
- Parents and professionals are not well versed in how to teach social cognitive lessons, as they usually acquired these skills in early childhood without direct teaching (e.g. children learn to relate to others and play without classroom based instruction on these concepts). Hence, as part of Social Thinking we need to teach a range of professionals how to deconstruct the complex social learning process in order for us to directly teach elements of it to our students who have social learning disabilities.
- Therefore, a large part of what we have developed lends itself to the adult parent/professional who we teach to think more deeply about the social learning process to help them more readily develop their own creative treatment ideas.
- Our students need to learn complex, synergistic information in more concrete ways. They need us to break down core concepts into a manner in which they can begin to digest the information in more simple ways and then slowly grow in how they can process and respond to the complexity of it.

- Students have different social communicative expectations placed on them by their community based on their age, hence lessons need to also be developmental (e.g. how one says "hi" to another person changes with age and situation).
- The most effective treatments are going to be the result of us understanding a student's social learning abilities rather than focusing on their diagnostic label.
- Parents and professionals need to have core information about social learning, which they can utilize across a range of situations and environments, in order to continue to create helpful lessons to the individuals they are teaching in a group.

WHAT SUPPORTED YOUR PROCESS?

My personal desire to provide treatment programs that align with my clients' needs was the most powerful motivator. I was consistently frustrated seeing my clients score well on tests but function far more poorly, which led me to think outside of the box. Their parents were also frustrated with this general feeling that no one really understood their kid.

In my learning process, I reached out to a number of diagnosticians in the local community to try to better understand my client's needs. One psychologist, in particular, who worked for Stanford University strongly encouraged me to develop treatments.

Once I began to develop treatment ideas and share them at meetings, etc. administrators, teachers and parents were very encouraging.

My students, many of whom were now seeking me out to spend time with me during their non-scheduled treatment appointment, also helped me to see that I was doing something really meaningful for them.

WHAT INHIBITED IT?

When I worked in the high school district, I was definitely outside of the box in my thinking. I challenged the assumption of many of our school psychologists that standardized tests were accurate measures of social, and even academic, functioning. This resulted in a number of heated professional discussions. I was not inhibited by less than enthusiastic responses to defining what we were observing in more creative ways, but I did have to deal with my own personal anxiety of not liking to be confrontational at a professional level. I learned it just takes time and practice to become more comfortable with discomfort, a lesson I also now teach my students.

DO YOU HAVE ANY PERSONAL PRACTICES
THAT YOU THINK SUPPORT YOUR CREATIVITY OR WORLD VIEWS?

My personal practices are forged, to some large degree, by my personality. I am my most comfortable considering what I have learned and then trying that information out in new and different ways. For example, I have never been one to feel that I needed to closely follow a recipe when cooking.

When it came to developing Social Thinking (something I never had planned to do), I was comfortable creating lessons based on new learning and new experiences. In my adult life, I have found that questioning our assumptions is important in all aspects of our life. I loved the book, Freakanomics by Levitt & Dubner, (2006), which teaches us that if you ask a different question with the same set of data you can get a radically different answer.

I felt our human service fields (educators, mental health, etc.) had accepted how we should all teach social skills without really asking a different question. Social Thinking evolved from me asking myself, "What are social skills and how do we teach them differently to people with different learning abilities?"

How Has the Experience Influenced Your Current Creativity?

I have been tremendously rewarded for my creativity. Parents and professionals are very enthusiastic and openly complimentary about how the teachings of Social Thinking have impacted them personally and professionally. Many people have sent me letters explaining how they were about to change careers as they were burnt out in their professional lives that were lacking in creativity, but they ended up staying in their work and taking on studying and teaching social thinking to their students/clients. In the past 15 years I have also traveled to over 15 countries teaching about this concept.

I continue to work with clients and evolve the teachings of Social Thinking.

What I have also noticed is that the community is really embracing that our lessons encourage their own creativity. With Social Thinking we provide a philosophy, core concepts, frameworks to structure our understanding of the social world, teaching strategies, guidance on how social learning relates to mental health, curriculum standards, etc. but then we tell them to take the information and apply it in their situation with their students. This has fostered a whole community of parents and professionals who are interested in learning more, since they have such direct input in how it is applied.

From my experience, I have seen that most people want to be creative; what kills their passion is when they are told they must teach or relate to a person in a very specific, contrived manner that removes all the "art" from the relationship.

Describe Your Experience with Creating ... Is It a Steady Process? Episodic? Manic? Drought? Does It Feel Like It Comes from "You" or Elsewhere?

Given the individuality of each client I see or each team I consult with, my creative process is steady and on-going. I have worried at times that this may stop, but it never has. Next year will be 20 years since I began to evolve this teaching methodology. The tools I need to foster my creativity include cognitive flexibility, a strong framework from which I can hinge my thinking, and a range of clients.

HOW DO YOU NURTURE OR NURSE FLEDGLING IDEAS?

I started by building a framework of understanding the social mind and as I try to make sense of new situations, which require creative thinking, I first try to understand how the situation I am facing aligns with or challenges my old thinking.

I find that it is important to not fear having been wrong in the past so that if I come upon a situation that provides clarity but requires me to discount a prior idea, I can do that. I think the willingness to think and re-think and to be unapologetically able to shift perspectives keeps one from getting stuck.

WHAT ROLES DOES/DID YOUR COMMUNITY/COLLEAGUES PLAY IN YOUR CREATIVE EXPERIENCE?

For many of my early years when I was actively evolving Social Thinking after leaving the public school system in 1999, I was the mentor to many and did not have anyone who really challenged or questioned me in a big way. In 2005 I met Dr. Pam Crooke who did some research on my work. When we went to dinner to discuss the research (she was not someone I knew previously), she asked me many good and challenging questions about why I decided to proceed in certain directions with Social Thinking. I really enjoyed that, and I convinced Pam to come work with me. Since that time I found the collaboration has allowed me to develop deeper thinking and to broaden the reach of Social Thinking.

In 2010 Pam and I then started a Social Thinking Training and Speakers' Collaborative. We now have about 10 people we hand-chose to work closely with us, and it is impressive to see how they are also helping to push the boundaries of Social Thinking.

WHAT WOULD YOU DO DIFFERENTLY?

I can't honestly say that I would have done anything differently, as it relates to the creation of Social Thinking and its on-going evolution.

There is also the business corporation I own that manages the growth of our products and conferences related to that idea; the place where I would do things differently is in how I have run the business. The business has successfully helped to launch the concept into a broader and growing community, but along the way I wish I had known how to treat some of the issues related to employees differently.

The reality is, if you have a creative idea, it will only get shared if you have a vehicle for sharing it. That vehicle is typically a business or a business deal. I grew up in an entrepreneurial family so I was perhaps better prepared than most SLPs or mental health professionals for running a business, but there is a still a lot to learn! As Social Thinking evolves, so does the business; dynamic, creative thinking now takes on many forms!

WHAT'S NEXT?

Giving Pam the time to coordinate research projects within our community, to show the evidence of our teachings in a more traditional manner.

To write out more of the ideas that are relatively easy to develop with a client but hard to describe to others in print.

WORDS OF WISDOM/INSPIRATION?

When you see barriers, ask a lot of questions. Avoid letting people tell you "no".

Creativity is not measured by IQ; IQ tests have no creative components. Don't limit your own abilities with pre-conceived notions about your intelligence or another's willingness to consider what you have to say, as long as you say it in a manner that connects to their own understanding of the world.

I have considered starting a website for people who are considered "successful" but felt dumb in school.

In: Fostering Creativity in Rehabilitation
Editor: Matthew J. Taylor

ISBN: 978-1-63485-118-3
© 2016 Nova Science Publishers, Inc.

Chapter 13

NURSING

Carey S. Clark, PhD, RN, AHN-BC

Assistant Professor, RN-BSN Program, University of Maine at Augusta, Augusta, US

WHAT CHALLENGES AND OPPORTUNITIES ARE SPECIFIC TO YOUR PROFESSION?

The challenges and opportunities in contemporary nursing are complex, and I have previously published a two part series on many of our professional issues (Clark, 2002; 2010). Challenges include complexity in the workplace, the nursing shortage, lack of autonomy, professional oppression, lateral violence, and over-medicalization of nursing care.

Nurses' work is technologically complex and the effectiveness of the nurse relies on his or her ability to make sound clinical decisions, while also maintaining a caring presence. Nurses work in stressful environments and failure to adequately manage our own professional stress has greatly impacted our ability to create the sort of caring-healing environments that we are ethically obligated to create (Clark, 2014). For many years we have strived to move toward autonomy in our professional practices, and yet we remain what might be called an oppressed group, our work being managed and driven by healthcare facility administrators and federal regulators (Clark, 2002).

While we have such amazing theorists to guide us toward creating caring-healing practices, there remains a prevalent gap between and amongst theory, research, evidence, and education. It is no wonder that our new graduate nurses leave their first jobs at the rate of 30% in the first year and 57% by the second year of practice (Twibell et al., 2014). New graduate nurses report higher levels of anxiety and stress versus the seasoned nurses who has gained the needed experience to make sound clinical decisions (Twibell et al.), and yet we continue for the most part to fail to address our ethical obligation to prepare nurses who are capable of managing stress in order to create sustainable caring-healing bedside practices (Clark, 2014).

With these challenges comes the polarity of opportunity for change and transformation. With the beginning workings of the affordable care act in place, I do believe there will begin to be a greater shift toward prevention and healing as cost containment issues come into greater play. As the holistic nursing movement has been growing over the past 40 years, the nursing profession is finally being afforded opportunities to enter into the era of caring-healing that Florence Nightingale proposed over 150 years ago. Patients are hungry for caring-healing modalities and holistic nurses are beginning to undertake the healing journey themselves as they strive to support the healing and health of those they care for.

WHAT DID/ARE YOU DO/DOING?

In addition to writing about our issues in nursing, in order to help usher in this new era of sustainable caring-healing practices, I have developed a holistic nursing curriculum for RN-BSN students that supports their ability to manage their own stress by supporting and valuing self-care throughout the curricular journey. Students have the opportunity to take academically sound upper level electives such as Integrative Yoga and Reiki, which they use to support their own healing journey and the journey of their colleagues and patients. I have written several articles about the curriculum and the emerging outcomes in hopes to disseminate the ideas (Clark, 2012; 2013). I present the findings from the curriculum implementation at conferences, I am actively involved in the American Holistic Nurses Association (AHNA), and I developed a student- faculty chapter of AHNA to support student growth in learning about holistic nursing and holistic modalities. Additionally, I strive each day to act as a role model for my students and my colleagues by engaging in self-care activities.

WHERE DID YOUR IDEAS/DESIRE COME FROM?

I found myself growing increasingly disenchanted with the healthcare system after only 3 years of floor nursing in the late 1990's. I longed to be able to care for my patients deeply and to be less engrossed in the medical-technical demands of nursing. I became a hospice nurse and recognized the potential of caring-healing bedside practices when the whole team is actively working together and the nurse has the opportunity outside of the stressful hospital environment to truly "be" with patients. To sit and witness, to be with patients and families through the end of life mystery was nourishing for my own soul. By being present, I learned that I could be an aspect of the healing environment during the suffering, love, and mystery of life's journey.

After many years in academia as both a student and a nursing faculty member, I eventually pursued a humanities doctoral degree at the California Institute of Integral Studies (CIIS). During my studies related to transformative learning and change, I was able to examine our professional nursing and academic issues through the lenses of the transdiscplinarity approach, which helped me to envision a new way to do the work of nursing academia that is integrally based in caring and healing. In addition to experiencing a new way of education through the integral approaches offered at CIIS, I had the opportunity to experience a caring-healing curriculum when I took a week-long course with the nurse theorist Dr. Jean Watson out of University of Colorado Health Sciences. I knew that creating caring circles was the way that I wanted to teach nursing, and my doctoral dissertation highlighted the movement toward this type of caring curriculum experience.

I have a strong desire to support nurses in caring for others, and I also now see myself as caring for and nursing the nurses, supporting them on their own healing journey. I desire a better world for my own children, and I strive to live a caring presence in my own life. I believe that many of my ideas and desires do not come from "me", but rather they emerge from the divine spirit and move through me. However, another polarity to this process is my ego that drives me to keep pushing for this transformation, to keep pushing and moving forward with the innovations and disseminating the ideas on a larger scale. I admittedly have a strong desire for recognition, being the human that I am. Over many years of practice, I have learned to quiet my mind each morning, and take some time for getting out of amygdala response and entering into relaxation response through meditation. This process coupled with taking time for rest, relaxation, and rejuvenation clears the clutter from my mind and allows for new ideas to emerge, allows for spirit to move through me and generate innovative ideas and enthusiasm to keep the spark of transformation alive.

WHAT SUPPORTED YOUR PROCESS?

Learning to meditate, practicing yoga, great mentors, fabulous colleagues, having a supportive and loving family, letting things go toward the greater good, striving to look at conflict and polarizations as needed events along the journey, and learning to practice self-care. I have begun to look at challenges to my beliefs as opportunities to learn how to address those challenges from the perspective of the challenger. One thing that continues to help me is to look at my own creations as belonging not to me, but to the universe at large; this takes some of the pressure for success of me and I am learning to trust the universe, to let go, to practice acceptance, and to know that I am guided, all is well, all is well.

WHAT INHIBITED IT?

I have a high number of adverse childhood events and traumas that shaped my brain in a way that my stress resilience is low. I tend to enter into anxiety and stress response easily, react fearfully to challengers of my ideas, and feelings of anxiety and depression can get in the way of the creative process.

One night of poor sleep can throw me off kilter for several days. Luckily for me, the science of psychoneuroimmunology supports the idea that we are neuroplastic beings, and my daily meditation practices and self-care activities such as yoga, meditation, and exercise support my development of greater stress resilience.

DO YOU HAVE ANY PERSONAL PRACTICES
THAT YOU THINK SUPPORT YOUR CREATIVITY OR WORLD VIEWS?

Meditation, yoga, moderate exercise 6-7 days/ week, spending quality time with loved ones, practicing Reiki, making time for rest, relaxation, and recreation.

HOW HAS THE EXPERIENCE INFLUENCED
YOUR CURRENT CREATIVITY?

My current creativity is focused on spreading the word of the positive and empowering outcomes from implementing a caring-healing curriculum. Many times when I am meditation or working out, new ideas emerge in a way that is beyond my Ego self. I also have been able to let go when ideas I think are headed one way end up in a differing direction or a dead end. For some reason, I am being guided in a different direction and that is okay.

DESCRIBE YOUR EXPERIENCE WITH CREATING ...
IS IT A STEADY PROCESS? EPISODIC? MANIC? DROUGHT?
DOES IT FEEL LIKE IT COMES FROM "YOU" OR ELSEWHERE?

The work I do with teaching is demanding, particularly at this time as I am well into progressing on the tenure track process. The demands of academia are such that little time is left for creative endeavors, so during the academic school year, I try and create snippets of time for creative outlets. When summer rolls around, I tend to get more creative work done. I suppose in this sense, my creative work tends to be episodic. I often try and commit myself to being creative on a daily basis (write something each day!), but I often become ensnared in my responsibilities as a faculty member and mother of two school aged daughters.

HOW DO YOU NURTURE OR NURSE FLEDGLING IDEAS?

Generally, I roll them around in my head and I try to get something down "on paper" as soon as possible. If this does not happen, then I find myself losing the ideas. However, I also believe that nothing is lost in the universe; did the idea go to a different person or back to the universe … or will it emerge again in the future? While it can be disappointing when the creative genius ideas float away, I try not to cling to the loss for long.

What Roles Does/Did Your Community/Colleagues Play in Your Creative Experience?

I have learned over time that the creative process is not about me, the Ego sense of me, and that I need others to make my dreams into reality. For instance, having a team to work with was essential in getting the innovative curriculum we developed through the rigorous accreditation process. I find inspiration from all of the amazing nursing theorists who have paved the way, the patients whose suffering lingered with me, the students who have transformed their lives, and the conferences of like-minded people who engage my ideas on a meaningful basis. I have had several mentors, both in and out of nursing who just let me know: I could do it, there are always possibilities! When I entered graduate school, I was so grateful that I could contact nurse leaders like Dr. Jean Watson and Dr. Peggy Chinn and dialog with them about emerging ideas. Also, in graduate school where much of my creative process was initiated, I was blessed to be supported with a like-minded group of colleagues and an amazing dissertation advisor; these people cheered me on; they created a space for holding and supporting my work in a way that it was destined for evolution.

What Would You Do Differently?

I would have started on a healing and creative journey at a younger age. I would reach out more during times of isolation and loneliness.

What's Next?

I want to continue to write and research with nurses and nursing students. I will continue to support nurses in their self-care and healing efforts on a larger scale, perhaps developing a graduate level holistic-integral nursing program that could be delivered on a larger scale. I want to take time each day for creativity to emerge, whether that is in my own creative writing process (I have a healing poetry blog) or looking for creative solutions to problems.

Words of Wisdom/Inspiration?

Take the time to nurture yourself, connect to spirit or your own inner wisdom, and meditate or enter into relaxation response daily through yoga, exercise, prayer, and/ or sacred chant. Remember, all is well, your life is unfolding exactly as it should be.

References

Clark, C. S. (2002). The nursing shortage as a community transformational opportunity. *Advances in Nursing Science, 25*(1), 18-31.

Clark, C. S. (2010). The nursing shortage as a community transformational opportunity: An update. *Advances in Nursing Science, 33*(10), 35-52.

Clark, C. S. (2012). Beyond holism: Incorporating an integral approach to support caring-healing-sustainable nursing practices. *Holistic Nursing Practice, 26*(2), 92-102.

Clark, C. S. (2013). An integral- caring science RN- BS nursing curriculum: Outcomes from fostering consciousness evolution. *International Journal for Human Caring, 17*(2).

Clark, C. S. (2014). Stress, psychoneuroimmunology, and self-care: What every nurse needs to know. *Journal of Nursing and Care, 3,* 146.

Twibell, R., St. Pierre, J., Johnson, D., Barton, D., Davis, C., Kidd, M., & Rook, G. (2012). Tripping over the welcome mat: Why new nurses don't stay and what the evidence says we can do about it. *American Nurse Today, 7*(6), electronic issue.

In: Fostering Creativity in Rehabilitation
Editor: Matthew J. Taylor

ISBN: 978-1-63485-118-3
© 2016 Nova Science Publishers, Inc.

Chapter 14

NUTRITION

Beverly Price, RD, MA, E-RYT

CEDS Director, Inner Door Center, Royal Oak, MI, US

A NUTRITION ENTREPRENEUR IS BORN, NOT MADE

> "Coming Full Circle"
> "O, what a tangled web we weave"
> *Ralph Waldo Emerson*

The most difficult part of my life's learning lesson and awakening were the years following the sale of my 13 year nutrition private practice. With no concrete plan going forward, the sale of my practice in May of 2001, and beginning of my new "consulting career" unfolded quickly into 9/11, a tragic tale in this nation's history. From there on, life changed for many as priorities changed and a way of life began to evolve. A heightened spirituality began to emerge resulting in individuals turning to prayer, meditation and/or their place of worship in search of a sense of community and belonging. The stress of working countless hours in my nutrition practice with challenging clients, coupled with a young child at home, fueled the sale of my practice into a slower and more spiritual way of life...or so I thought....

So, here I was, October 2001, with a consulting career in the medical supply industry that I had fallen into, while also developing my own practice management firm for dietitians and other healthcare professionals. Life was different, I was in "change mode," working as many hours as usual, but could not understand why I still felt so stressed. After all, didn't I just give up what was stressing me... my patient practice?

In the winter of 2002 I reconnected with my oldest childhood friend and now colleague, Dawn Singer. We were instrumental as a networking partners in the growth of each other's businesses in the early 1990s and she had come to town for business, staying at my house. I was in full gear with both of my endeavors and looked as haggard as ever with all of the traveling and late night hours. Dawn came into town on a Friday evening from Boston, her new home, and literally dragged me out of bed the next morning to go to a yoga class with our favorite local "guru," Jonny Kest at the Center for Yoga, Birmingham, Michigan. I thought I would strangle Dawn with my bare hands.

Jonny was an old friend and colleague who was introduced to me by Dawn in the early 1990s at a healthcare professionals' networking program. Jonny brought yoga to Michigan and was starting classes in suburban Detroit while I was just starting my nutrition counseling business when Jonny and I met. I attended yoga, on a fairly regular basis in the 90's, but didn't quite understand what it meant to be committed to the yoga lifestyle. I didn't quite have that concept of balance in my life!

It was in the winter of 2002, when I found myself in the middle of the most intense yoga class with Jonny Kest, now quite polished with over 10 years of teaching and a tremendous following. What was I missing all of these years? Through Dawn and Jonny's encouragement, I became a devoted "yogini." Ironically, Dawn left the corporate healthcare world in Boston and moved across country to southern California and opened a successful donation-based yoga studio in a yurt.

In September of 2003, I was encouraged by one of Jonny's yoga teachers to enroll in Jonny Kest's teacher training. Skeptical but intrigued, I followed through. Although I did not have any plans to become a full-fledged yoga teacher, of all things, but thought I would use the course to deepen my yoga practice and immerse myself into Jonny's teachings.

A requirement of the yoga teacher training program was to complete a special project—it was anything that spoke to us. I chose to research yoga and its impact on the treatment of eating disorders. A large frustration of my former private practice was that I was treating so many individuals with eating disorders, from a nutrition standpoint, along with an outpatient treatment team of a therapist and physician. However, I always felt that there was something missing in the treatment component. As I delved into yoga, the messages from my teachers in relation to the practice became crystal clear that yoga was the missing link in eating disorder treatment. As someone who personally struggled in my high school and college years, this "yoga" that I found was the true healer—beyond a therapist, physician and dietitian.

I then connected with Gretchen Newmark, a dietitian and yoga teacher in Portland, Oregon who wrote an article on yoga and eating disorders years ago in the Yoga Journal. She was a mentor and guided me in the science behind yoga. In addition, Jonny Kest put me in touch with his brother Bryan Kest in Santa Monica, California. Bryan shared with me one of his first careers in teaching yoga was working with individuals who struggled with anorexia nervosa in conjunction with their psychotherapist.

Following the completion of my Yoga teacher training, I knew what I needed to do…and that was go back into private nutrition practice with a new outlook and updated method. I needed to combine yoga in the treatment of eating disorders…and that I did…. On January 2, 2004, I opened up my doors again. I started out incorporating the physical and spiritual practice of yoga into my nutrition sessions and also held "yoga and eating disorder" support groups. In these two-hour support groups, I taught a yoga class interspersed with a message that continued into the support/discussion portion of the program. The name of the program emerged one day, following yoga class that I attended. Jonny had weaved a theme into this particular yoga class regarding the "disconnect" that so many individuals have with food. Inspired by this class, my program became known as "Reconnect with Food."

I traveled near and far with my Reconnect with Food program, holding it at various yoga studios in the metro-Detroit area along with studios and conferences across the country.

The two hour support program grew into a weekend intensive and then a week intensive featuring not just yoga but mindful eating, art therapy, music therapy and more…with a variety of other professionals. The program finally needed a center of its own vs. a one room school house. My vision was to surround myself with other professionals in a multi-disciplinary program to bring healing to many who struggle with eating disorders across the spectrum—anorexia, bulimia, binge eating and co-occurring disorders including substance abuse.

In 2008, I found a place to house my vision -- a 3,000 square foot building just off downtown Royal Oak, Michigan. Serendipitously, I had also rented space at this location in my early return to private practice following yoga teacher training. The therapists, who ran their psychotherapy practice at this building, dispersed and left the building sitting for over a year. I negotiated a sweet deal with the landlord who also agreed to renovate the building. Royal Oak is an eclectic and cool town just outside of Detroit. It offers an area to shop and eat, providing great opportunities for patient experientials for restaurant eating, people exposure for those who struggle with social anxiety, field trip opportunities with meaning and walks in nature outside of the downtown area.

During the first year at this center, I did not have as clear of a business model as I thought…I had first opened this center to other eating disorder therapists to rent space from me and conduct their own psychotherapy practice, along with subcontracting their services for my now two week long yoga and eating disorder intensive. In addition, we held no insurance contracts. In the history of my private nutrition practice, there was never any insurance coverage offered for nutrition services by Michigan insurance companies, but I built my business in the midst of a community with disposable income in the height of the 1990's. My business model in 2008-2009 failed because patients in our area, undergoing psychotherapy, generally relied on insurance…especially in the current economic time. In addition, the therapists currently renting space at my clinic not only did not know how to market themselves, nor did they care to, nor did they have the where-with-all to build their business….they wanted instant booming results. Therefore, I was supporting the huge building myself and surprisingly making it in this tumultuous economic year. One of the therapists on board suggested that we all look into insurance contracts, including contracting of our intensive day treatment program as a partial hospitalization program (PHP).

A Michigan licensed and credentialed PHP consists of at least six hours per day of therapeutic programming, a meal, snacks and individual along with family therapy. Along with my young office manager, I continued to investigate the insurance payer mix in Michigan and began to invite provider contracting representatives to our office to learn about eating disorders, along with the vision for our program. Because there were no other day treatment programs in the area, insurances were willing to contract with our program as a carve out for eating disorders although we were treating the host of co-occurring disorders that come with the disease including OCD, anxiety, depression, PTSD, and substance abuse.

We needed a license to contract with insurance companies, so the Michigan mental health licensing board granted us a substance abuse license. At this time, we were told to hold off on a designated PHP license based on our size. He also felt that an eating disorder itself was congruent with a substance addiction so the license was fitting. The head of the license bureau was a little skeptical of the yoga, but we weaved the yoga right into the PHP programming - from the physical practice through each therapeutic modality requirement - while keeping in line with the medical model requirements. We ultimately obtained our Michigan partial hospitalization license and became accredited by the Joint Commission - the healthcare gold standard for safety, quality and efficacy.

We also contracted with insurance companies for outpatient psychotherapy services. For those therapists who ended up staying at the clinic, we absorbed them as part of our staff. Our outpatient therapy program grew slowly (a slow build as my yoga teacher says, as a metaphor for the yoga practice) as did our partial hospitalization program, each a feeder to the other. Eventually, the entire business was named Inner Door Center—again inspired by Jonny Kest as he said in class one day, "You have to go in that door, before you come out," meaning... you have to go deep inside to access yourself.

In addition, as our insurance contracts were solidifying in 2009, a generous benefactor who supported my programs from their inception and throughout the years, funded a pilot program to immerse selected patients in our PHP and give it a whirl. The pilot program was a huge success, and various insurance contracts kicked in gradually in 2010. At first the program was scarily slow...I remember in early January of 2010 in the freezing winter months of Michigan, there were days that my office manager and I were the only two people in the entire building. One day, she looked at me and exclaimed, "Are we just PLAYING office?" Funny and scary as it was, it was true. However, within the year the flood gates opened.

Our partial hospitalization program doesn't just offer a yoga class in which we begin our day. The yoga teacher does not walk in, conduct her class and then leave as in other eating disorder treatment programs that have caught on to using yoga. Our yoga teachers, who are currently trained yoga therapists in eating disorder treatment by our charter member school of the International Association of Yoga Therapists (IAYT), are an integral part of our treatment team. They function on the same level as our doctoral and master's level psychotherapists and registered dietitians, headed up by our medical director psychiatrist and adjunct medical director internist, along with physician assistants and psychiatric nurse practitioners. Our registered yoga teachers (RYTs)/yoga therapists (YTs) oversee meals and also conduct therapeutic groups. They also document in our electronic medical record. All have tremendous connections, as you can imagine, with our patients. The RYT/YTs also are instrumental in staff training and development along with running a good portion of our yoga therapy/yoga certification program in eating disorders.

Our program integrates the chakras and eight limbs of yoga in a circular theme, also woven into our patient treatment plans. For therapeutic practitioners, the chakras parallel the wellness domains along with Maslow's Hierarchy of Needs. Not all of our patients are familiar nor have been exposed to yoga prior to entering our program, although it is a draw for many who have struggled for years with no avail. The yoga benefits those who struggle with eating disorders by helping them discover roots and messages contributing to thought processes, delay impulses, promote enjoyment of their body, eat mindfully, heal negative body image and develop self-acceptance, avoid using food or starvation to numb painful emotions and encourage integration of techniques into a daily yoga practice. Family therapy is also a significant part of our treatment program, for if the families do not heal, the patient cannot move forward. We dig deep and uncover layers that go way beyond food...food is just a symptom of the emotional roots....it is how the whole ball of wax manifests.

Studies have shown that Mindful Yoga and meditation can affect the cerebral cortex, improving focus and awareness. The cerebral cortex is the center of the brain that is responsible for impulses, irrational thoughts and behaviors. Activating the cerebral cortex can diminish the impulsivity along with irrational thoughts and behaviors involved in eating disorders, substance abuse and related addictions. Our program does a great job of integrating eating disorder and substance abuse treatment, as most who access our program struggle with both concerns. We also treat a variety of psychological concerns in our outpatient program.

The Reconnect with Food® Mindfulness Yoga-based treatment program that is conducted at the Inner Door Center® is congruent with the more progressive therapies used in eating disorder treatment, described above, including DBT, MBCT and ACT.

The patients and their families on the whole, who we treat, are absolutely wonderful to work with. The staff each brings their uniqueness and wisdom to the program - they are the cream of the eating disorder crop. As the program has evolved and grown throughout the years, we have implemented a formal human resources, marketing and accounting departments. We recently remodeled, softening color scheme and adding fireplaces in both lobby and yoga space, while taking over an additional building on our property to house a spectacular, "home-like" area for our intensive treatment program, along with additional administrative offices.

My husband, David Price, and I run the center. David is the detail person, where I am known to "wing it." We are a good team. My husband is an amazing substance abuse therapist. Tawana Jackson, the fearless "T" as she is referred to as, entered my life in 2011 and is one amazing woman. A former automotive manager brought her skill and style (in addition to the style of her clothing and shoes) to the Inner Door Center. She often talks in automotive manager language, but it is good for our business. She now functions as our office manager...but is beyond that role...she can do anything and everything. She was largely instrumental in helping us become accredited by the Joint Commission and then our official Partial Hospitalization license by the state of Michigan. I am so grateful to T and everything she does for our center. Her beautiful energy is contagious.

For those of you reading this who may not be aware, Detroit is still auto-town regardless of its rocky history. If you work in the Detroit area, you are generally connected to or affected by the auto industry or you work for Quicken Loans and/or a family of companies founded and/or owned by Dan Gilbert, the "Donald Trump" of Detroit. Detroit has made a huge comeback, and oddly enough we receive resumes daily from individuals that want to relocate to Detroit...still blows my mind...but we are happening according to a recent New York Times article!!

But I am digressing….the Inner Door Center, with close to 30 staff members currently, is growing faster than we can keep up with ourselves. Over the years, I have transitioned away from direct patient contact. Currently, my role is to hold the space and intention for the business, while staying connected to its core and belief in the support of our divine mission. I work ON the business more so than working IN the business.

What does the future hold for this yoga and eating disorder treatment center?

Lately there has been a frenzy of fascination with and hope for the economic recovery of Detroit. This undeniable buzz is positive, infectious and has provoked people to think in new ways about reclaiming the prosperity of the Motor City. Yet, while the city is being physically recovered, there is an underlying need for personal recovery both physically and mentally.

Contributing to many influential and stable cities across the country is the mental health stability encouraged in recovery communities for its residents. The Fix identified the 10 Best Sober Living Cities in America. For individuals searching for new beginnings to move beyond their addiction and emotional strife, these cities boast unique recovery communities offering intensive treatment, sober living, cultural awareness and social outlets.

For instance, Boston boasts a "commitment exchange" program, similar to an AA group, which focuses on building a sobriety network. Delray has a coffeehouse with its own therapy group, a radio show and even a recovery motorcycle club. Houston dedicates "clubhouses" as venues for recovery. Minneapolis features public sober high schools. Nashville has many community events including homemade ice cream contests, spring flings and cookouts. San Francisco is quite diverse and open-minded in its communities, including LGBT support groups, and Spanish-speaking groups. These communities offer ways for people to be connected not only physically to others, but also virtually through social media sites. There is a great deal of energy found in youth undergoing recovery and communities provide alternate ways to have a good time. People find comfort within a wider range of recovery around people facing similar struggles as well as successes. Many are inspired to provide service to give back to those in need during thousands of weekly support meetings and AA groups. In addition, communities promote sober living experiences, raise community awareness of recovery and stimulate the economy, offering jobs to locals.

It may be beneficial for Detroit to learn a lesson or two from these iconic and lucrative cities. A relationship clearly exists between a healthy population and a resultant prosperous city. How can people take pride in Detroit if they do not take pride in themselves? The Inner Door Foundation, the non-profit arm of Inner Door Center, has identified a definite need in the Metro-Detroit area for a Recovery Community. While the city is being physically rebuilt, we hope to grow a recovery community for people facing eating disorders, substance abuse and a variety of mental health concerns. Here at the Inner Door Center®, we plan to simulate the efforts of the programs around the country within Detroit and the surrounding communities. Our wish is to spread positivity and provide hope for those suffering, past sufferers, and those in recovery.

WHAT WE ARE DOING

The mission of the Inner Door Center and Foundation is to raise public awareness of eating disorders and to promote the education of holistic treatment. The rebuilding of Detroit and the renovation of the Inner Door Center® mirror the physical and mental stabilization of those in recovery.

The Inner Door Center® provides eating disorder treatment, substance abuse treatment and outpatient therapy for a variety of other mental health concerns, along with the renowned Mindfulness Yoga-Based treatment system.

We offer support groups, including Reconnect with Recovery and Reconnect with Food®. Reconnect with Recovery is a free community support program open to the public every 3rd Saturday of the month and includes group support & yoga-based healing. We also started an alumni program to connect our alumni in a recovery community.

WHAT ARE MY/OUR CHALLENGES?

The biggest challenge that I personally have is being able to trust and delegate. I often find myself on one extreme micromanaging and then on the other hand letting important stuff slip by, such as when our recent dietitian appeared to be slipping into her own eating disorder and restricting food and she resigned. I was told all along by our lead therapist to start looking for a new dietitian. I didn't listen and found myself working as the staff dietitian for three of the longest weeks of my summer…I was the new sheriff, the meanie, the bad mom who had to force the patients to eat foods like pizza, French fries, etc. This was not a new philosophy to our company, but me rejuvenating the old that has been there and gotten lost. Ayurvedic nutrition, although a sister-science to yoga, unfortunately has no place in our treatment center as it promotes a rigidity that we are trying to move away from. Nor is vegetarianism congruent with an eating disorder, although I once thought otherwise. Any food plan that puts restrictions on or eliminates food groups promotes the disorder. We have since hired on a new dietitian. Yay, back to running the company.

As new opportunities emerge, we look towards expanding to into other areas of Michigan with satellite outreach and support programs, along with full blown intensive treatment programs using our model. This means more training programs for professionals in the field, in order to carry out our model. Our training programs also extend to middle and high schools, colleges and universities along with corporations.

Another huge challenge is moving our PHP away from insurance contracts. As the new contracts are presented, we have chosen not to sign at this point in time. Our outpatient therapy clientele relies on insurance, and we have no plans to move away from insurance contracts on the outpatient side. However, on the program side as insurance changes and requires frequent authorization for continued stay, it is hard to keep up with changes, regulations, payments, etc. This has forced us to move more to a healthy combination of out of network self-pay for program or non-covered levels of our program, combined with insurance coverage to help the patient as an adjunct for payment. This allows our patients to feel invested in their treatment, while maintaining our ability to sustain our program along with focus on the intent of our program.

MY PERSONAL GROWTH EDGE

Our relationship with food parallels all other relationships in our lives. My work in healing my own eating disorder did not just end with my comfort with acceptance of all foods. Through yoga, I learned that my relationship with food extended into my personal relationships with others, my work, the way I interacted with others, along with how I conducted myself in all aspects of my life. It was my yoga that stripped me down, chewed me up, spit me out and allowed me to look at myself from all angles. The binge, purge, restrict cycle extends way beyond food. Through my regular yoga practice, I can catch myself falling into a cycle and can pull myself out before I am taken under.

There was a man who dug for water…

My yoga teacher, Jonny Kest, tells a story about a man who was digging for water. When he did not find any water right way, he quickly moved on. After digging many holes, and not finding any water, he became discouraged. What he did not realize is that he did not take the time to dig deep enough. So when it comes to forming a business, take the time to focus and don't give up so easily! It is easy to become distracted when matters are not going the speed in which you would like them to advance. You then get involved in more projects, and more projects to try and create success. If you just keep the focus, the "slow build" takes place. Before you know it, you too have a large and thriving business.

One more jewel to remember is that Love and Trust are mutually exclusive of Fear and Doubt. If you approach your endeavors with an abundance of love and passion, trusting that the universe will guide you in a healthy direction, then fear and doubt cannot intervene.

"Success is Attitude, not Aptitude".

In: Fostering Creativity in Rehabilitation
Editor: Matthew J. Taylor

ISBN: 978-1-63485-118-3
© 2016 Nova Science Publishers, Inc.

Chapter 15

ART THERAPY

Renée van der Vennet PhD, LCAT, LMHC, ATR-BC, CGP

Assistant Professor of Creative Arts Therapy, Nazareth College,
Rochester, NY, US

WHAT CHALLENGES AND OPPORTUNITIES ARE SPECIFIC TO YOUR PROFESSION?

In the field of art therapy, there are a number of challenges and opportunities that inhibit or support creativity, but the potential for burnout is one of the greatest challenges for the art therapist. My experience has been unusual, because burnout led me to switch between two very different fields, coming from a scientific background to become an art therapist. I made this change partially because I was burned out by working as a scientist in industry, but also because I was driven and inspired to become an art therapist. In making this switch, I knew I was entering a field in human services where burnout was also a concern. Therefore, I did my dissertation on burnout with the personal goal of making sure I had coping strategies in place for myself as I made this career change. I learned that people in the field of art therapy value creativity and artistic abilities. If I could develop strategies to support my own creativity, my own artistic self, then perhaps I could deal with the challenge of not getting burned out as an art therapist. As a clinician, I also learned that I have an ethical obligation and responsibility for my own self-care. As an academic, I have the responsibility to model this behavior of balancing my workload with my creative outlets. I am constantly aware of this fine tightrope I walk between overload and creative expression.

In addition, I learned with this career change that the art therapy profession values creativity so much that it is seen as a cornerstone of the field. The concept of creativity is listed as a component of required course content for art therapy training. Also, in the field of art therapy, one's identity as an artist is always present. Thus as an artist, you might say by definition, we are assumed to be creative individuals. Ironically, the challenge in the art therapy profession regarding developing one's creativity is to find the time, space, and inspiration to be artistic and to be creative. The art therapy literature discusses this challenge in asking the question, do art therapists have time to create art? We are expected to be artists.

We are expected to be creative. Do we have time to create art while doing our jobs as art therapists?

Also, we work with clients using art as therapy, using art for therapy, and practicing art psychotherapy. Is using art this way with clients the same as us being creative and artistic ourselves? For me the answer is no. I am an art therapist so I want to use art with clients in this way to help my clients. I also want to be the artist that I am. I also want to be the creative artist that I am. Can I do both? Yes. I believe I can. I know I can. I just struggle with finding the time and space to be the creative artist that I know I am. Yet is my art for product and show? Or is my art for my own processing? I create art for product as well as process. And for me, both avenues are creative, yet the results are not something I am always willing to show.

In the field of art therapy, because we are supposed to be artists, there are opportunities to participate in art shows and sell art when it is produced for the purpose of product and show. However, when the art is produced for process, then the opportunity is for my own personal use and self-growth.

WHAT DID/ARE YOU DO/DOING?

In the field of art therapy, there is a constant debate about using art for product versus process. I came into this field because I discovered on my own journey that using art to process my own life experiences worked. I also discovered that my experience of using art for product was different than using art for process; although both avenues can be very creative expressions.

Since I was a child, I have always been interested in developing artistic skills in painting, drawing, clay, and sculpture, and I have always taken classes to improve on techniques. The pre-requisites for the field of art therapy require competencies in basic use of art media: drawing, painting, and sculpture. I thrived when taking studio art courses to develop my skills for refining the product in order to meet the pre-requisite requirements for art therapy. Watercolor painting became my medium of choice. Therefore, with respect to my focus on product, I paint watercolors. When I work on a watercolor painting, I focus on the skills to render the best product I can produce. I can be creative in this process of focusing on the product and some of my paintings have been good enough to show and sell. Yet, it has been years since I have been inspired to paint a watercolor. I feel like I have been in a drought when it comes to watercolor painting. I miss it.

In contrast, because of my own life experiences and drive for self understanding and personal growth, I discovered what Carl Jung calls the process of "individuation." In this process, I was drawn to the use of creative media, e.g. drawing, painting, and the use of clay, to explore my own unconscious. I was drawn to use my nightly dreams to guide my way. I discovered Jung's process of "active imagination" that calls for the use of these creative media to explore the dreamscape and one's unconscious realms. Active imagination is an enactment technique developed by Carl Jung for direct interaction with the unconscious. The enactment technique involves the use of an unstructured situation, experience, nighttime dream, or material. The material may be clay, painting material, a sand tray, music, or writing, so that the images may be expressed in a concrete way. In other words, I discovered how to use art to process my own life experiences while being guided by my nighttime dreams. I seek out places, workshops, experiential trainings and classes to build on this process in support of my own personal growth. I also utilize personal therapy to support my process.

In these experiential workshops, I use collage, clay, paint, sand tray, movement, and music to create, to explore, and to delve into my being. Again, I gravitate to process painting using a 24-color palette of tempera paints on 20 X 26" white paper (or larger) to explore my unconscious and to be creative.

Process-painting is an opportunity for me to get in touch with my creative self. I paint in a safe environment where there is no judgment, no lecture on skills, no critique, comparison or criticism offered. I face the white void of the paper with the palette of paint and a variety of brushes. Anything goes and there are no rules about what I want to paint. There are no mistakes and no accidents. When I understand that the product is not the goal, the colors and forms flow from the unconscious in a very natural way (Cassou & Cubley, 1995). When I give myself permission that no one need see the painting, I have the opportunity to be in touch with my own source, my own essence, my own flow. This moment is difficult to explain. Painting for process connects one to the source (Cassou & Cubly, 1995; Gold, 1998). Getting into the process involves facing the void, choosing colors, and feeling the flow of the paint on the paper (Cassou & Cubley, 1995). I have no plans. I just paint. I am drawn to a color. I paint a line, a dot, or a shape. I just paint.

I have created a space in my house that is permanently set up so I can process-paint. I also search out workshops in magical settings like Taos, New Mexico or Brevens Bruk, Sweden to spend days painting in studio space dedicated to process-painting with like-minded individuals. I work hard at meeting the needs and fulfilling the responsibilities of my profession, so I am committed to treating myself to creative workshops where I can play with just as much drive and commitment.

WHERE DID YOUR IDEAS/DESIRE COME FROM?

Again, to answer this question I need to talk separately about product and process. For product, I paint watercolors. I am very inspired by the travel vacations I take, the places I visit, and the pictures I take on these journeys. When I travel, I take a lot of photographs to inspire myself, and I also take a drawing journal to sketch and make quick watercolors.

What supports my process? It may sound trite to say my dreams, my actual nighttime dreams support my process, but they are an important source for my creativity. I have the same belief as McNiff (1992) who stressed that the uses of dreams are themselves works of art; I find myself continually drawn to their wealth of images, symbols, and content for my creative endeavors. In Jungian theory, dreams are the symbolic representation of the psyche. Dreams are self-portraits, which open the door to the person's unconscious via imagery and symbols that are the language of the unconscious (Sharp, 1998). Dreams support the process of individuation by requiring the waking conscious ego to face itself more objectively and consciously (Hall, 1986). Hall (1983) recommends following the dream series in order to follow the process of individuation. In this way, I use my nightly dreams to create in support of my own individuation process. I journal my dreams daily, my soul's language, which guides me. For example, the following dream is one I had at the beginning of my journey to become an art therapist.

In the dream, I am watching a group of people from the front of a high-powered speedboat. I want to turn around to see where we are going, but I cannot. I feel the motion of the boat, the energy of the people, and the excitement of moving forward. A swimming pool, my pool, is on the hill, and there is a slide from my swimming pool that leads down to the river. My pool is being filled up from the slide, and the water is moving uphill! I stand outside of my pool on the opposite, downhill side of the slide where I am inundated in the waters surrounding the pool. I reach to move the pool slide down, knowing that the water from the flood will engulf my pool. Even though this motion was precarious, I do it anyway. Then the forces of the floodwaters take me down the slide. I am scared at first; then I brace myself for fun.

In the dream, the pool is my unconscious; the floodwaters are the collective unconscious; and I am making a connection to a higher source. Although I am frightened because I cannot see where I am going on the speedboat into this new field of art therapy, and I know the power of the flooding water, I feel in tune. I feel the motion, and I am ready for fun. This dream was a guidepost that convinced me that doing this dream work, this process work, and making this career change would be challenging, fun, and an opportunity for personal growth and creative expression. I have never been focused on regrets or looking backwards, but I continue to regularly journal my dreams to be in tune with myself in the present.

I also want to note that my husband supports my process. Being married takes work and commitment, especially as each partner is growing and maturing individually as well as a couple. I feel the love, commitment, encouragement and support from this man, so that I can take this personal journey through my dreams and process-painting. It is the sense of safety, love and support from him that gives me the grounding in a positive relationship that I need in order to explore my life and grow both personally and professionally as an artist and an art therapist. Without this man in my life, I could not be the creative person I am.

WHAT INHIBITED IT?

The inhibitors are work schedules, workload, deadlines, and meetings. To put it simply, I get overwhelmed by the lack of enough time to do it all. Is there enough time to do my work as well as schedule time for my own self-care? It is the same question I posed to myself when I started in this field of art therapy: How do I maintain a balance with my work and my own self-care so that I do not get burned out? I still struggle with this balance.

DO YOU HAVE ANY PERSONAL PRACTICES THAT YOU THINK SUPPORT YOUR CREATIVITY OR WORLDVIEWS?

I do have many personal practices that support my creativity: specifically, they are daily journaling and exercise. My daily journaling includes journaling my nightly dreams. I often use the dream series in my daily journaling in support of my process.

At times I go beyond the use of verbal discourse in my daily journal and employ the use of a creative journal. The creative journal employs art as a tool for personal growth to express feelings and thoughts, to sort out life experiences, and to deal with creative blocks and negative patterns (Capacchione, 1989). I keep the creative journal open and ready to be worked on in my studio space in the basement. I often use it to make collages, create watercolors, and even poems.

How Has the Experience Influenced Your Current Creativity?

This question is like asking me why I became an art therapist. I became an art therapist because art therapy works. It worked for me. The experience of remembering my dreams, journaling my dreams, and then drawing or painting my dreams keeps me tapped into my own creative process. I dream; I journal; and I paint to be alive. For example, my individuation process of change and transition continues today as I describe in the dream series in the following paragraphs and in the drawing titled "Struggle" that I created years ago (22 x 28" Charcoal, pastels, mix media, 1999).

In the first dream, I am in a life-drawing class. My family, four of them, joins me for the exercise as my instructor arrives. She puts her head through the door to say hello to me as I eat with my family at a picnic table, and then she continues her activities with a throng of her people. When she returns, I introduce her to my family, which includes two sisters, my mom, and dad. My instructor has them gather around her so she can explain the lesson for tomorrow. They will have a head start on the others by getting the explanation today. My family seems to be interested in the drawing activity.

In another dream I am again in art class, and my instructor is going over instructions. She hands out large pieces of tapestry and finished paintings because she wants us to do similar things. She realizes she has not given us the painting materials to work with and then she realizes that I am confused by her assignment. She tries to explain in better detail.

In the third dream it is a dark Friday evening. I make my way to the regular life drawing session at the art school. When I need to get my drawing board out of the office, I am asked if I have ever been here before. "Yes, once about three years ago," I respond. The nude female model sits in poor light on the front porch. I want to draw her like my colleague does, but I can hardly see the model. She keeps moving even though she said she would pose for five minutes. I cannot see. Now there are tree limbs in my way.

In the fourth dream, I prepare to leave for art class, but I would like to go to Canada for dinner first. My cousin asks me if I want to join them on their trip to Canada this afternoon. "Are you staying for dinner?" I inquire. Since the answer is no, I would rather not go. They plan to return around 6:30 pm without eating. If I were not going to get dinner, I would rather remain and go to my art class at 7:00 pm. After my art instructor brings some new plants and flowers to the studio, and she asks if some of the new ones are mine. I see some beautiful ,exotic plants that I do not recognize, but I know they will need to be replanted and watered or they will die. They do not belong to me, but I can help her.

In the final dream I find myself in my instructor's last art class. Again the life-drawing model sits in the dark. She is clothed and sitting up. When I draw my picture, I pick up vine charcoal for my last gesture in the last class. My instructor looks at me and tells me, "It's over."

At the time of the dream series and when the drawing, "Struggle," was produced, I was "struggling" to finish up my work obligations at the company where I worked so I could return to graduate school to become an art therapist. I was in a life drawing art class, with an instructor whom I dreamt about frequently. I really enjoyed the class, which not only gave me an opportunity to develop my art skills, but also provided balance to my corporate world responsibilities. In addition, the instructor provided a safe, challenging art studio environment to encourage creativity. The third dream in the dream series pointed to my need for safety, free from criticism in the art class in order for me to develop myself artistically and creatively.

The "beautiful exotic plants," that I did not recognize in the fourth dream, I interpret as my own potential that I have yet to tap. Because I knew in the dream that the plants needed "to be replanted and watered or they will die," I know I need to nurture this artistic side of myself with art endeavors such as drawing, painting, and sculpture or I will "perish," so to speak. These art endeavors are important for my soul. The fourth dream also focused on my need for actual food, i.e. dinner, to nurture myself. The dream theme for the series is that I have a need to nurture myself creatively or I will die.

The last art class in the final dream corresponded to the final class, and it was at the same time that I left the corporation. As the instructor said in the dream, "It's over," I knew I would have to deal with the process of letting go. The dreams pointed me in the direction to let go of my identity as the scientist in the corporation and embrace this new direction as an artist and an art therapist. At that time, I needed to nurture and grow into my new identity as an artist and an art therapist. I still need to pay attention to my dream series, draw and paint them, and allow myself the time and space to be creative in order to continue to grow as an artist and an art therapist. I still need to do this to be in tune with my creative being and to be in tune with my creative process.

DESCRIBE YOUR EXPERIENCE WITH CREATING...IS IT A STEADY PROCESS? EPISODIC? MANIC? DROUGHT? DOES IT FEEL LIKE IT COMES FROM "YOU" OR ELSEWHERE?

I love to be in the process of creating—to be in the flow, to be in that moment when time stands still, to create. Yes, to be in the process of creating is a steady process, once I am in it. Yet, there are times when I feel as if I am in a drought to find the time, the place, and the energy to be in this flow. Yes, when I am in the creative process, the energy comes from elsewhere but also from within. Jung would call this tapping into the collective unconscious via the personal unconscious.

The process-painting workshop experience is an experience I use to get in touch with my creative process (Cassou & Cubley, 1995). A safe environment to paint creatively without judgment, comparison, or criticism is offered. Flattery and praise can be as destructive to creativity as criticism, therefore they are not allowed. Anything goes. I listen to my inner critic and tell him/her to shut up.

The process in the workshop starts with a 24-color palette of tempera paints, a blank white sheet of paper, and a comment from a facilitator, "If you had a color what would you use?"

I then give myself permission to play, and I open myself to the moment.

When facing the white void of the paper, I simply paint. When in doubt, I paint dots, as long as I keep my brush moving (Cassou & Cubley, 1995).

Another facilitator says, "What would you not want to paint? Now paint it."

"If you want to paint an ugly picture, paint an ugly picture," another facilitator says. I note more permission to proceed with my process. I note other comments that help my process as I paint; comments like:

"Proportions do not matter!"

"If you think you are done with the painting, you are not."

"What do you feel? Take the feeling from your gut and your heart and put them on the paper."

"Do not interpret the picture."

"Do not focus on the end result."

The process—there is always a moment in every painting where I get stuck. It is in these difficult moments that I keep painting. I know it is important to keep my brush moving because I am tapping into something new deep within me (Cassou & Cubley, 1995).

"Don't worry about ruining the picture," I am told.

"If you had a color to add, what would it be? Now paint it."

I begin the process based on the dream I call "The Scream." In the dream, the huge gorilla has returned. This demanding gorilla devours the other gorillas and they land in her gut. I watch this horrifying process. I need to get away from this gorilla, and there is a train coming. The gorilla and other family members await. Will I be able to get on the train?

The dream continues with the elevator door that opens and becomes an opening to the train. "Don't mess with the moving train car!" I scream at my young friend Stan but he is playing with little Renée. The two are engrossed with each other's company and oblivious of me.

At this same time, a dancing competition is about to start. Irish dancers are all in line, ready to begin their performance. They resemble cattle being taken to market. I recognize Stan and his little sister, Lucy, in the line, and I want to watch those two perform. I take a seat.

Stan's sister's girlfriend dances her hard shoe dance. She is wonderful. Her shuffles are so fined tuned, quick, and precise. She dances right over my head as I watch from the pit. When she is done she is relieved. She dances only so that she can hang around Lucy. The two are the best of friends, and one now is ready to go off to college; but it is not Lucy. Lucy hugs her when she is done. She did a spectacular performance for someone who is not very interested in the dancing activity. The next dancer is about ready to begin and she carries two wasps over to the stage. She must dance with the wasps. Lucy's friend did too, although I had not noticed the wasps when she danced. The girl carries the two wasps to me. "They are very aggressive towards one another," she comments as she brings them closer to my nose. I do not want anything to do with them. I run into my friend but she ignores my presence. She is upset with all these people around, because she feels these people are invading her space. The dream ends at mom and dad's house where the quintuplets play - three girls and two boys. The babies are about one year old. Will they notice my presence, I wonder? "How does one take care of all these babies?" I wonder aloud. I am mesmerized as I watch them all play. Each child seems engrossed in its own world.

I paint this night's dream, "The Scream." I paint the dream that has the dancers, the wasps, the babies, my friend, the music, and the noise. I pick the ugly colors that I do not like

- pink and baby blue. I paint with the pink and baby blue, and now I add grey and purple. I never use these colors but I am using them now. "Bomb bomb bomb bomb," I hear the noise in my head as I paint. "Bomb bomb bomb bomb." The dream. The song. The scream. "Shut Up!" I scream in my head as I paint. The music. How do I paint SHUT UP? I do not want to write out the words. I paint the female figure. The female figure covers up the rest of the picture, the dream. The words need to be screaming from her mouth. The song. The music. The dream. The noise of the children yelling. How do I paint SHUT UP? How do I stop the noise in my head? "Bomb bomb bomb bomb." When will I be done? The process. "Shut up ... SHUT UP.... STOOOOPPPP ITTTTTT!!!!" Yellow, white, and finally RED streaming out of her mouth. I paint yellow, white, and finally red. RED IS SHUT UP! I paint red. The noise is gone in my head. I am done. Silence.

When the painting is really finished, Cassou and Cubley (1995) say that there is a very precise and deep feeling of satisfaction, whatever the painting looks like. I feel that satisfaction. This is my process. I have no plans. I just paint. I paint a line, a dot, or a shape.

HOW DO YOU NURTURE OR NURSE FLEDGLING IDEAS?

To nurture my fledging ideas, I continue with my daily practices of journaling and exercise. In addition to the journaling of dreams, the journal provides a space to brainstorm. I also use the approach described by Julia Cameron in *The Artist's Way* (2002). She describes a 12-week journey of ideas, activities, and challenges, which can jumpstart anyone's creative process. I have used her 12-week process on at least five different occasions to jumpstart myself, especially when I have been feeling stuck and in need of nursing fledging ideas.

My exercise routine also helps in this process. I thrive when I can feel my body running along the Erie Canal as the sun rises. To get outside no matter what time of year and be one with nature is also fuel for my soul. I get many ideas and let my mind wander as I run. I then return home to journal with a good cup of coffee at the kitchen table.

WHAT ROLES DOES/DID YOUR COMMUNITY/COLLEAGUES PLAY IN YOUR CREATIVE EXPERIENCE?

The biggest role my colleagues play in my creative experience is that in the field of art therapy, creativity is valued and artistic expression is expected. Because creativity is valued and artistic expression expected, people do allow their colleagues time and space for such expression when requested. For example, taking sabbatical time can be a great opportunity to focus on such endeavors. Also taking time out for process-painting experiential workshops is supported.

WHAT WOULD YOU DO DIFFERENTLY?

I think I am ready to engage in another 12-week *The Artist's Way* experience as defined by Cameron (2002). I feel blocked now. I need to make time to balance my workload, and I need to make time to be creative. What I would do differently overall is to schedule more creative time for myself on a regular basis. This is easier said than done.

WHAT'S NEXT?

On a daily basis, I continue journaling and exercise. To keep the momentum going regarding my actual process painting, in the next six weeks I am scheduled to attend an eight-day process-painting workshop in Taos, New Mexico.

WORDS OF WISDOM/INSPIRATION?

For me, my dreams are my best and most creative time of day. Remembering my dreams and journaling them are the most important sources of creativity to me. I create to connect with myself. I create to feel alive. I am grateful to be alive. My philosophy on life is as a chemist August Kékulé said, "Let us dream, gentleman, perhaps then we can learn the truth." I dream. I journal. I paint. I live.

REFERENCES

Cameron, J. (2002). *The artist's way: A spiritual path to higher creativity (10th ed.).* New York: Tarcher.

Capacchione, L. (1989). *The creative journal: The art of finding yourself.* North Hollywood, CA: Newcastle Publishing Co.

Cassou, M., & Cubley, S. (1995). *Life, paint and passion—Reclaiming the magic of spontaneous expression.* New York: Jeremy Tarcher / Putman Book, G.P. Putman and Sons.

Gold, A. (1998). *Painting from the source.* New York: Harper Collins Books.

Hall, J. A. (1983). *Jungian dream interpretation: A handbook of theory and practice.* Toronto, Canada: Inner City Books.

Hall, J. A. (1986). *The Jungian experience: Analysis and individuation.* Toronto, Canada: Inner City Books.

McNiff, S. (1992). *Art as medicine. Creating a therapy of the imagination.* Boston: Shambhala.

Sharp, D. (1998). *Jungian Psychology unplugged: My life as an elephant.* Toronto, Canada: Inner City Books.

In: Fostering Creativity in Rehabilitation
Editor: Matthew J. Taylor

ISBN: 978-1-63485-118-3
© 2016 Nova Science Publishers, Inc.

Chapter 16

RECREATIONAL THERAPY

Marieke Van Puymbroeck, PhD, CTRS, FDRT

Associate Professor,
Recreational Therapy Coordinator Clemson University, Clemson, SC, US

"We cannot solve our problems with the same thinking
we used when we created them."

–Albert Einstein

Recreational therapists use leisure and recreation to improve function and well-being in individuals with disease and disability. Our treatment goals focus not only on enhancing functional skills, but also include assisting the individual in getting back to active participation in enjoyable roles in his or her life. Our society often views free-time, leisure, and recreation as secondary or even superfluous to "more important" tasks. This can make treatment challenging, and may also lead to other health professionals not valuing the contribution of recreational therapy. Prior to engaging in treatment with recreational therapists, some patients also tell us that they don't need to have fun, they need to get better. Although after engaging in recreational therapy the patients understand that functional improvement can be enjoyable, these are the types of pervasive negative societal attitudes about recreation and leisure that need to be changed. In the United States, we tend to value work over enjoyment, financial success over happiness, and material status over well-being. Bhutan, a country with a Gross National Happiness index (instead of the Gross National Product), incorporates song and dance into every major local or national event. In the 2013 rankings of quality of life by country, the United States ranked 17, after countries that have mandatory and/or long vacations available to their citizens. It is time in the United States that we recognize the positive impact that recreation and leisure can have on the health of an individual and society. Taking time to re-create, or recreate, is essential to learning, to creativity, and to improved health and quality of life.

That being said, there are many health professionals who support, recommend, and advocate for recreational therapy services at their place of work. These peers know that when delivered with passion and creativity, recreational therapy has the potential to enhance function, well-being and quality of life for our patients and their families. It is not only in my work where free-time, recreation and leisure is important, but it is through my recreation and leisure time pursuits that I am able to tap into my creativity.

While I loved working in clinical practice, I decided to go back to graduate school to pursue degrees that would allow me to teach students. My intent was two-fold: I was working in a rural area of the country that, at that time at least, did not value advanced academic degrees for women. The thinking was that work was a place for women only until they found a good husband and started having children. This environment was stifling, and I knew I needed to find a path to counter those views. Also, while I knew my work was making a big difference in my patients' lives, I felt that I could have greater impact if I could teach people how to be good therapists, so the ripple effect that my experiences could create would be much more than if I remained as a therapist. After about 10 years in clinical practice, I received my Ph.D. in rehabilitation science and became an educator of recreational therapy, with a dual focus on research and teaching. When I started my first academic position, I struggled to become an autonomous researcher and teacher. After 5 years of working primarily on bringing others' ideas to fruition, it was time to determine my own path. I was literally aching with a need for grounding, growth, and creativity, but I did not know how or where to begin. Having given up many leisure activities during my graduate school years, I decided to enroll in a yoga class. In downward dog during my first yoga class, I felt a flash of insight (or creativity?) that yoga may be both a personal and professional path to pursue. I felt so much different, better, and expanded (physically and mentally) after that class that I started to explore the possibilities of researching yoga as a therapeutic tool to improve function and well-being.

Studying yoga, both professionally and personally, has helped me to sow seeds of creativity. The space that yoga creates in my heart and head allows me to think differently about opportunities or challenges. I love the above quote by Albert Einstein because I have realized this same sentiment often, by hitting roadblocks in problem-solving by attempting to use the same path in which the obstacle was created. By considering different, non-traditional and more experiential learning approaches, I believe that my teaching has also improved. I have actively sought to help my students find the passion in their chosen field by seeking creative ways to teach content. For example, I teach a broad medical terminology class to students. This content can be superbly dry and hard to get through, so I often incorporate movement and/or song into teaching the words, particularly the difficult words. You can imagine that my undergraduates are often reticent to start moving around or raising their voice in the classroom, but just like the YMCA song that has associated movements, we do similar things for words like homonymous hemianopsia and anhedonia. Once the students start moving and singing, they really appreciate the kinesthetic incorporation into learning. I believe that incorporating creativity into the classroom has been one of the best inspirations I've had, and happily, my teaching evaluations support that.

It has been my experience that creativity is not a steady stream of inspiration and novelty. In fact, creativity is an episodic process for me. It is easy for me to get caught up in doing what I've always done. During these times, my tasks and duties are not teeming with creativity. In fact, these periods can be an impediment to creativity. I often have to make a conscientious effort to think differently about the opportunity or task at hand. When I'm really stumped, bored, or challenged, I find that seeking inspiration is really important. In addition to yoga, I do this by visiting the local botanical garden or even walking around neighborhoods to admire other's gardens. For me, there is something really creative that happens by spending time in gardens that I often can translate to other ideas. I'm not sure if it is seeing how gardeners challenge the norms by choosing unusual groupings or unusual plants, but these walks often help me consider things differently. This process is often similar to marinating food for a delicious meal. I like to think about an issue or opportunity and let it marinate for a while. The best opportunities for creativity and growth come when I am marinating an idea by letting the idea take a back seat in my mind, and explore outdoor, natural areas or through yoga practice. Often, ideas float to the surface during, or shortly after these experiences.

I once went to a talk for junior researchers by a really well-respected and well-funded aging researcher. As he was discussing his team's approach to developing new ideas and plans, he said, "My best ideas are margarita-laced." My best friend is also my closest research collaborator, and we have taken those words to heart! Aside from the obvious benefits from drinking a margarita together, other activities implicit in this experience are that they occur during free-time and are often in a low to non-stressful environment. Although we are now thousands of miles away, and our visits are unfortunately far between, we FaceTime every 1-2 weeks so that we can maintain our close friendship, and these meetings are so lovely because all we need is an internet connection to make it happen! Coupled with spending time with a valued colleague and friend, these "meetings" have certainly helped to facilitate a broader approach to thinking about opportunities.

If I were to do something differently, it would likely be to reduce the number of tasks that I say "yes" to. Feeling stressed and overwhelmed certainly limits my creativity. I moved to a new state a year ago, and am still working to get my life ordered in such a way that creativity can thrive! As a type 'A' personality, it is important for me to feel order prior to tapping into much creativity. I have started tending my new garden, and this has opened my mind and ideas to bringing creativity to my new home. This has also opened new avenues when thinking about my work. There is something so therapeutic about having my hands in the dirt, weeding and creating new beautiful spaces, that during this time while I am so focused on the tasks at hand, it seems that my mind opens to new opportunities. The concept of *flow*, first described by Mihaly Csikszentmihalyi, describes this experience: it is when an individual is so ensconced in an activity, with abounding feelings of joy, focus, and energy, that all else is secondary at the time. I believe that it is in these flow states (which, incidentally can occur in any recreation or leisure activity) that the mind is broadened to allow for other opportunities and ideas to flourish.

Much of my creativity flourishes during, or is enhanced by, my free-time and recreation/leisure pursuits. I enjoy the process often as much as the product, and feel my best when my creativity is flowing. I believe that there are many areas that health care could be enhanced by increased creativity. I'm inspired by the other chapters in this book, and look forward to continued discussions in this area. I hope that my colleagues in recreational therapy and other allied health disciplines can work together to think outside the typical medical model box, and explore new, collaborative, and creative ways to provide creative, person-centered health care. The practices in Part IV of this book may be a good place for all of us to start.

In: Fostering Creativity in Rehabilitation
Editor: Matthew J. Taylor

ISBN: 978-1-63485-118-3
© 2016 Nova Science Publishers, Inc.

Chapter 17

MUSIC THERAPY

Robin Rio MA, MT-BC

Associate Professor, Music Therapy
Arizona State University, Tempe AZ, US

INTRODUCTION

Music therapy is the intentional use of music, sounds, words and movement, facilitated by a credentialed music therapist (MT), to bring about desired change in a person or group of people with an ultimate goal or goals in mind. It is a discipline that combines the clinical approaches of the social sciences with the art form of creative music experiences, within the context of the healing relationship. One of my favorite definitions is written by Kenneth Bruscia, *Music therapy is a systematic process of intervention wherein the therapist helps the client to promote health, using music experiences and the relationships that develop through them as dynamic forces of change.* (1989, pg. 20). Much of my clinical work has been in dementia and end of life care.

At the very beginning of my music therapy career, I had the privilege of helping a child with a developmental delay say his first word, "blue"! I wrote a song for the child, "What is the Name of this Color?" The tune was simple, and I left a noticeable pause (musical prompt) where there was a space for the child to fill in the answer. And he did fill in the answer! Not right away, and I'm sure many, many others contributed to the skill building he needed to reach the point where he *could* speak the answer, but I had the honor of being the therapist who was present at the right moment to elicit the response, using a creative problem-solving technique. This individualized, simple song had helped a young child to achieve a very important goal. This was a first in the many rewarding moments that would inspire and teach me, through experience, how to be a music therapist.

WHAT CHALLENGES AND OPPORTUNITIES ARE SPECIFIC TO YOUR PROFESSION?

Challenges and opportunities in music therapy abound. Challenges faced earlier in one's career can be academic and music-performance obstacles. Gaining entrance into a bachelor's program in music usually requires an audition in addition to the typical standardized test scores, high school grades and essays. The applicant auditions on his or her main instrument, which can be an orchestral instrument, voice, or anything that requires formal (and usually classical) training. Professional music therapists need to "diversify" their talents, so that they are able to sing, play guitar, and play piano/keyboard and represent a variety of styles, as well as improvise and write songs.

After professional training, challenges for music therapists are similar to those with colleagues in related disciplines, with a common concern being funding. Hospitals, schools and arts businesses experienced many cuts during the recent recession, and music therapy, just like our close relatives in music education and therapeutic recreation, were often the first to be cut. Medical insurance pays for some music therapy services, but as of yet, it is not the norm.

Fortunately, the opportunities in music therapy are endless, and I believe it's the creativity of the therapists that have allowed for the proliferation of music therapy within so many diverse settings. Often there are more available jobs than can be filled, and there are enough opportunities available so that a music therapist may use his or her particular strengths. Many MT's, particularly pioneers from the first years of the profession in the 1950's-1980's, needed to create positions or departments where none existed. Some looked for positions within organized structures, such as Veteran's Affairs medical centers and large residential psychiatric facilities, aligning with medical staff, psychiatric professionals, social workers and other rehab therapists already within the system. Others created new paths, such as in wellness and community building. Today, there are many opportunities available as private practice, neurologic music therapy and hospice music therapy programs are growing rapidly. Specializations in Guided Imagery and Music, Neonatal ICU Music Therapy and other approaches provide trainings and certifications specific to therapists' interests.

WHAT DID/ARE YOU DO/DOING?

My work was first clinical, and now is primarily educating music therapists in the university and clinical setting. The first skilled nursing facility I worked in strengthened my understanding of the care team. Supporting spiritual connections among clients, honoring their unique religious history and traditions, and finding friendship and collegiality from the diverse departments in the care team expanded my views on professional roles and responsibilities, truly informing the holistic nature of music therapy. I worked closely with art therapists and therapeutic recreation specialists to provide combined art and music programs, and saw how individuals responded dramatically to these experiences. I then learned what it was like to start at ground level when I moved to a new center for extended care and rehabilitation. The staff of nursing, social work, rehab, therapeutic recreation and medical staff bonded over that first year of opening. Nursing personnel might come with me, singing or talking with residents, encouraging them to make a sound on a percussion instrument, to ask for a song of choice, or to introduce me to a person who was not responding to any other treatments. One dramatic encounter was with a resident who was in a coma. He had been lying in bed for weeks, receiving personal care, family visits and sensory stimulation. I sang with him, playing guitar at his bedside. After weeks of no response, he began to moan and yell. Later words came out- yelling in pain and confusion. His lurching movements seemed aggressive, but they weren't. My small caseload made it easy to provide music therapy daily or every other day. Further along he began recovering volitional movement and coherency, he regained his ability to talk, opened his eyes, and eventually sat up purposefully and ultimately returned home. He remembered hearing the music when he was transitioning from unresponsiveness to a very painful awareness. He said, "How could you keep coming back, when I was yelling like that?" After relying on encouragement from the care team and blind faith, I was amazed and grateful to learn that he could hear even though he couldn't respond…a truly miraculous feeling for me.

I returned to school in a powerful program that honored self-reflection and introspection and "back to the source" experiential learning. There I was introduced to clinical improvisation. At my workplace, I started an internship program with students from two universities, and interacted with other local music therapists who supported and challenged me. My understanding of psychology bloomed, more creative uses of music were discovered as my formal education focused on improvisation, group dynamics, and music psychotherapy.

Following ten years of clinical experience and four years of part time teaching at community college, entering a position as an assistant professor seemed like the natural progression. There I learned what creativity is in the academic setting without having a full clinical caseload. I was excited about being the director of the university music therapy clinic, and found that applied and descriptive research were most suited to my abilities and interests. Academic creativity is different than clinical creativity. Creating songs, assignments, and structures for college students requires a separate skill set, but can be grounded in being a therapist, just as research and creative activity outside the classroom can be grounded in clinical work.

Here I share opportunities with my students that I found most helpful in my learning. I've continued developing my own peer group with professional music therapists, and collaborated with a colleague to birth a new program called *Strength Based Improvisation* (SBI). The SBI training is a three-day intensive where therapists improvise music, using individual, musical and interpersonal strengths and support of peer group members. Each person is supported in composing and playing their personal music life-story. Through sharing these important life stories, therapists are able to nurture their own creativity and expand their version of what it is to use improvisation in therapy and in life.

WHERE DID YOUR IDEAS/DESIRE COME FROM?

My ideas and desires have primarily come from seeing a *need*. There are so many needs in the world: need for peace, need for wholeness, need to connect with others, the need to be heard. There is the need to be a part of something bigger than oneself: a team, a special event, a community.

My desire is partly innate- I have this capacity to care and to transform. Occasionally I become a bit zealous- and want to share this with others. My desire to be a helper rather than a "help-ee" has to do with feeling a sense of having enough, or being a leader, and sometimes my desire to be in control. This common desire for control or structure in our lives doesn't match what we may see or be "born into" especially when personal freedom is missing. My desires are a balancing act, finding freedom within structure and also security within the changes inherent in the creative process.

My upbringing fuels my desire to be of service with music. It is a sustaining process rooted in seeing the pride my mom took whenever she told someone that she was a nurse and the example of my dad being a "fixer" and problem solver. Music throughout my upbringing helped me connect with my family members through singing sacred and secular music, connecting with friends in school, and later on, colleagues and my own students.

WHAT SUPPORTED YOUR PROCESS?

My limitations initially gave me the most direction. Turning from what I didn't excel at doing, I did see myself as being good at singing and being with people. The repetition and structure found in music and performance ensembles supported my process. I would sing and play the same things over and over until they sounded pleasing, practicing what I enjoyed with others who also en*joy*ed the music. A tremendous support in my process as a musician has been this focus on joy, finding joy and exploring it, which is taken seriously by musicians and beloved composers and authors. Collaboration supports my process. The support of mentors, of family, of seminars, attending and participating in conferences; of the special moments and events, like seeing tone chimes played by beautifully by children with disabilities, supported by music therapy pioneers Clive and Carol Robbins, founders of Nordoff-Robbins Music Therapy. Staying connected to music in all the phases of my life, from marching band playing tuba, then percussion, and learning piano and guitar. Listening to the rich harmonies of Crosby Stills and Nash, the unique female perspectives of Joni Mitchell. Attending concerts given by folk music activists Pete Seeger and Arlo Guthrie where the whole crowd sang along. In college, being in a huge choir performance with soloists and orchestras, singing Beethoven's Ninth Symphony, which includes "Ode to Joy". By living my depths of emotion in the music I am supported. I find joy in the darkest moments that can lead to triumph and redemption discovering the beauty of all of humanity being magnified in the drama and sensory experience of living in the music.

I was particularly supported at a retreat for our chanting group, *Daughters of Harriet*. As equals, we used music and improvising to relax, connect and go inward, with the intention of articulating our personal mission and mission for our chant group. During this creative music making process I realized that as a group we had "it." Being able to recognize and trust that I know what "it" is has come from experience and repetition. Translating my inner world through music to my outer world, in relationship with others, supports process. Finally, my interactions with students and interns have been enormously inspiring. Their insights, compassion and determination support my process every day.

WHAT INHIBITED IT?

My biggest inhibitor has been a lack of confidence. This inhibition may be partially due to the lack of support for women in leadership roles while growing up. As a woman I have noticed that today we are much more aware of the stigma young women feel when labeled "bossy" and have made many moves to rectify the imbalance of power for women. Having no mentor at key growing points in my life, I felt inhibited from developing or expressing my opinion. I suspect grounded in the fear of being wrong this whole idea of being perfect, being the best, or being in a competition where only the top achievers win, inhibited the trial and error needed for invention.

Music therapy is a fledgling profession that is both artsy and scientific, which can lead me to sometimes feel as if I'm an outsider in both the fine arts world *and* in the world of science. As an outsider in the world of professional music performers, I often get a "pat on the head-isn't that sweet" condescending attitude; music performers are given a lot of credence in our culture. Sometimes I have felt that my work is not taken seriously, so I've gone overboard by being super "professional" (whatever that means) and risked my exceptional talent of combining music-one of the most powerful and sacred capacities we have to offer another- being lost by lack of musicality in the gain of intellectual-only, polished and business-like pursuits.

Finally, aggressive actions by others tend to inhibit me. Whether it's yelling, posturing, being rude, demeaning the profession or ideas, it took me a long time to learn how to push back. I have learned from other kind scholars who are used to argumentative discourse not as malice, but an opportunity to present a position. Finding allies in all professions, not just my own, greatly combats these inhibitions.

DO YOU HAVE ANY PERSONAL PRACTICES THAT YOU THINK SUPPORT YOUR CREATIVITY OR WORLD VIEWS?

My involvement in a variety of spiritual, therapeutic, artistic and music practices support my creativity and worldview. This provides me a healthier mind and body, and connects me with others who are also on a spiritual path of creativity with relationship as its center. Organized religion with its' own traditions and rituals and awe-inspiring music has been a support, too.

My performance and guest artist schedule helps me stay in touch with the artistry in music and the newness of other disciplines. Yoga and chanting with students, clients and the *Daughters of Harriet* facilitation group have had a big impact on connecting mind and body for wellness. Other music therapists who improvise and sing chants as part of a mindfulness practice has supported my song writing and relationships, and apprised me of the modern peace movement and use of music in social justice. Staying as politically active as possible, through voting and attending grass roots political meetings (Valley Interfaith Project.), shapes my worldview and how to negotiate with legislators for desperately needed changes in education and healthcare. Setting boundaries on family time and work for work-life balance and time for myself is a challenging but a crucial and rewarding daily practice. The self-care of regular exercise with my "exercise buddy" and a good night's sleep are other key personal practices.

How Has the Experience Influenced Your Current Creativity?

My confidence has improved with experience and age, reducing my need for reassurance and acceptance from others, as I know and trust myself better now. Repetition is how I have come to notice patterns, and through patterns and familiarity come stability and security, with which to try new things, improvise, and take risks. Experience has allowed me to relax into who I am and repeat the processes that work. Once I established myself and put my work "out there" to the world, people have liked my ideas and approached me. I create with these like-minded people, and we influence each other from a place of admiration, and then through the alike-ness, share the differences that make us more creative.

If I repeat a processes that doesn't work or make a mistake multiple times, I am gentle with myself and remember the times things went well. I try to treat myself the same way I would a client or a friend: with compassion and affirming feedback, and gentle support when something isn't working. Listening openly without judgment can keep open the lines of communication with my creative self. I lighten up when I am being too harsh, realizing I have some control over how I talk to myself as my own coach.

I've learned to recognize when I am suggesting or directing an intervention in a way that allows the client to be as independent and in charge as much as possible. As with myself, their own experiences can help guide them, and I can fill the role of supportive and trusting team member, allowing as much self-direction in their recovery as possible.

Describe Your Experience with Creating...is It a Steady Process? Episodic? Manic? Drought? Does it Feel Like it Comes From "You" or Elsewhere?

Creating is an ongoing process that moves in spirals over time. As I develop my music therapy practice and writing voice, I circle back to original beliefs and ideas, coming around the spiral to interact and learn new ways, back again to the familiar and traditional, setting out on a new spiral, with the new direction remaining connected to it's past. When I create, it's often in some kind of an interactive human experience. In addition to the spiral, it is a going back and forth between people and places, inner world and outer world, like a wandering garden that journeys but always leads home. It is that ever circling back to the source that seems to work best for me.

My creativity is most flowing when it seems to come from a higher power or the collective of all humankind. Fully immersed in creating, I am unaware of time and in what I call an "alternate state of consciousness." Still aware of where I am and who I am, but more connected to my inner self. I also enjoy creating with a small group of trusted "creatives" who are in the same state. Together we are connected to a larger source greater than ourselves. It is not unconscious, but connected consciousness. These "peak experiences" cause me to feel very open and ideas and music come easily.

Sound and relationships develop and evolve without a set structure when time and safe space are set for creativity. Something always evolves from this void and lack of structure, even if only that "stuck" space. But the stuck space is a reminder that the creative process isn't always easy and accessible, and even in the stuck space we learn. It gives me something to measure the peak experience against, and from which a new song or relationship can emerge, and enhancing empathy for the individual who may be stuck.

I share this approach to nurturing creativity by "holding the space" for students or clients to create, allowing time to experience the void, the chaos, and sometimes, the catharsis that comes from creating that original act together, be it words, movement, musical sound, or something unexpected. I trust my skills to take over, with no real need for conscious connection to intellect. When I know that thing so well I don't need a leader or a teacher, I can let go the same way a young child dances. By repeating the scenarios that open me up to process, working with that scary empty space or that cluttered distracted place, and repeating the mantras and rhythms of my genuine inner voice, I can reach outward to the collective of "kindred spirits" to share in this divine sourcing. When I've been open, I find my soul mates on the path to the self, mirrored in my search for true community.

HOW DO YOU NURTURE OR NURSE FLEDGLING IDEAS?

Giving time and patience to develop ideas is important. Writing down and audio recording help me to remember the ideas as they are developing, and then sharing them with a trusted friend or colleague makes them real. It usually takes me three to four times longer to complete something than I initially expect. When it comes to writing or making a recording, it may take even longer, because there is that sense of finality that once it is in print or recorded and pressed, it can't be changed.

Sometimes knowing the end result at the beginning of the process and having a "big picture" can be helpful. With the end goal in mind, I break it down into steps. Nursing an infant is a fine analogy, because while nursing should be natural and easy, in actuality it may not be simple at all, depending on the circumstances. My first daughter was premature and didn't know how to nurse, and as my first child, I didn't know how to nurse her and only had the "big picture" view of nursing. A lactation specialist showed me how the process really was a series of baby steps and with calm reassurance from this person who had a lot of experience, paired with a lot of repetition, trial and error, I was finally able to nurse my infant. I also need a certain amount of privacy, for just like a new idea, you may not want to open it to criticism from the world. I shut out the intrusion of naysayers, "you will need to give her formula- she's too small!" and persevere, listening to the wisdom of the lactation specialist by my side. Once competent in nursing, I was able to take the criticism of those who didn't agree or were embarrassed, and was free to be myself.

Conference presentations and writing opportunities and having an expectation to publish all nurse new ideas, despite their extrinsic nature. Without a deadline I tend to put things off. I also find it helpful to share my ideas with people who know very little about my topic but who like me as a person. These people are often more supportive and don't have any hidden agendas. I have had to ask for help from people to edit my work or with a new form of research, or to support my learning a new technology or regain motivation.

Reading what others have written on a similar idea and listening to their talks or music has also spurred my beginning ideas to maturity. *Free Play: Improvisation in Art and Life* by Stephen Nachmonovitch (1990), and *The Mythic Artery* by Carolyn Kenny (1982) are both books that provided me with deep inspiration and passion. Hearing the true stories from a patient, for example, the recovery of Jason Crigler (2013), inspires me to try harder, knowing that there is always hope.

WHAT ROLES DOES/DID YOUR COMMUNITY/COLLEAGUES PLAY IN YOUR CREATIVE EXPERIENCE?

The greatest discovery gifted to me from my community has been learning improvisation, which is creating in the moment. I needed to improvise over and over to feel comfortable, as do many of my colleagues. I first learned about improvisation from jazz musicians, but later learned that clinical improvisation in music therapy is quite different from jazz.

I started leading improvisation groups after learning how to improvise with a small group of peers in graduate school for a class, and my community was a big part of this experience. I brought clinical improvisation to my older, highly musical nursing home clients who had severe memory loss and cognitive delays. Modifying the approach with the group dynamics in play and the musical and environmental structure, the residents in the long-term care facility were able to benefit from the group improvisation. (Rio, 2002).

In my earlier years as a university professor, I found some of the greatest creative support through the camaraderie and structure of *playback theater*. Essential Theater (Southard, 2014) uses improvised drama, taking the stories of the audience and in the moment, "playing back" and dramatically and symbolically reenacting the story through sound, words and movement. I learned the approach with other actors and musicians, and was the only music therapist. Some of the audience members from our community had disabilities, while others were homeless; some were refugees, and we also led workshops with juvenile offenders. In this improvisational theater, we tried what we were afraid to try, developing trusting bonds with the members of the troupe, very much like the therapy process.

Through active mentoring and giving me space, the director of the music therapy program at ASU "protected me" and supported me throughout the tenure process. She gave me suggestions and basically stayed out of my way, writing letters of support, finding others from her vast experience within the academic network to write letters on my behalf. Music therapy and soulmaking: Toward a new theory of music therapy (Crowe, 2004) was especially inspiring, because my own mentor and program director was taking on new and exciting material, complexity science.

Supporting student and colleague's fledgling ideas also helps me personally and creatively. I am so inspired by the creativity of the university students I mentor, and the professionals with whom I collaborate. I learn so much about how to tackle projects and as a byproduct, gain new insights into my creative process. When others ask me for help, I feel a sense of responsibility and dedication to their work, and become engaged and energetic in their process. Those sparks can ignite work that I am engaged in and shed light on other projects that may at first seem unrelated.

WHAT WOULD YOU DO DIFFERENTLY?

Speak up. Push back. Too many times I have taken longer than I would have liked to share my opinion, and I wish I would have, even when it was unpopular or not grounded in quantitative research. I would write down more client stories, good and bad, sooner so I could remember them. I would procrastinate less on the note writing, and be more creative in how I recorded sessions and time with students, perhaps putting them in a form other than writing.

I feel pretty fortunate that things have gone the way that they have. I have always had an innate desire to discover and to rest, and that back and forth action is what gives me the impetus to continue. Many things have fallen in place for me, and when I was ready to make my next move the opportunity that presented itself could be taken, because I had done the background work to be ready for that next step. I would have learned the *Tennessee Waltz* sooner. A client in long-term care requested the song and I didn't learn it before she died. I have lived with that, but been spurred to remember that I must do it if I say I will, and be careful about what I say I will do.

WHAT'S NEXT?

For me the next step is in the direction of wellness in music therapy, through chant circles and interactive performance, shared outside the therapy rooms as well as in clinical practice and with my university students to reduce stress and build community.

I am excited to complete my audio recording to accompany "Connecting through Music with People with Dementia: A Guide for Caregivers," so that others may use the tools together. I am working with my colleague on developing levels two and three of "Strength-Based Improvisation" training for therapists, and we hope to offer this to other professionals. Continuing formal research in music therapy practices for dementia care is ongoing and embraces multiple disciplines in healthcare and the arts.

WORDS OF WISDOM/INSPIRATION?

Embrace the chaos. Working with other humans is a messy, complicated business. Your theory and practice are the safety net, so that when you take a leap, you don't need to be as worried about falling. In therapy all of the insecurities surface for each party, and the therapist is working from a place of mystery, not knowing a lot about the history and the inner beliefs and workings of the client. Being vulnerable and present with the client can bring you together in the chaos and help you become a unified team.

Try not to be too terribly concerned if others like or approve of what you are doing, or how you are doing it. Often there is no proof for the best way, so don't become too dependent that something has been proven and you must do it one way. "The proof is in the pudding."

Be silly whenever you can. Maybe it means volunteering with kids in a preschool once a month so you can get into a bubble blowing mood, or learning a new game, or going out to hear standup or karaoke, or trying a dance that you really don't know and being OK with looking ridiculous. Don't take it all too seriously. Being silly is a refreshing change to all the problem solving and intensity we encounter in our professional lives.

Take time for yourself and your own creative endeavors. Sometimes we may forget why we were originally drawn to the work. Our culture seems to have become so focused on productivity that there isn't much time in a day to get away from the messages, requests, beeping and sound pollution, and constant input of information, to focus on the inner self and personal development. You know what turns you on creatively, and if you have lost touch or evolved into a new self that is desiring something different or new, take time to discover what that is.

Ask questions and be persistent; notice when there is an unfair practice that you can improve. Why can't we sing at our music therapy meetings? In a workplace I may ask, who do I need to speak to so that I can try this out? A general, more political question: Why are there systems that devalue the traditional roles of women and domestic care-taking needs of those in the home? And a question to ask an institution administrator: How can the individual have more of a voice in this institution? Who is the advocate for the direct care staff? A question for our educational systems and other programs where the majority of the workforce is female and the head of a household: Why isn't there childcare at this school when so many of the teachers have young children? I don't believe we can solve all the systemic dilemmas in institutions, but with our creativity and education, we can be a part of the answers and solutions to questions we ask.

Receive what others have to give. We are notorious for not being able to receive help. It is OK to take back sometimes. The vulnerability of receiving gives us the opportunity to understand how to be helped.

Be aware of what you want and make your desires known. Move in the direction of what you want, be patient, and, you will get results. Once others understand your desires, they may help you to achieve them.

Repetition helps everyone. We need repetition to remember movement and sounds. We need to repeat the most important concepts if we wanted them remembered.

IN CLOSING

As rehab professionals, we help our clients find their deepest connection to health and wellness, encouraging them, providing hope and companionship in the struggle to be whole. Whole does not mean perfect. We need to hold on to the song for the other and for ourselves, in despair and depression, in isolation and fear, just as traditional healers hold the spirit world and present world to help connect the gap between the two spaces of time and energy. We need to keep our own song present, whether it's loud and clear or soft and gentle, and keep the fire burning, smoldering under the embers of our creation, so that when the flame is needed, it can light into action.

In my work with people who have Alzheimer's disease, I realize the impact of my work by being the memory for those who have forgotten or are unable to express themselves. Keep a recorder or video camera or tablet handy for your great moments- they are fleeting and daily work can distract from remembering those moments. Ask yourself, what am I the keeper of? Are you a keeper of the dance? The nourishment? Our song becomes a metaphor for life. The nutritionist becomes the nourisher of the soul. The physical therapist is the nourisher of the body. Such huge responsibilities we are entrusted with! I encourage you to write more poems and dance more dances. Those who want to listen and watch will come to you, and maybe they'll even join you.

> We are the keepers of the song.
> Retrieving memories from the lost and found
> A beacon when you're all alone
> A nightlight when there's no one home
> Keepers of the song.

You may want to substitute other words for the lyrics above. Are you a keeper of the flame? A keeper of the story? I am a keeper of the _____. You fill it in.

REFERENCES

Bruscia, K. (1989). *Defining music therapy* (1st Ed.). Gilsum, NH: Barcelona Publishers.

Crigler, J. & Crigler, M. (2013). *Stroke Recovery: A True Story.* Music Care Conference, University of Toronto, Canada.

Crowe, B. (2004). *Music and soulmaking: Toward a new theory of music therapy.* Lanham, MD: Scarecrowe.

Daughters of Harriet. (2010). *You are a Song.* Audio Recording.

Daughers of Harriet. (2013). *From the Heart.* Audio Recording.

Jackert, L. (2006). Developing my music self-the prelude to strength-based improvisation and the joy of collaboration [contribution to moderated discussions]. Voices: A world forum for music therapy. Retrieved from http://www.voices.no/discussions/discm53_01.html

Kenny, C. (1982). *The mythic artery: The magic of music therapy.* Atascadero, CA: Ridgeview Publishing Company.

Nachmanovitch, S. (1990). *Free play: Improvisation in life and art. New York: St. Martin's Press.*

Rio, R. (2009). *Connecting through music with people with dementia: A guide for caregivers.* London: Jessica Kingsley Publishers.

Rio, R. (2002). Improvisation with the elderly: Moving from creative activities to process-oriented therapy. *The Arts in Psychotherapy, (29),* 191-201.

Southard, S. (2014) Essential Theater retrieved Jul 24, 2014. http://www.susansouthard.com/essentialTheatre.html

Valley Interfaith Project. (2014). Retrieved Jul 24, 2014 http://valleyinterfaithprojectaz.com/

In: Fostering Creativity in Rehabilitation
Editor: Matthew J. Taylor

ISBN: 978-1-63485-118-3
© 2016 Nova Science Publishers, Inc.

Chapter 18

DANCE/PERFORMANCE REHABILITATION

Staffan Elgelid, PT, PhD, GCFP

Associate Professor, Physical Therapy, Nazareth College, Rochester, NY, US

WHAT CHALLENGES AND OPPORTUNITIES ARE SPECIFIC TO YOUR PROFESSION?

In the physical therapy (PT) profession, as well as in most of health care today the challenges are numerous, but so are the opportunities. Everything from insurance issues, time pressure, mergers of big hospitals squeezing out the smaller private practice, as well as a whole host of other issues can be considered challenges. On the other hand insurance issues, time pressures and merger of big hospitals squeezing out the small private practice, as well as a whole host of other issues can be considered opportunities. Yes, it all depends on how one looks at the issues.

Working with performers I see these challenges mostly as opportunities. Performers are concerned about one thing – Performance. If you can demonstrate that your work with the performer will improve their performance- whether that is the musician, athlete, dancer, or weekend athlete- then they will seek you out.

It was easier to break into the performance field in 1985 when I started working with runners after graduation from PT school. The big hospitals had not figured out that catering to the performer was something that was profitable and that working with high level performers would raise their profile in the community. I was lucky in that I was a runner, so I connected to the running community in Spokane, WA and started working with runners. Some of those runners reached world-class level, and they and their sponsors invited me to travel to races with them. At that time college and high school athletics were still not influenced by money. It was local people that took care of the athletes, often for free, during practices and games. Something has happened since then though.

The hospitals and "performance clinics" have realized there is money and prestige in working with performers. Large, multi-million dollar facilities have sprouted up. Performance centers, institutes for athletes, performing artists etc. can now be found in most towns. These institutes have money behind them and often actually pay the team, college, etc. to work exclusively with them. Yes incredible as it might seem, often teams and colleges will sell the right to work with their athletes. This has made it more difficult to get started working with the high-level athlete and performer. The person breaking in today must have either a background in performance, connections and/or a bit of luck. Once the rehab professional has gotten started working with a few high level performers though, the playing field is level. The athlete/performer will more than likely first go to whatever institute is sponsoring the team, or to the big fancy clinic, but in the end they will go to the practitioner that will improve their performance. The performance is the only thing that matters to the performer! The practitioner with the knowledge of performance, the skill to observe and suggest ways to improve, and who has the flexibility to cater to the performer's schedule will come out ahead. There is not a doubt in my mind that the insurance issues, time pressure, mergers of big hospitals squeezing out the smaller private practice, as well as a whole host of other issues are great opportunities for the creative and skilled practitioner. The non-creative and non-skilled practitioner will not survive in today's climate as their practice will be usurped by either the larger organizations that can buy themselves clients or by the creative and skillful practitioner. The big advantage of the creative, skillful practitioner is their ability and flexibility to really create something that is unique and valuable to each performer and that is less likely to happen in a larger "we will buy out or competition" driven institution. In my case, I was more driven than the therapists in the larger institutions due to the fact that I owned my clinic and did not have high volumes. I also had the freedom to increase treatment times according to the client's needs and did not have to follow a set schedule or a certain productivity quota. These are freedoms that are less likely to happen in the bigger practices and therefore the smaller private clinics can have an advantage in their ability to be flexible. So yes there are challenges for the physical therapist that wants to work with performers, but for the therapist that is creative and skillful there are more opportunities than ever.

WHAT DID/ARE YOU DO/DOING?

For many years I had a private PT clinic in Spokane WA. In addition to the clinic, I also worked on the road so that I could take time off and travel with athletes and spend time in Sweden. It was a fantastic opportunity to see how PT was practiced across the US and a wide variety of settings. I was not pleased with how conventional PT was practiced and felt like something was missing, so I went through a 4-year professional Feldenkrais® training program. I graduated from that in 1996. I went to the University of Central Arkansas to get my PhD in 1998. That is when I really started working with performers other than athletes. I started working with musicians at the University and eventually started working with actors too. I went back to the University because I felt as though I wanted to give back to future generations of PTs what I had learned in my unique practice opportunities.

I was somewhat surprised how little interest there was at the University for practical knowledge compared to in the clinical community and running community. Having been a runner my whole life and having worked with the very best in the world I was stunned that I was not even invited to share my knowledge about running. The person who lectured on running injuries there had no practical knowledge of running, but had read books and research. When I spoke to and worked with therapists in the field and coaches, they were more interested in my practical experiences of working with high level runners and what interventions had worked in individual cases. At the University an individual case was often written off as "anecdotal evidence." Anecdotal evidence is another term for "that is interesting and cute, but we really don't need to pay attention for this since not all variables were controlled."

Since my first university teaching experience I have taught at several schools and find the same situation in most schools. Real world knowledge is not valued as much as having the right degrees and research knowledge. I eventually finished my PhD and have been in academia ever since. I am lucky in that I am now teaching at a small private college and have more freedom in what I teach. I have also been very involved with yoga during the last few years and have completed 800 hours of yoga therapy training. I still see clients in my spare time and combine yoga therapy, and Feldenkrais with PT when I work with my clients.

WHERE DID YOUR IDEAS/DESIRE COME FROM?

When I entered PT school my ideas where shaped by my background growing up in Sweden. I had always taken an interest in what was not considered mainstream medicine modalities such as Acupuncture, Homeopathy and other alternative schools of thought, and combined that knowledge with my knowledge from athletics. When I graduated with my PT degree, I put those alternative ideas on the backburner for a while and was strongly influenced by my PT training, manual therapy, soft tissue work and exercise. As I continued to develop my skills, I realized that most of my new ideas came from complementary treatment ideas and from readings outside of PT. Sad to say, none of my ideas came from the mainstream medical/PT journals since I felt that the research published did not apply to my clients that were high level performers or had multiple medical conditions. I was much more inspired reading about martial arts and other movement practices. Since graduating from the Feldenkrais training in 1996, I have been greatly influenced by the Feldenkrais Method. Exploring my own movements and looking at habits changed the way I looked at not only PT, but the way I looked at everything in society. Still I felt like there was something missing in the Feldenkrais Method. I had been on the outskirts of Yoga for many years. In 2011 I attended a Yoga Therapy conference and saw the full force of good Yoga Therapy. I realized that comprehensive yoga therapy deals not only with postures and breathing but also with emotions, wisdom and spirituality – the areas that I felt were lacking in the Feldenkrais Method. I immediately started a Yoga Therapy training program and now I combine Feldenkrais and Yoga Therapy as a way for my clients and myself to inquiry into who we are.

WHAT SUPPORTED YOUR PROCESS?

I could not have done this without the support of my family, clients and wonderful friends. I have always traveled a lot from place to place, but I have managed to have 10-15 friends that have supported me in various ways. They have supported me through good times and bad times, including when I have been sick, and they always been great sounding boards. They have always supported my ideas, but they have also forced me to think about alternatives. Barnes and Noble has also supported me…. Yes I have spent many days and evenings buying a cup of tea while reading numerous magazines and books and taking notes. There is so much to read and I am thankful for all the people who put their thoughts down on a page. It takes courage to publish, but I am so thankful that people share their ideas since I have received such benefits from reading an article in a magazine whether a sports, spiritual, news or rock and roll magazines. The ideas that flow from the pages often become incorporated in my practice and way of being.

WHAT INHIBITED IT?

What inhibited it/me? That is a good question! I inhibited myself! Or maybe I should say I allowed others to inhibit me. I had the support of my friends, my clients and the results I saw. Still I allowed influences from the outside to inhibit me. I allowed the MD's who would refer to clinics that were seeing a patient every 15-30 minutes, and who followed the "normal" protocols to inhibit me. I saw a patient every 60 minutes and sometimes wondered if I was ineffective. Once I entered academia I allowed myself to become even more doubtful, and allowed individual faculty members to inhibit me. I read the journals and listened to faculty who could rattle off research studies. My arguments that the research did not apply to my real patients with multiple conditions fell on deaf ears. I allowed the faculty to plant seeds of doubt in my mind. These were successful people with many degrees who I felt represented the pinnacle of our profession. After many years of teaching, I now know that many of these people are brilliant, but they have not seen many, if any, patients. They are teachers of theory and research, but so much more goes into treating a client. So no one inhibited me, I allowed myself to be inhibited by the "norms!"

DO YOU HAVE ANY PERSONAL PRACTICES THAT YOU THINK SUPPORT YOUR CREATIVITY OR WORLD VIEWS?

Absolutely. One of the weakest aspects of modern healthcare including physical therapy is the lack of a personal practice to deepen our understanding of ourselves. Throughout history the personal practice was important and part of your medical education. This is true for Chinese Medicine, Ayurveda, Shamanism, and other medical people trained in traditional societies. In modern health care we do not see that the connection between the depth of your understanding of yourself and your sensitivity to yourself has a direct correlation to how well you can sense and understand your client. We still have the belief that there is a subject and an object and that the two do not interact. This is slowly changing but it has not yet penetrated into the academic institutions where health care professionals are taught. I spoke more about the slow changes in academia in Chapter 5. For me the biggest change came when I started my Feldenkrais Training. This forced me to look at my habits and why I did and believed what I did. Exploring movement options through the Feldenkrais Method also opened up my brain for changes in how I viewed health care, performance and other aspects of society. The Feldenkrais Method did this through introducing movement options. Then adding the yoga therapy training to my Feldenkrais practice has added a layer of emotional and spiritual understanding to my interaction with my clients. I still mostly work through the body and it's habits when I work with myself and others, but I am relating what I notice in the organization of the body more and more frequently to the emotional and spiritual status of the that person I am working with. This way of relating the organization of the body to emotions and spirit has definitely made my life and the life of my clients richer. While I believe a personal practice is crucial for creativity and an understanding of our clients, and ourselves maintaining a personal practice is not an easy thing to do. The discipline it takes to maintain a personal practice is not easy, but the biggest obstacle to a personal practice is what we find out about ourselves. Not everything one finds out about oneself is pleasant!!!

HOW HAS THE EXPERIENCE INFLUENCED YOUR CURRENT CREATIVITY?

My creativity comes from working with clients, my personal practice and contact with my mentors and fellow creative practitioners. If I don't do my personal practice then my creativity dries up. Since I mostly intervene through movement patterns, whether the concern of the performer is physical, emotional, spiritual, or energetic, it is crucial for me to have my own movement practice. It is through and during my movement practices that the ideas come up about what options might be appropriate with clients, writing etc. I might do my personal practice in the evening before bed, in the AM, or in between clients. As a matter of fact, I almost always do some movements or go deep within myself in between clients to allow options in approaches to the next client emerge. Often that is then the approach I follow, but it also happens that once I am in front of the client something else emerges based on the present interaction between the client and me. What is important though is that I have all those movement ideas/options within me, which I allow ideas to emerge when I am with the client and that I maintain an internal silence and awareness that allows this to happen. I hesitate to call this process creativity, since I don't feel like I am doing something and creativity is about creating something. I just allow thing/ideas/ contexts to emerge. I feel quite passive when I am in the moment of working with clients.

My experiences with Feldenkrais and yoga has also allowed me to relate body organizations and emotions. As a somatic practitioner I do believe that each emotional state has a corresponding body organization. Working with musicians, I found that they tended to be excellent at certain pieces. Pieces that had a certain tempo, mood or emotion, that matched the performers tempo, mood or emotion. This was especially obvious when a talented young musician was playing an emotional piece and the music just didn't seem congruent with the performer. After doing some reading and sensing it dawned on me that maybe the musician could not reach the emotional body organization that was needed for the piece. I found the same with actors trying to project an emotion on stage. It is more than just changing the voice or changing the body, you must also sense the emotion in your self and find the organization that evokes that emotion. Of course this is more difficult for a younger actor or musician since they have had less time to experience various emotions. Most of the time when I am dealing with a performer trying to access a certain emotion, I take them through a Feldenkrais lesson or a yoga asana that evokes that emotion. Then I have the person stay in that organization/emotion for a while and then go in and out of the body organization that evokes the emotion. That way the performer learns how to consciously go in and out of the body organization that evokes the specific emotion.

An athlete is similarly limited by their habitual body organization. I work with creating options for the athlete so that they can improve their performance. An athlete will only reach a certain level of a success with a certain body organization. In the case of an endurance athlete it might be a movement that interferes and is not congruent with the direction that the body is moving. In the case of a "multi directional athlete, such as a basketball player, it might be a lack of ability to develop differentiation and/or integration of body parts that stops the athlete from developing a variety of moves on the court.

To the reader this might sound like an approach that is a straight biomechanical function, especially when it comes to the endurance athlete. I will claim that it demands creativity and personal practice to help the athlete reach a higher level of performance, as well as some knowledge of anatomy and biomechanics. By first guiding the athlete to a place where they can recognize their habitual movements, the athlete will recognize the benefits and limitations of the habits. From a biomechanics perspective it is usually about replacing a habit with another movement. From the somatic education perspective that is very linear and not a very creative way to think. An athlete has developed a movement that is efficient based on his individual body and nervous system. His nervous system developed the best solution to the movement demands that it could. My job as a practitioner is to develop options to the movement habit to allow the athlete to perform better. It is not about removing a movement habit, since the movement the athlete has works for many contexts. It is more about adding options to the habitual movement. For the endurance athlete adding some options of combinations between hip, ankle and knee positions, or between the shoulder and hip will then allow the nervous system to incorporate that option to the previous movement pattern and the result will be a more efficient body organization that will allow the athlete to reach the next level. For the basketball player it might be about teaching the body to be organized in a way that it turns with equal ease in both directions, or differentiate the pelvis from the eyes thereby giving the player the option to trick the opposing player that he is going in the direction of the eyes, but he is really going in the direction that the pelvis is going. By having my personal practice I play with how to differentiate and then integrate various movements. When I am with the athlete I can then draw on those experiences in the sessions. As you can imagine there are 100's of ways to differentiate, and learning them all from a textbook is not possible. By having a personal practice those differentiations are present in my body. I can sense them in my self as I teach them to the athlete. My personal practice informs everything I do with performers.

DESCRIBE YOUR EXPERIENCE WITH CREATING, ...IS IT A STEADY PROCESS? EPISODIC? MANIC? DROUGHT? DOES IT FEEL LIKE IT COMES FROM "YOU" OR ELSEWHERE?

I am not sure I am creating as much as allowing something to emerge. So then the question is, is it coming from me or elsewhere? Well to some extent it is coming from me. It is emerging from inside of me, and it is clearly based on my personal movement practices whether it is Feldenkrais, Yoga, Tai Chi or Meditation. So yes it is coming from me, because without the personal practice I doubt that anything would emerge. On the other hand the combination of movement and ideas that emerge from me might not be of my own making. At least I can't say that I consciously combine the elements that emerge during sessions. Sometimes I almost laugh when I am with clients and I see what emerges. They will ask me if I have done that before, and I sheepishly have to admit that I have no idea where it came from but it was an interesting combination of movements.

Creating for me is not a steady process. Many times I don't do anything for a long time. I do my personal practice and see some performers, but I can't seem to get anything really moving. During those times I sleep a lot and read a lot of murder mysteries, or go see mindless movies, or do anything else that does not require brainpower. Then all of a sudden these mindless activities bore me out of my mind and then the creativity comes back. It is like I need to hibernate every now and then. Just shut off my mind and be mindless in my mindfulness. I have no doubt that ideas are stirring somewhere deep inside of me while I am going through these mindless states. Maybe by not reading or doing anything creative for short periods of time, the ideas that are humming along get time to incubate and develop before they emerge. So my creativity is more sporadic, or at least they emerge sporadically but there is probably always some development of ideas going on. Of course, when I am going through these stages of not using much brainpower I am still seeing clients. I sometimes feel like I am cheating the clients, since I find my sessions to be subpar, but it seems like the clients are just as happy. Maybe my brain gets out of the way at these times and my hands work without interference. Who knows??

How Do You Nurture or Nurse Fledgling Ideas?

I don't nurse fledging ideas!! I let ideas emerge while engaging in personal practice, while with clients, while writing and while reading. I have no idea why a certain idea will come to mind at a certain time. Some ideas I develop and some of them will sink back to the depths again. I have no doubt that I have dropped many good ideas because I did not write them down or nurture them. BUT I have full faith that I knew at some deeper level that the time was not right, and when the time is right the ideas will emerge again. Not in the same form, but in combination with something else that makes it a better more appropriate concept. There is a time and context for everything and that comes for ideas too.

Creative people have so many ideas. Some people put them down on paper and then logically make a decision on what to act on. I am a bit different. I allow the ideas to emerge and then act on what sticks in my mind and that I just can't get rid off. The ideas may hang out and stir in the back of my mind for a long time, and then they come out more or less fully formed when the time is right.

When I work with performers, I think there is a communication of what I have stirring in the back of my mind and what is stirring in the back of the performers mind. We work and create together. Performers are creative people. Many times they are more creative than me. I listen to the person I am working with. Listen to the reason they are there to see me. Since I am doing a combination of Feldenkrais, Yoga Therapy and Physical Therapy I see all kinds of conditions, including straight musculoskeletal injuries, to emotional turmoil, to performance anxiety/stress and on and on. Many times I sense an underlying perceived sense of a "lack" in the performer that manifests in a condition. It could be a lack of self-confidence, a perceived lack of support, talent, nurturing etc. I usually have an idea about what is going on, but I guide my client towards finding the answer instead of providing answers. Part of my goal is to get the performer to trust their internal senses, just as I trust my internal senses when it comes to what direction to guide the client in.

I believe a big part of creativity is to trust the internal senses. I want the performers to become more sensitive to their internal senses and then follow what emerges from there. If the performer can trust the internal senses and then combine this with a solid education in their craft then their performance will have an authenticity and a uniqueness that will become the trademark of that performer. A trademark that no other performer can copy, because they don't have the same background and identical growth of their nervous system. A performer who only has the solid education but does not listen internally will be a competent performer but will never develop the uniqueness or reach the height that the performer who combines solid training with internal listening can reach.

WHAT ROLES DOES/DID YOUR COMMUNITY/COLLEAGUES PLAY IN YOUR CREATIVE EXPERIENCE?

As I mentioned before, my friends are crucial for my creative experience. Just knowing what they are creating is inspiring. Some of their ideas will influence and improve the ideas I am thinking about. Cross-pollination (I prefer to call it cross-pollination rather than stealing) is a constantly on-going thing for me while creating. It might be from something that a friend or someone in the community (and here I include list serves, Facebook, and other communities) wrote, said, texted, tweeted etc. There are so many influences.

I have also learned that some people's role is to shoot down anything that is not "normal" according to their standards. The lesson from that is that some people you should avoid. You need people who question and dialogue with you, but nobody needs people who question and cut you down due to their insecurity and unhappiness. Creative people need to be careful whom they share their time with. Come to think of it, everyone needs to be careful about whom they share their time with! We don't need to spend time with people that try to bring us down to their level of unhappiness. We need to spend time with people that support us and that will bring us up!

WHAT WOULD YOU DO DIFFERENTLY?

I would like to say be more committed to one idea or movement practice, but… When I first got out of school all I wanted to do was to work with athletes doing massage, exercise and manual therapy. If I had committed to that one idea I would still be doing that. Maybe I would be very satisfied doing that, but I would not be where I am now. The next thing was the Feldenkrais Training. I could have stopped there and become a fabulous Feldenkrais disciple, but where would I have developed the emotional and spiritual aspect of the work and in myself? I then entered Yoga Therapy Training and I found those aspects. I have also been greatly enriched by meeting and sharing ideas with members of the Feldenkrais and Yoga

Therapy communities, people I would not have met if I had rigidly held on to my initial vision after graduating from PT school.

In the same vein I wish I had stayed in one place for a long period of time to develop a larger practice. I wish I had stayed in Spokane and developed my practice, but then I would not have met my friends in the Midwest, and my mentors on the east coast. I wish.... Nah, my life is the way it is and my practice today is a combination of everything I have experienced. Some practitioners will be better off developing one approach to its fullest and stay with that. I chose a different path and like to integrate approaches into something that feels right to me. So even if I wish I had done some of those other things, I am perfectly pleased with where I am and would not have anything different. We follow the path we are called to.

WHAT'S NEXT?

Well here is the contradiction; it is time to stop training in new and different approaches. It is time to start putting the approaches I have already trained in together a bit tighter and then prune. Remove the peripheral ideas and come down to the essentials. What are the essential components in what I do? How have I combined Feldenkrais, yoga therapy and physical therapy? I need to prune back some of the branches to get more clarity for myself, for my clients and for my fellow practitioners. It is time to write about my approach and encourage others to take what I have learned, mix it up with what they are doing and then watch something interesting emerge. To do that I need to prune, clarify and simplify. I need to find the essence in what I do. This is difficult for me since I am curious about different approaches and ideas, so I need to really discipline myself and not investigate more interesting approaches. I trust that I have what I need. Now I need to use some logic to organize these pieces. A combination of the logic of the body and the logic of the brain! Stay tuned!

WORDS OF WISDOM/INSPIRATION?

Go in the direction that feels right for you.

Stay away from negative non-supportive people, and surround yourself with people that are supportive of you!

Keep up your personal practice and the ideas will emerge up from inside of you. Don't doubt your true inner wisdom!

Know when to add and when to prune, but never doubt your internal sensations for when you need to do what.

In: Fostering Creativity in Rehabilitation
Editor: Matthew J. Taylor

ISBN: 978-1-63485-118-3
© 2016 Nova Science Publishers, Inc.

Chapter 19

WOMEN'S HEALTH

Diana Munger, PT, DPT

Desert Physical Therapy, Phoenix, AZ, US

Creative is not a word I have ever used to describe myself. I was quite surprised when asked to contribute a chapter to a book on creativity. However, once I stood back and reflected upon the development and progression of my career, I began to recognize how it truly has been a personal journey of creation. I established a job for myself that did not previously exist and my methods of rehabilitation rarely resemble those I was taught in school. Apparently, some creation has occurred, but how? With gratitude for this opportunity to explore the creative process, I offer my story in hope that it may shine a light upon and inspire your personal creative journey.

I always knew I wanted to work in a field where I could be of service to others. Coming from a family of medical practitioners, the world of healthcare seemed a natural fit. However, in exploring my options, I became frustrated with the myopic view of modern medicine. I eventually chose physical therapy (PT) because I appreciated the opportunity to work with the whole body.

While in graduate school, I was lucky enough to be introduced to yoga at my local fitness club. As a dancer of many years, the postures of the practice came naturally, but I quickly sensed there was something different taking place. The concepts of breath control and meditation were new to me. Learning to quiet my spinning thoughts, bringing my mind and body into the same place at the same time, was life changing. Not only did this practice support me through the rigors of PT school, it also sparked ideas about the entire human experience. It was a wide view and I was intrigued.

EXTENDING MY SPINE AND MY HORIZONS

I began to take more classes including Advanced Power Yoga because I was getting to be 'good' at this yoga thing. My new teacher was impressed with my flexibility and introduced me to more challenging postures. Scorpion pose quickly became a favorite because of the "oohs" and "ahhs" I could elicit from my peers as I flung my spine into extreme extension. Yeah, yoga is pretty cool. But why am I beginning to get back pain . . . and how come I don't leave class with that peaceful feeling anymore? I knew there was much for yoga to teach me, but it was time to reach out beyond the offerings of the small town where I was living. Internet, here I come.

There are so many interesting characters one can meet on the Internet. I happened to find Matthew J. Taylor, a PT in Galena, IL who was already integrating yoga into his orthopedic rehabilitation practice. Through a few emails exchanges, I expressed my interest in the therapeutic applications of yoga. He directed me toward a yoga teacher-training program called Integrative Yoga Therapy. Not being one to turn down an adventure, I juggled my summer schedule between the second and third years of PT school, and signed-up for their 200-hour training program. It began with a two week intensive at an ashram in the mountains of Pennsylvania.

SHIFTING PARADIGMS

Some experiences change you; others ignite a transformation beyond anything you could previously conceive. What began as an expanding awareness in those first gentle yoga classes, accelerated into a foundation crumbling, alternate-reality opening, paradigm shift from which there was no return. I learned a new way of studying the body, incorporating the physical along with the mental, emotional, energetic, and spiritual aspects. I came to recognize that one part of a human could not be addressed without every other part also being affected. I experienced the insight and growth that comes along with a personal practice. "Yes, *this* is it!" I thought, "Forget PT school. I finally know what I want to be when I grow up: a yoga teacher!" Yes, I have a tendency toward the extreme at times. Thankfully, a wise teacher encouraged me to stick with my schooling. While it may be a fractionalized view of the whole human experience, the knowledge base physical therapy training provided would be of great value to me. Sometimes you have to spend time studying the pieces before you are able to assemble the larger puzzle. Additionally, those little initials that would come after my name upon graduation and board certification could open doors in the medical community that may be less accessible to those outside of the healthcare club. But I wasn't ready to head home yet. Maintaining my commitment to PT school, I also arranged to stay at the ashram for another two weeks to attend their next training session on yoga therapy.

A TWIST OF FATE

The extension of my yoga training interfered with a scheduled PT class on Orthopedic Strength and Conditioning. A call to the school office informed me that there was another class available a few weeks later that could fill my requisite hours: Women's Health. Not only did I accept their gracious offer to switch classes, but a spark of intrigue into this not seemingly coincidental opportunity arose. The Women's Health specialty had not interested me before. In fact, I thought it was a weird undertaking for a physical therapist; too personal, too close to bodily functions. Yet, my curiosity grew and I focused my attention over the next two weeks on the topic of women's health. From the energetic anatomy of the pelvis and reproductive organs, to pregnancy, hormonal shifts, and emotional holding patterns, I was fascinated to explore the feminine through my new lens.

The whirlwind month lasted forever and went by in a blink, placing me squarely back in reality. Filled with a combination of excitement and apprehension, I returned to school and began the Women's Health course. Straightaway, I knew I had found my niche. Every concept the knowledgeable visiting instructor presented, fit brilliantly with my emerging holistic paradigm. She taught the importance of looking locally at the symptoms, but also considering patterns in the entire body. She spoke of emotional trauma and cycles of thought contributing to physical symptoms. She expressed the importance of a social support system. She encouraged us to recognize that pain is real to the patient regardless of whether a cause can be found. While I may have heard these things before, my time delving into the depths of yoga had allowed me to understand them on another level. When the time came to explore case studies, I found myself not regurgitating the 'right' answers based on what we had just learned (as I had done so well through all of my years of schooling), but instead considered the whole complex system and discovered I had ideas of my own. I saw an opportunity to bring my experiential knowledge of yoga into the practice of rehabilitation. With joy, I embarked on my journey as a Women's Health Physical Therapist.

TEACHERS, TEACHERS EVERYWHERE

Heading into my third and final year of PT school, I sought out an internship in Women's Health (WH). Without an option pre-arranged through my university, I reached out into the community to find an opportunity. I found a small group of WH PTs who met quarterly. They graciously accepted this eager student into their circle and allowed me to fill the role of secretary to earn my keep. As I got to know these wonderful women and heard about their approaches to patient care, I gained clarity as to with whom I wanted to study. Two of them agreed to be my clinical instructor. One became a dear mentor who I continue to learn from till this day.

My WH mentor appreciated my knowledge of and passion for yoga, yet she did not share this practice. I felt a need to find someone else to talk to about ways to merge my worlds of yoga and rehabilitation. Fate was in my favor. I heard through the grapevine that my previous contact, Matt Taylor, had moved to my home state of Arizona and was planning to open an integrative rehabilitation clinic. Not only would I have local access to another exceptional mentor, but also a potential place to work. In yet another synchronicity, my WH mentor connected with Matt via a different channel, and agreed to move her practice to his clinic as an independent contractor. I arranged a meeting with Matt and his lovely wife and partner, Jennifer. They placed their faith in my offerings and opened a space in their practice to me upon my licensure. A dream opportunity, right?! Two brilliant teachers, along with multiple other open-minded, creative rehabilitation specialists, were under one roof. I hit the jackpot.

ROAD BLOCKS AND TRAFFIC

The dream job lasted about six months. My experience at the clinic was significant and insightful. The easy access to seasoned colleagues was tremendously valuable to continue my professional edification. I had freedom to dictate my schedule as an independent contractor, a rare liberty for a new graduate. I loved being part of a community that valued personal growth. It was a group of innovative, like-minded individuals and I was a part of it . . . sort of. While I tried my best to hide it, I was a kid. A bright-eyed, bushy tailed kid, who felt more like an intern than a peer. There are challenges working with the best of the best. My schedule began to fill up, but I couldn't shake the feeling that many of my patients would be better off with one of the other therapists. Marketing meetings with potential referring physicians were awkward at best as I struggled to find something clever to say. This insecure version of myself was far from creative. With so much energy spent trying to be qualified, not to mention the fatigue of a terrible commute across the large metropolitan area, I was spent. Any new therapist experiences exhaustion by the end of a day, but mine was becoming excessive. I also carried the weight of my patients' suffering, yet to understand that I could not be everything to everybody. My husband missed me even when we were together; there was not much 'me' left. It was too much. I reluctantly told Matt I needed a change.

A TIME TO GROW

Have you ever gotten everything you ever wanted only to realize you were not ready for it yet? Recognizing that *you* are the limiting factor in your dreams can be tough. But I'm the type of gal that was taught to pull myself up by my bootstraps. I got back to work, starting with myself. My meditation practice, along with journaling and heart-felt discussions with my confidants, helped me clarify my situation. What do I really want? How can I get the experience needed to feel qualified? What would an ideal day at work look like at this point in my life? How long of a commute can I handle?

Once I regained my footing and knew my general course, I hit the streets to find my place (within a 10 mile radius of home this time). I knew my independent spirit would be happier with the freedoms of contracting versus employment. I set up interviews at multiple rehabilitation facilities to discuss leasing space. I found a private, female-owned outpatient orthopedic and aquatic physical therapy clinic that fit the bill. They had a private room that was rarely used in which I could see my Women's Health patients. Additionally, they offered to let me treat their orthopedic patients for a contract rate as I built up my WH clientele. I was able to get well-needed experience in various types of physical therapy practice. The owner was a strong advocate of my specialty and generously included me in their marketing efforts. Most of the PTs there had less than five years' experience. It was a light-hearted environment and we all had a good time together. I got plenty of practice redirecting, with ninja-like reflexes, the tacky poop jokes and innuendo with regards to my specialty. My business grew swiftly, along with my confidence.

AN ABUNDANT FIELD

The niche of Women's Health was ripe with opportunity for creativity. While the specialty developed over 35 years ago, it was just beginning to gain mainstream attention. Being a 'new' therapy meant many incoming patients did not know what to expect. Most often, women entered my office with an open, beginner's mind. This was an excellent opportunity to introduce a new model of integrative rehabilitation. Patients frustrated by previous failed therapy attempts were eager to try a different way. I joyfully watched as they began to release some of their long-held fractionalized ideas about their bodies. Of course, there were others who came in expecting their rehabilitation to fit into an established schema of what PT *should* look like. Why are you looking at my feet when I told you it hurts here? What does breathing have to do with my inability to pee? Education became key.

The intimate subjects broached in my office could be difficult for some patients to discuss. During the evaluative process, I would keep close to the conventional model, giving a sense of familiarity to the process. I discovered that my willingness to listen to someone's sensitive story and be consistently present through their roller-coaster journey of healing, fostered a deep connection. As mutual trust developed, the intimacy of our talk became fuel for transformation. We became a team, trusting one another to take steps that may be new to both of us. Creativity flowed from all sides, shifting old patterns, and allowing for authentic healing.

A PLACE TO CALL HOME

Eventually, I felt ready to open a clinic of my own. However, this was by no means a one-woman show. I leaned heavily upon the previously mentioned mentors extraordinaire as well as another skilled WH PT. And I cannot forget the significant financial and emotional support provided by my beloved husband. The clinic was modeled after Matt's inspired practice, with a collection of independent contractors all sharing space and office support. Our practice was specifically designed to focus on Women's Health rehabilitation services. We lovingly refer to it as our 'co-op'. It has been a place for collaboration, commiseration, and sweet compassion.

Opening a business often feels like being thrown into the middle of the ocean without a raft; I had to learn how to swim with haste. I learned about leasing space, setting up LLCs, the many different types of insurance coverage, and the expensive, circular path of working with attorneys. I learned how to set-up Medicare billing, and later how to shift to a cash-based practice. I learned how to save up during the high profit months in order to survive the summers and multiple maternity leaves (mine and others). I learned about hiring, and unfortunately, firing employees. I learned the difference between cash and accrual accounting. Most of all, I learned how to ask for help.

I ran the business for six and a half years. Last month I handed over the reins to my trusted colleague. I recognized it was time to loosen my grip on the business and all the future planning that went with it. Releasing some of my responsibilities has opened my time and mental space. I have more energy to direct toward my greatest professional passion: patient care.

Today, my days consist of weaving together my physical therapy skills and therapeutic yoga knowledge to serve women and men with pelvic health challenges. Yes, men have pelvic floors too and we opened our doors to their knocking about the time the paint dried on the 'Women's Health Center' sign out front. Apparently, the creative flow has a sense of humor. The majority of my practice addresses conditions involving discomfort or dysfunction of the pelvic floor muscles. While the focus is on the pelvis, treatments are rooted in a philosophy of whole-being wellness. Additionally, I teach weekly prenatal yoga classes and prenatal partners workshops, as well as various educational talks in the fields of pelvic health and therapeutic yoga.

PRACTICE MAKES . . . MORE PRACTICE

I love the word practice. Physical therapy practice, yoga practice - the term reminds me that there is no destination. The process, in each new moment, is at the heart of any endeavor. As soon as you feel like you are getting to be 'good', as Scorpion pose taught me so long ago, life smacks you with a new lesson. Here are a few of my on-going lessons:

Chasing Knowledge

I am a life-long learner. Being in a field that requires continuing education is like telling a kid that they are *required* to have dessert. I ravenously attended continuing education courses early on trying to acquire as much knowledge as possible. Every time I was stumped by a complex patient, I would seek out a training to fill the void. I wanted to be an expert. In all honesty, I still do. But a deeper, wiser part of me knows that 'expert' is a fallacy. We all possess everything we need to do what we are meant to do. It is nice to have fancy anatomical or Sanskrit words for it, but I have come to recognize that I don't have to try so hard. Spending more time exploring the movements of my body and mind, and sitting in stillness are just as informative, if not more. As with most things in life, it is both. Training is necessary to gain competence in a specialized field; *and* integration, time, and experience are necessary to really get it. Each day is a practice of accepting that there is nothing to *become*; it is simply the act of being mindful in each new moment.

Healing Hands

Many patients have called me a healer over the years. While the term strokes my ego, I have always known it to be false. And yet, I have fallen into this trap again and again. I'll call it the 'Fix Me' trap. My hands are most often the culprits. They have spent many hours being fine-tuned to sense the slightest changes in muscle tone, fascial mobility, and blood flow. They are skilled manual therapists. As a patient describes their symptoms, I can feel energy flowing to my eager hands ready for palpation. It is easy to jump into manual therapy techniques knowing I can, most often, get a painful, spasming muscle to release. Who doesn't love the quick fix, right? But while this fix makes them feel better and makes me feel like a hero, it does nothing to empower the patient. It teaches them reliance on an outside source to fix their body. Much like my desire to quickly tie my four year old's shoes for him when we are running out the door, I am robbing them of an opportunity to learn to help themselves. Manual therapy is an integral part of my practice, but I cannot let myself get into the comfortable rut of, "Oh here, let me do that for you." My ongoing yoga practice and philosophical studies shine a light on this pattern of mine. I'm nowhere near 'good' yet.

CAPTURING CREATIVITY

Trying to be creative is an amusing, but futile task for me. This is probably why I have never considered myself to be creative. It does not come on command. Nor does it come wrapped in a pretty package, alerting me to its arrival. Creativity seems to arise as a practical possibility to a challenge. For example, when available options are not a fit for me, a creative solution often emerges. This seems to be a key pattern in my professional journey. The same pattern can be seen in my treatment room. Patients are my muses. They enter with their list of challenges and we begin to play. The volley of open-hearted conversation with a patient can reveal a deep well of creativity. In those inspired moments, I am able to synthesize knowledge and experience from diverse fields to come up with novel, customized approaches to rehabilitation. It is an exhilarating co-creation. And in the next hour, I may find myself falling back into the 'Fix Me' trap. There is an ongoing flow that does not seem to be graspable. Thus, I continue to practice.

FINAL THOUGHTS

This process of reflecting upon my own creative journey has helped me gain a new understanding of creativity. Being a creative therapist does not mean you must have a trademarked method, a series of continuing education classes, and your own YouTube channel. Creativity is available to everyone in every setting. It simply means showing up for each patient, your whole-being present with their whole-being. It means opening to what the world offers you each day, in each moment. It means both taking knowledge in and freely sharing ideas. Creativity flows with the process of self-discovery; understanding who you are and what you have to offer is vital. Know your strengths and focus on them; it is far more effective than trying to 'fix' your short-comings. And remember that we are all already in a constant state of creation. Take a wide view, and ask yourself, is this what I want to be creating?

My yoga practice has been a great source of inspiration for me, but it is not necessarily about yoga. Find what inspires you. It is not the type of practice, but the practice itself. Return to something day after day that teaches you about you, your relationships, and life itself. It could be running, gardening, or origami. Find what brings you joy and do it with an open heart and clear mind. Many blessings along your chosen path of creation.

In: Fostering Creativity in Rehabilitation
Editor: Matthew J. Taylor
ISBN: 978-1-63485-118-3

Chapter 20

SOCIAL WORK

Jennifer Collins Taylor,[1] MSW and Charles Trull,[2] PhD

[1]Living Life Dying Death, Scottsdale, AZ, US
[2]US Naval Hospital, Camp Pendleton, CA, US

We, Charlie Trull, PhD (CLT) and Jennifer Collins Taylor, MSW (JCT), embarked as two unique individuals on a shared writing experience. Where would we connect? Where would we diverge? Early in our first phone conversation we decided to "Live the Questions" separately for at least the first month, with weekly check-in support phone conversations as we explored deeper levels of insight. As most life experiences have taught us, our first responses were quite different from what appears here in the published text. We decided to "begin to begin" and allow the organic process to emerge. We agreed to be mindful of ourselves, each other and of creativity, life itself. Full disclosure: we are friends with respect and curiosity to learn from one another and honor the process. We also believe that chaos and complexity is an integral part of the creative process. Sensitivity, deep listening, and open, gentle questioning of a friend, mirrored our professional relationship with clients; a synergistic collaboration. In this way, each of us was allowed to explore what we truly believe about fostering creativity in the social work profession. Ultimately, in this mirroring process we came to see our authentic selves, our authentic friendship and a vision of the social work profession filled with passion, innovation and transformation.

Social workers are all individuals that seek to create meaningful change in the world. We meet the client with standardized core knowledge, values, ethics and skills. As empowering social workers, we believe in the self-determination of the individual that seeks a social worker's compassionate and resourceful support in life challenges. Social work is poised to support the entire lifespan of people, being available to be utilized from pregnancy to end-of-life care. Additionally, we have the flexibility to impact the micro (individuals and families) to the macro (such as organizations, communities and national institutions).

Inherent in the interaction between the two individuals, a creative practice begins of deep listening, clarification, and honest communication. We create a safe space that holds possibilities for the desired outcomes. Credibility, connection, and unconditional positive regard created in this safe space is essential for the therapeutic alliance. The alliance within this space fosters a freedom to emerge for both the client and therapist to explore creative opportunities. Overall, the social work profession has traditionally accepted and appreciated creativity in the scope of practice. When the therapist is properly trained, the five aspects of the whole person (mental, emotional, physical, spiritual and sexual) are available in the social work scope of practice. The entire human experience can be explored primarily, through each other's culture, minds, emotions, and spirits with occasionally a physical component such as play therapy or dance. Different clients respond to different doorways towards their therapeutic goals, such as movement, sound or touch. Most often the goal(s) is to bring growth, joy, purpose, and/or peacefulness to the human experience. It is our opinion that it is imperative that the social worker has a personal practice that develops their own human potential in all aspects of their being, as well as a creative outlook, to bring credibility and freshness to the therapeutic alliance. Creative collaboration occurs when both parties are active participants.

As social workers we share similar challenges with other health care rehabilitation careers such as financial feasibility for both private practice and within organizational settings due to many factors. However, the most limiting force is the current insurance dictatorship, umm we mean constraint (the word constraint being a social work technique of reframing!) which has substantially impacted all of health care. Time restrictions, reimbursement minefields, and paperwork nightmares contribute to the current third party reimbursement situation. There are no easy answers on how to go forward for our national healthcare, but one thing is for certain, the health of our nation is at risk. This entire insurance driven atmosphere within Sardar's post- normal times impedes creativity.

Health care administrations that devalue the social worker's role are problematic because the social work professional also then loses the respect of the entire interdisciplinary team. Quite often social workers are the clean up crew to be the quick fix and move or discharge patients/clients as quickly and quietly as possible. Usually this is due to power hierarchies and fear-based management within the organization. The administration is reacting to the significant pressures from third party reimbursement. Consequently, social workers are highly encouraged to discharge the commodified clients due to having either met the "goal" in the recommended sessions or discharge the client because they are not showing the signs of potential for meeting their goal. These pressures of course devalue creativity.

Another challenge that the social work profession faces is that some of the patients/clients have been through trauma......sometimes unimaginable pain and suffering which compounds the need for time, compassion and resources for the patient to move towards health. Additionally, through the current system of classification, these individuals may have been labeled 'pathological' and assigned a DSM-5 diagnosis that carries its own stigmatism. This anguish is sometimes further compounded through decades and generations of grief and shame. These situations can smother any flicker of creativity in what has come to be seen by clients as an apparently hopeless circumstance.

Social workers ourselves, as with many professions, become our own worst enemy to living and working creatively. Living in a demanding world that brings its own set of burdens to the therapist greatly impacts the therapeutic relationship. Mindfulness, the act of being aware of the present moment and sensing emotions and thoughts has not been taught in the traditional social work school settings. Nor have social workers traditionally been encouraged to learn supportive mindful, personal practices. The social work professional that has limiting thoughts and behaviors impedes a reflective relationship as therapists themselves get stuck in rote responses and solutions. This lack of reflection and introspection as a part of our clinical mastery development generates a lifestyle that hinders creativity by the reactionary behavior patterns it sustains.

The social worker profession is often misunderstood and generalized. This dilemma is not unique to the social work field, but a contributing challenge to creativity in our career. We face the reputation of being domineering individuals that think we know what is best for another individual. For instance, the misrepresentation or caricature of the social worker who appears "kind" but has the "power" to take children away from their parent. Very problematic is the social worker that IS overbearing and actually DO believe they know what is best for another person! This disempowering attitude further diminishes the emergence of creativity.

Creativity isn't a bullet point event, but a rippling process that continually circles both outward and inward. It is a paradoxical exchange of opportunities and possibilities weaved into challenges and chaos.

Life is this dynamic rippling. Nature is both beautiful and seemingly cruel, however, it teems with possibility, even in chaos and uncertainty. Within the unknowing of life, lives the opportunity for social workers as well as all rehabilitation professionals and those they serve, to be mindfully aware and prepared to respond with life-honoring solutions. Patients/clients seek out their own truth, and when the therapist has listened to the personal call to continue to grow and learn, they both will be available for a creative therapeutic relationship. This is possible through innovation and creativity. From the micro individual to the macro cultural shift, the passion of the social worker and rehabilitative professional transforms life's experiences. The creative reward is that, while the social worker aims to make a difference in another's life, so does the client make a difference in the social worker's life. It is our belief that creative responses and renewals are essential to a life well-lived. In the following sections, we would like to share a little bit of our personal and professional creative responses.

CLT

My own evolution as a social worker began as a response to my desire to effect positive change in my clients in an environment that was challenging to creative approaches, and that evolution has been nurtured by my spiritual path. While established modalities of service are employed with success by many social workers I found myself feeling less effective than I wanted to be in helping my clients. My own healing experience through an unconventional therapeutic process was an affirmation that there were untapped opportunities to explore in the universe of helping and healing.

When I returned from Viet Nam I found that I was hyper-vigilant, I had difficulty sleeping, explosive anger, and was depressed. In short I was suffering the effects of PTSD. It ruined my first marriage, made it difficult to create friendships, and cost me several jobs. I began to drink so I could not feel so raw. I sought individual counseling and group therapy. Nothing was helping, until an old shaman arranged for me to have a Warriors Sweat Lodge Ceremony. Following that experience I began to heal. I have found that ceremony engages the whole of me: mental, physical, spiritual, emotional and sexual. As opposed to psychotherapy which is mostly mental. I believe that by engaging the whole person the healing process is accelerated. I went to graduate school and became a social worker, at the same time I apprenticed to a Shaman to understand the ceremonial process more thoroughly. Having experienced first-hand the power of ceremonial experience I was convinced it could help my clients, but I was at a loss as to how I could tap into that power to help them.

One answer to this question came when I met a Lakota woman in Phoenix AZ. She worked with drug and alcohol dependency among the Native American population on parole. I was fascinated by her use of traditional ceremony such as the sweat lodge ceremony to treat her clients, as well as the support she was receiving from government entities. The funding she received was for interventions limited to clients with a cultural background that that was supportive of the modality. She called upon the client to connect with his heritage and accept his own power as a warrior of his people. Her interventions were alternative but culturally grounded. Many conversations with her about her own creative process brought me closer to realizing my creative path. I have come to find that collaborative work with creative practitioners is helpful in priming the pump of creativity.

One of the tenets of Social Work ethics is client self-determination. I see this as the source of great opportunity and great challenge in the practice of Social Work. The human psyche, much like the human body is a self-healing entity. For the purposes of this discussion I refer to the emotional and mental aspects of the client as the psyche. If given the proper environment and nurturing the psyche will heal itself. The focus of the social worker is to create such an environment and support the healing process. I have found that creating such an environment can be challenging. Many clients are resistant to the concept of healing themselves. There is an obstacle to creating the healing opportunity that I think of as a learned helplessness. This is the belief that someone is going to fix me. The willingness to take responsibility for our own healing can be difficult to assume. It can seem like a foreign concept to us.

Engaging with opportunities to heal can be frightening to the client if he or she is wedded to the role of helpless victim. This resistance can be a starting point in the process of empowering the client to begin the healing process.

Creating a safe environment for the healing process begins with establishing a relationship that is based on unconditional positive regard. The client must trust that the social worker is on their side in supporting their best interests. The client must view the social worker as competent and connected. This requires all the skills that the social worker has for communication, active listening and displaying compassion. In my experience practices such as Buddhist Psychology and Positive Psychology and mindfulness are most helpful.

Having reviewed the literature on the above and seeing the results in others practices I began a dedicated investigation of them in 2011. I had explored mindfulness in my own spiritual practice and found it helpful in my own healing process so I was excited to see how it could fit in my professional practice as a tool to facilitate the healing process in others. The acceptance of what is and seeing what is as what needs to be here and now releases the client from judgment and guilt that accompany many modalities. The doorways to mindfulness practice can be varied. Sound, aroma, movement, tactile experiences, can all be used to assist the client in achieving the experience of being in the present moment

I now work as the geriatric specialist and discharge planner at the Naval Hospital Camp Pendleton. My clients include active duty military personnel returning from deployment and their families, as well as retired veterans from WWII to the present and their families. Many suffer from PTSD, Traumatic Brain Injury, and a whole host of other medical issues. Some are facing the end of life. Even today I have mentors and co-workers with whom I share cases. I ask for their feedback about my approach and solicit their suggestions for improvement. My work at the Naval Hospital Camp Pendleton is enhanced by the fact that it is a teaching hospital and open to new approaches in healing. Nurses here practice therapeutic touch. We have a full time acupuncturist, and several staff doctors trained in acupuncture. Our chaplain department has fostered a yoga class each day at noon. As a senior social worker I have been given a great deal of autonomy, but also the support to work with a large inter-disciplinary team. These collaborations are not only informative but inspirational. With this background I began to explore the world of alternative interventions.

I begin my day by opening my chakras. This allows my energy to vibrate at a frequency that lifts all with whom I interact. I use a simple meditation technique to open the chakras using mudras (hand positions) and sounds. I begin by bringing my awareness to the 1st or root chakra which is between the anus and genitals. With my awareness there and touching the tip of my index finger to my thumb I chant "LAM". I do this until I feel the chakra vibrate as it awakens. I then go up to my sacral chakra and with the appropriate mudra I chant "VAM" until it also vibrates as it awakens. I continue up the chakras using the appropriate sound and mudras as I open each. Sometimes I find a chakra that resists opening. This is an opportunity to explore what may be blocking me is some way. For example: if my throat chakra is resisting opening, am I not willing to say something that needs to be said. Or if my heart chakra is resistant, am I withholding love where it needs to be given.

I begin each interaction whether with a group or individual with a silent prayer: "May you be blessed. May we be blessed. May we all be blessed." I do not speak it aloud and it is only for me to know. I have found that this simple prayer often changes the very atmosphere in the room, creating a peaceful environment for heart to heart communication. As I engage the client or group I listen actively and closely to whatever they share with me, while using as few as possible of my own words to encourage them to go deeper into their own experiences.

Having time alone in nature is my way of allowing the creative process to flow within me. I will strive to go into a park or wilderness and find a place where I can neither see nor hear other humans. I have found that when I can be truly alone with nature I shed inhibitions and constraints and become my natural self. It is this natural self that is truly free to express creativity. Many of my ceremonial practices take place in nature. I find that it is a powerful way to shift focus. When my clients shift focus they become aware of new perspectives and possibilities. It is in the possibilities that healing abides.

On my spiritual path I have been taught that the creative process occurs in 10 steps. This is called the Zero to Nine Law of creation. The steps are: focus, substance, form, determination, understanding, imagination, freedom, pattern, chaos. The tenth step is the void or dissolution.

An example of how I use this in practice is the following. As I am thinking about the next therapy group I will be facilitating I am considering some device that will assist me in generating the group discussion. The process is:

Step 1: focus.
Step 2: substance. I decide to take a walk with the goal of finding a token I can use to begin the discussion.
Step 3: form. While walking I am open to everything around me, sights, smells, sounds, my own internal dialogue etc.

Step 4: Determination. I see a broken branch lying on the ground with bright green leaves that have just emerged after a long winter. I pick it up.

Step 5: understanding. As I walk and contemplate the leaves I am aware of the symbolism. A new leaf can represent new beginnings; turning over a new leaf means a change in behaviors that no longer serve me, etc.

Step 6: imagination. I bring the leaf to the group and ask them to examine it, touch it, smell it, engage with whatever comes up for them and share with the group.

Step 7: freedom. The discussion within the group flows in whatever direction and at its own speed.

Step 8: pattern. I assist the process by gently questioning and suggesting in ways that link this discussion to positive results from past group sessions.

Step 9: chaos. The energy of the group for the discussion begins to fade, or gets stuck in nonproductive process and the cohesiveness of the topic begins to unravel, I recapitulate the main ideas brought forth and summarize the progress we have made. We go our separate ways with instructions about how to integrate the progress we have made.

My experience with this process is that it is enhanced by and guided by my own attentiveness to both my interior and exterior environment. This requires that I am diligent in my own practice and that I am mindful my own process. Mindfulness is encouraged in the group process described above in the imagination step. The clients are told to engage with whatever comes up for them as they encounter the object I brought to group. Their encounter in this example is based not only on sight but also on each of the senses they can bring to their awareness. As the facilitator I guide them through the process. "How does this feel as you receive it? Is it light or heavy? How would you describe the texture? Does the feel remind you anything else, or another experience you may have had. Smell is a potent carrier of memories. Is there a fragrance to it? What comes to mind when you inhale? What is happening within your body as you engage with this? Is there tension or release or lightness or heaviness?"

Opening the client to each sense as they narrow their awareness to the object at hand opens their mind to allow what needs to present itself to them to come forth. Each client is invited to share a thought or word that describes what is present for them. When each has shared I read the words from the entire group back to the group in a story form. Since I studied with a shaman the narrative form is engrained in my being. This has been the form used to pass on information for millennia. One very familiar example in western culture of this is the parables of Jesus. Stories are much easier to remember and retrieve than just a list of facts or instructions. Narrative therapy is an accepted and effective psychotherapy tool and I have often used it successfully. Encouraging the client to understand that much of his or her emotional pain comes from the story he or she is telling about what has happened in life and then teaching the client to change that story in a way that alleviates pain brings about positive action is a powerful therapeutic tool. The client understands that he or she is the author of their life and can then assume authority.

I see my role in the therapeutic process as that of creating a safe space and bringing to the client an awareness of possibility. Many of my clients believe that they have exhausted their options and are faced with no way out of a painful situation. A part of my job is to encourage them to see that there are other possibilities. I tell them that for every problem there are a minimum of five solutions. Then I assist them to explore the solutions available to them.

At this stage of my career I am limited by my tendency to get stuck using the same tools with which I am already familiar. I must challenge myself constantly to seek out new therapy tools and fresh perspectives. Complacency is my enemy. Early in my education from the Shaman I was taught that enemies exist to make us better and stronger. So I see my tendency toward complacency as a spur to drive me to explore new opportunities. The question for me is always: What new and creative way can I use to bring the awareness of possibility to my clients? How can I become more self-responsible and assume more authority in my own life so I can assist my clients to do the same in theirs? How can I increase my own compassion for myself and others, and translate that into my practice?

JCT

Elevator speeches are always interesting when your subject matter includes the topic of death. I usually riff on the sentence, "I encourage, educate and inspire healthy conversations about death, dying and grief to empower living life fully today." However here-in lies some of my inspiration. Most people lean in and share their personal experience with death, dying and grief, relieved someone has a sympathetic ear to their story. I have self-published two books and recorded an instrumental harp CD for relaxation and comfort which supports my mission. I have supported many individuals through the dying process and others with their life grief journeys, bringing experienced compassion during a challenging life experience. As I believe all of life is a creative act, I love to cook, organize, decorate, support my family and friends, garden, dance, arrange flowers, and listen to music.

Creativity for me is a deep calling. As an expression of my life, it is seems that it is continually in my conscious and subconscious mind. This includes my nighttime and daytime dreams. However, creative living is a little different from creating a "product". This experience for me is an ebb and flow wave-like activity, which includes the spectrum of anticipation (excitement and joy of a new expression) to the release of ideas (with the usual trepidation to say my thoughts and ideas out loud to others and truly be "finished"). I have learned that I need to give time for the avalanche of ideas and be gentle with myself as I savor the beginning moments of new ideas. It is cruel to myself to crush the idea right away!

I believe that my personal history has deeply influenced my creativity. Since childhood I have held an inner belief that I am "creative" and I believe so are you... it is universal! However, the suffering of my brother dying when I was 21 years old, brought me down a path of discovery in which I asked myself, what was "dying" and what was "living life fully" which ultimately led me to end-of-life social work. This personal experience, leading to professional experiences being with the dying and those that they love inspired me to create books and music to guide people. I believe our culture diminishes the dying process and I am certain it is a vital aspect of life. As an empowering social worker, I believe that ultimately individuals can find their personal answer within themselves of what it means to live well and die well.

Personal practices which support my creativity are:

1. Connection, reflection, and silence/solitude in Nature & beauty (art, etc.)
2. Yoga/ meditation (especially savasana)

3.   Reading/learning/curiosity/listening
4.   Self-discovery
5.   Native American Prayer to the Four Directions as taught by CLT
6.   Travel
7.   Listening to dreams, intuition, & Spirit
8.   Playing and listening to music
9.   Acupuncture.
10. Planning and honoring the time and energy it takes to create.

As I hone my creative expression from this list of activities I have come to appreciate the paradox of *both* respecting my need for solitude and social connection with others. A new personal practice is that I take time to "hang out" with my Laughing Buddha statue trying to learn that laughter is the ultimate response to my wanting to "control" Life! I consciously try not to allow fear to paralyze my ideas, following the same encouragement I give others: remember the joy within.

The support from others is a wonderful aspect of creating. I have an incredible husband (see editor!), wonderful children, parents, siblings and friends that allow me to be me! Ultimately I think that I myself am the strongest impediment to creativity: myself, also known as ego, self-consciousness and self-limiting inner dialogue. For me it is fear & anxiety masquerading as perfectionism and over-analyzing. I truly believe that no one inhibited my creativity except myself. Of course I did have some push backs from organizations. While creating my Masters of Social Work thesis, the Institutional Review Board didn't want me to study death attitudes (meaning they probably had death anxiety), but I found research to prove my methodologies and it was granted approval. Also, there was a hospice that wanted to claim my creative expressions as their own. But in some ways, push backs encourage me to re-examine my passion for the project which then catapults me ahead.

My past experiences have taught me to act more quickly and courageously, let go of perfectionism and expectations, and create and create again, remembering that the work is not about me, but the larger picture of Life. Through age and experiences I have become more open, peaceful, joyful and confident with "creating" an artifact. The many experiences of individuals telling me the difference that the book or music has made in their life enlivens me. Those conversations remind me of the fact that I am connected to a larger purpose. I am grateful for the opportunity to contribute to the world. I have learned that success is not defined by financial success. Ultimately, I have learned that I need to put my ideas out into the world. From this experience I believe we all have this opportunity and responsibility from our shared human condition that when we create, the rest of humankind can benefit from our insight.

I am currently writing a children's book about life and death. The three main themes are that life is impermanent, we are all connected, and love remains. I also am creating a participatory art installation project about the ways our culture *does* talk about death. Travel, flowers, playing (harp, dance,) add to my daily creative acts. However, along the way most importantly I am continuing to learn how to best support my friends and families through the aging, dying and grief experiences.

I have two main quotes that inspire me.

"I meant to write about death but life came crashing in, as usual.'"
                              -Virginia Woolf, diary entry, 17 February 1922

What do you intend on doing?......what keeps "crashing in"?

"Life is about not knowing, ...having to change, taking the moment and making the best of it, without knowing what's going to happen next.
    Delicious Ambiguity."

                                                              -Gilda Radner

How can you let go of expectations? Can unknowing be peaceful and/or fun?
Life is short. Celebrate life. What is YOUR answer to this very personal statement?
In the end, only _____ matters.

CLT & JCT

The social work professional has daily opportunities to respond creatively to both their patients' needs as well as to their own personal needs. We envision that the grassroots efforts of those writing this book and reading this book, along with individuals that quietly go about the daily creative rehabilitative "work" will transform rehabilitative health care. These professionals serving those with physical, emotional, mental, and spiritual distress are both wise and inspirational. Creativity in the social work profession allows the strength, beauty and courage of the human spirit to shine.

In: Fostering Creativity in Rehabilitation
Editor: Matthew J. Taylor

ISBN: 978-1-63485-118-3
© 2016 Nova Science Publishers, Inc.

Chapter 21

PSYCHOLOGY

Sari Roth-Roemer, PhD

Intuitive Psychology, PLC Scottsdale, AZ, US

INTUITIVE PSYCHOLOGY IN REHABILITATION

I sat in my first rehab case conference listening intently to the foreign language that was being spoken around me. As a novice psychologist, having come straight from my residency at a cancer research hospital to my new role as a rehab psychologist, I had no clue what they were talking about when they discussed the patient's ability to "move from supine to sit with mod assist." Luckily, after asking lots of questions of my kind colleagues over the next few months, I quickly acculturated and noticed that the hospital patients I was caring for needed more than cognitive evaluation, they also needed assistance with understanding their new surroundings. My job was to serve as a guide to this new transition point in my patients' lives.

WHAT CHALLENGES AND OPPORTUNITIES ARE SPECIFIC TO YOUR PROFESSION?

Psychologists are interpreters. Our specialty in the hospital is often referred to as "consult-liaison", getting at the need to link and translate between our patients and their care providers. Psychologists are skilled at helping people understand themselves and others. In a rehab setting, psychologists are often interpreters between their patients and the rehab team. The challenge and the opportunity in this are really the same…walking between different ideological worlds, and learning to speak and then translate different vocabularies for patients and the rehab team members. This was not just the "supine to sit" I mentioned earlier, but also being able to inform a physician that a patient pulling a catheter out wasn't angry defiance or depression but instead a delirium episode with severe confusion that needed to be treated. Helping a team member understand that angry non-cooperation from a patient refusing to participate in therapy was not an act of out-and-out belligerence, but rather an attempt to get back in control while feeling afraid, and that simply empathizing with compassion and offering limited choices could turn the situation around. Educating a patient that being asked to practice repetitive cognitive exercises was not meant to be personally demeaning, but a rather an effective way to relearn, strengthen and heal. And there is always the challenge of helping those patients who feel alone and cornered to see that the whole rehab team is actually on their side, working towards the same goal of helping them feel better and regain independence. The challenge is in the translating, but the opportunity is in facilitating the comprehension.

Psychology, of course, also shares many of the same challenges listed in Chapter One. Additionally, sometimes the challenge involves education for those who forget that psychology can make a difference in whether or not a patient participates fully in their rehab. Depression, anxiety, confusion and fear can all block the way of engaging in activities that can help a person heal. Opportunity comes when we are put in the position of helping a patient move through the emotional and cognitive blocks to their recovery and assisting them with connecting to the healing rehab environment.

WHAT ARE YOU DOING?

I have begun to practice what I am now calling Intuitive Psychology. After 20 years of working with patients recovering from medical illness, and witnessing the miracle of human resiliency over and over again, I began to wonder how to share what I was witnessing with the people who needed it most…my patients.

I knew from a young age how to listen and guide those who needed my assistance. As early on as the fourth grade my friends were coming to me for advice, and for some reason I felt happily comfortable giving it to them. In high school and college I developed a love for the study and practice of psychology. I volunteered for internship after internship and followed around as many psychologists as would let me; many of whom are still my dear friends and mentors. After graduate school and residency, I learned formal theory and technique to add to my innate ability. Following years of practice I realized that the formal and innate had blended. However, it was my openness to trusting myself and trusting my intuition that was the key to the work that I did, and more importantly, the key to the recovery of my patients.

It would always start like this… A patient would come into my office and tell me their tale of struggle, to which my internal voice would almost always say, "*Wow. That is really difficult. How will I ever be able to help them with that?*" After which I would smile at myself with an internal response of "*Just listen, there will be a way, the answers will come…*" This millisecond dialogue would take place like clockwork and never failed to open the doorway for intuition and guidance. The next step, of course, was to let the person in front of me know that not only was there hope, but that the answer and solace they sought resided within them and not me. This, to my mind, is the foundation of psychological healing - faith in ourselves as well as faith in our ability to heal, to learn, and to grow from adversity. Relying on our intuition - that personal and unique inner voice that connects us to some greater wisdom - provides us all with the insight we need to guide us forward on our paths. That is the inherent simplicity and complexity of Intuitive Psychology, helping people to learn to listen more clearly to their own inner wisdom. Simple in its obvious validity, yet, complex in the difficulty that we often have listening to and trusting ourselves. As we become aware of our own intuition, that inner voice that connects us to something greater than ourselves, we learn to make better choices about what to do with our thoughts, our judgments, and our perspectives, and ultimately how to positively impact our mind, body, and spirit. To be clear, Intuitive Psychology is not about knowing the future, it is about knowing the *now*.

WHERE DID YOUR IDEAS/DESIRE COME FROM?

From the time I was about 10, friends were coming to me for a listening ear. By the time I hit high school I knew I wanted to help people. My father was a physician, so initially I thought medical school would be my path…until I took my first psychology course…and my first organic chemistry course! The choice was clear for me. Psychology just made sense. It fit the way that I thought. Simply put, it was my *calling*…something I knew I had to do, and something that I was meant to do.

Perhaps because of my father's medical background, I found myself drawn to working with people coping with illness. All my internships, all my papers, all my study was aimed in the direction of learning how to help people with medical issues cope with this major transition in their life. My dissertation was on the health protective aspects of marriage for women with rheumatoid arthritis. My post-doctoral residency was time spent working with and researching the experiences of bone marrow transplant patients and helping them cope with the pain and the cognitive changes associated with their difficult treatment course. My first job was a consulting psychologist on a rehab unit. Over and over again I witnessed people face huge physical challenges. Bodies that had turned on them, illnesses over which they had no control, but minds and hearts that could be helped to remember what strong and resilient people they all were. Aesop's Fable about the tortoise and the hare became my salve for those impatient to recover. The ability to witness resiliency and the natural human ability to cope with even the roughest of circumstances became my daily reward. By helping them to learn to tune into their own answers, my patients began to trust themselves and their intuition. They began to see that they had a choice about how they coped with the awfulness that had befallen them.

I practiced like this for almost 20 years…and then I encountered magic. I was raised to be open-minded to alternative and non-traditional methods of healing. When an associate first introduced me to a well-respected medical intuitive, I didn't bat an eye. He linked a recent injury with some significant emotional stress in my life and I agreed. After all, as a medical psychologist, that beautifully intricate dance between mind, body and spirit was what I talked to people about all day long. However, when it dawned on me that his seemingly magical intuitive powers came from a source bigger than him, I realized that my own abilities, as well as *all* of our abilities emanated from that same source. Call it what you will - God, Universe, Nature, the Unknown - but this energy bigger than all of us, containing a wellspring of wisdom, could be tapped into with our own individual intuition.

It was then I realized that intuition is available to all of us, in our own unique way. The trick is simply…*to listen to it*. Sometimes we unintentionally block it. Emotions like fear, anger, sadness, shame, to name just a few, can cover it up, as similarly described in Chapter Three's discussion of the affective and insight domains that prime creativity. When people came to me with these emotional blocks, I learned I could teach them how to move through these emotions and come up with their own answers. The reward in this for them, and for me, was unfathomable. When you watch someone realize that they indeed have the answers they need to live a happy life, the world just seems to smile a little brighter.

WHAT SUPPORTED YOUR PROCESS? WHAT INHIBITED IT?

Of course I have to say it was intuition that led me to where I am now. There has always been a *knowing* that this was the path I had to travel on, and I have watched it unfold in front of me. I have learned with time to have faith in myself and to trust the creative ideas that come my way. Of course, there were times when I was afraid. Financial constraints, fears that others would think I was too *woo-woo*, concerns that I would be redundant without anything new to say, all blocked my forward motion at times. But ultimately, it came back to trusting the faith that I had in what I was doing and knowing that it needed to be done. I was determined, and remain determined to move forward on this path to help people learn to listen and trust to their own inner voice. At times it takes a bit of bravery and a lot of good old fashioned elbow grease to keep moving forward.

When I was first exploring working in this way with my patients, I was a little apprehensive initially to broach the subject of intuition. *What would they think? Would it make them uncomfortable?* I remember asking an 80 year old retired combat marine who was struggling with the realities of an aging body about his experience with intuition in his life. "*You were a marine? Did you ever use your intuition to get you through any of the difficult combat situations you encountered?*" He said that yes, he did - that there was a voice deep inside him that led the way to safety many times. And then he asked me, "*Where do you think that came from, Doc?*" before pointing upward with a wry smile and concluding for himself, "*...from the Big Guy?*" We talked about what that meant to him, since he had such a strong spiritual center. As we talked it dawned on him that perhaps he could use that same inner wisdom to help him through this difficult time in his life. I remember smiling and thinking to myself that perhaps I was on the right track after all.

And then there is mindfulness. Mindfulness helped provide me with the language to speak about Intuitive Psychology in a way that people could comprehend. I learned about mindfulness well after graduate school. Psychodynamic theory, cognitive behavioral therapy, existentialism, humanistic theory, and Gestalt were all the foundational roots of my graduate school theoretical education. I noticed that while each of these theories carried their own nomenclature, the overlap between them was surprising. To blend them into a beautiful integrative approach that psychologists lovingly refer to as *eclecticism*, was easy. We took the parts we found useful and left the parts we didn't. When I encountered mindfulness through books and workshops 15 years into my practice of psychology, I discovered a kinder, gentler, more meaningful vocabulary that resonated well with me, as it did with my patients. As I began to play with the concepts of Intuitive Psychology, I found that mindfulness concepts of awareness and purposeful attention lent themselves nicely to the idea of tuning into our own intuition. By adding an exploration of personal spirituality and openness to personal intuition, mindfulness could be broadened. More answers to personal questions could be found with even greater ease by purposefully paying attention to our own answers.

The popularization of neuroplasticity, the idea that our thoughts can literally make changes in the neural connections within our brain, gave scientific credence to the work I was doing. Neuropsychologists like Rick Hanson, Sara Lazar, Richard Davidson, Daniel Amen and others opened up doors to exploring how mindful awareness could not only help people feel better, but with practice could change the landscape of the brain so that we could become more resilient and better able to tolerate difficulty. In this same fashion, when we approach intuition with mindful awareness and intuitive psychological approaches, perhaps we can also rewire our brains to more fully utilize this natural resource.

WHAT ROLES DOES/DID YOUR COMMUNITY/COLLEAGUES PLAY IN YOUR CREATIVE EXPERIENCE?

Luckily, supportive friends and like-minded colleagues have made this creative road a friendlier one to travel. Being able to share ideas, and see how creative thought can exponentially increase not just our own creative process, but also improve the healing process of our patients, brings an excitement all of its own. I have been known to refer to our respected and beloved editor of this book, Matthew Taylor, as "*Magic Matt,*" a name, I have been told by my patients, he may not be entirely comfortable with. But I use it with my patients for a reason. As a colleague, Matt is extraordinary. He takes a psychological approach to his work as physical therapist (what he describes as the embodiment domain) that fully complements the work that I am doing with the patients we both treat. It's as if we are speaking a similar language using slightly different dialects. The magic happens in the intersection between the compassionate, healing approach he takes with his patients and the respect he has for the psychological aspects of their recovery. Being able to work with a colleague who shares a like-minded perspective, but who brings a different skill-set to treat the problem at hand, expands the successfulness of both our treatment practices. I have been so fortunate to have found a wide array of highly skilled colleagues from within my local healing community - cardiologists, primary care physicians, rehab physicians, neurologists, naturopaths, physical therapists, social workers, craniosacral therapists, acupuncturists, dieticians, massage therapists, natural healers and other mental health professionals who have all helped me to further my work by offering to share their insights and skill sets with me and my patients. I believe this is how we truly grow beyond ourselves.

DO YOU HAVE ANY PERSONAL PRACTICES THAT YOU THINK SUPPORT YOUR CREATIVITY OR WORLD VIEWS? HOW HAS THE EXPERIENCE INFLUENCED YOUR CURRENT CREATIVITY?

I was raised in a family that honored creativity. I was taught to believe that different was not just okay, but that different was actually *better*. I learned early in life that creative storytelling and later, creative writing, was a valuable pursuit. Additionally, I was part of a loving family that had strong spiritual roots. I always felt part of something greater than myself that I could not only draw strength from but also connect to regularly. As I got older, I discovered yoga and meditation. I found that taking regular time to quiet my mind and connect to something larger than myself opened up a space for creative flow. I also found that when I didn't take the time, my creativity would flounder and my effort level would increase dramatically. So now I walk every morning with the singing birds and let my mind be quiet, connecting to the natural world around me; I have a simple daily yoga practice; and I take time to sit quietly for a few moments to meditate and listen to my answers for the day. Sometimes it's just me listening to the natural rhythm of my breathing. Usually, though, the simple message of the day is right there waiting for me to hear it in the midst of the stillness.

DESCRIBE YOUR EXPERIENCE WITH CREATING,...IS IT A STEADY PROCESS? EPISODIC? MANIC? DROUGHT? DOES IT FEEL LIKE IT COMES FROM "YOU" OR ELSEWHERE?

Creative time is playtime. It's effortless and fun. Unfortunately, I forget that at times. I forget that when I sit down at the computer or sit in front of a patient or an audience, that all I have to do is purposefully flip the switch and enjoy. When I forget, procrastination blocks my creative process...but when I remember, it's all about stepping into the flow. I tell myself I am ready, as if I am getting ready to sit down on a raft at the top of a big waterslide and just GO...hands up, smiling most of the way down...unless I hit a bump of self-doubt or self-judgment on a rare occasion. When that happens I go flying off the raft and have to climb back up those metaphorical stairs and start again with more compassion.

This is my process: Turn on the computer. Take a deep cleansing breath. Notice a feeling of curiosity and wonder come over me. Find joy in the anticipation of, *"what will come today?"* Think of the topic I want to approach, then open up and let it flow through. My rule is, *no judgment* as it comes. Just let it flow directly from my mind, writing it down as it comes. Sometimes even looking away from the computer screen as I write to avoid the distraction of what I am seeing in front of my eyes. Tidying up after all of it has flowed through. Then I read it and wonder, *"Where did this come from?"*

I have to admit that sometimes I feel like the words that I am typing on the page are not entirely my own. While the ideas seem to be coming from my brain, I have begun to believe that perhaps they are coming through my brain. In my work with intuition I have learned to view our beautiful brain as more of an intricate receiver finely tuned into the specific pulse of the universe that each brain is uniquely set to receive. While that may sound a little whacky, it nevertheless feels true. In any case, I am grateful for the creative flow that is there for me to tap into whenever I make a purposeful point of doing so.

Discipline is both my friend and my enemy when it comes to creativity. I have always found discipline a bit constraining, so I will often procrastinate like a champion to avoid it. Luckily, my reasonable adult mind is there to remind me that discipline is all in my perception, and that when I take purposeful time to devote to my creative efforts, discipline is in fact my greatest ally!

HOW DO YOU NURTURE OR NURSE FLEDGLING IDEAS?

I love new ideas! They come running into my head whenever I take the time to be quiet. They almost always make me excited and I almost always think that this will be *absolutely the best idea I have ever had*! I run quickly to write the thoughts down so as not to forget them. And then I just let them sit there and percolate in the background until they let me know they are ready to be worked on. Sometimes I am inpatient and I check back in on them from time to time like a batch of oatmeal chocolate chip cookies to see if they are done. When they are not yet ready, I remind myself to be patient. Creativity comes in its own time. Then, when they are close to done, I take them out to play with them a bit…yes, I am one of those people who likes her cookies soft in the middle. I write the ideas down and I share them with a trusted few to get feedback. I may put them back in the oven of my mind for a little while to let them bake more fully, I may put them on the pretty platter of my blog and serve them to the general public, or I may end up throwing them in the trash and modifying the recipe. And then, if I am lucky enough, and quiet enough, I'll be ready for another batch soon again.

WHAT WOULD YOU DO DIFFERENTLY?

In theory, I would be more patient, more compassionate and less judgmental. Impatience, judgment and fear are the killers of creativity and hinder our intuition. And in theory, I would be more disciplined and carve out more time to devote to writing and creative pursuits. Without purposefully devoted time for creativity, as well as time for quiet stillness, creativity can slow to a trickle. But in truth, I would do nothing differently, because this is the path that I am on, and I learn, and therefore create, from the mistakes that I make.

WHAT'S NEXT?

Catch me on the Intuitive Psychology World Tour! My goal has always been to help others. I have practiced with individuals for many years in my private practice and in rehab hospitals. Most recently I have begun offering regularly scheduled educational workshops on Intuitive Psychology and wellness topics. These round table workshops have turned into wonderful forums for discussion and learning among an always diverse group of participants. My blog on Intuitive Psychology (intuitivepsychology.wordpress.com) was started as an introduction to Intuitive Psychology topics; it eventually turned into a writing workshop for my upcoming book. The book will explain the theory of Intuitive Psychology in greater detail and will operationalize its concepts. I am developing a curriculum to train counselors and helping professionals to use their own intuition to in turn teach those they work with how to use their intuition to heal and find their own answers. My objective is two-fold - to help people to learn to listen more clearly to their own inner wisdom and to train helping professionals learn how to help others do just that. As always, I hope to have some fun and learn a lot along the way.

WORDS OF WISDOM/INSPIRATION?

Anyone who knows me has heard me say a million times…*have faith in yourself*. Know that there is no problem that you cannot face when you tell yourself that you *can*. It may not be easy, but it will be possible. The key is quite simply paying close attention to what you are saying to yourself. What you say to yourself really makes a difference. There is power in your words. Make sure that you are giving yourself the message that you are creative…because indeed you are. The trick is to be accepting of the gifts you were given. Use what you've got instead of wishing you had something else. When you own the type of creativity that is uniquely yours, you can become an expert, grow your own voice, and brighten the lives of those around you. That is certainly a gift worth developing, utilizing, and sharing…

In: Fostering Creativity in Rehabilitation
Editor: Matthew J. Taylor

ISBN: 978-1-63485-118-3
© 2016 Nova Science Publishers, Inc.

Chapter 22

GUIDED BY THE MUSE INTO THE UNCERTAIN

Cheryl Van Demark, PT, MA
Director, Health In Motion, Chino Valley, AZ, US

It is said that what is most memorable for people is how you made them feel, so I would like to share with you an inspiring story of the day my Rehab Muse appeared.

The story begins somewhere around my twentieth year of clinical practice, on a busy weekday morning in the clinic. This was a beautiful, spacious physical therapist owned private practice dedicated to physical excellence. To this end, our clinician group trained together with some of the finest manual therapists and met regularly in study group to stay current on emerging research in evidence-based practice in rehabilitation. Consistent with the pursuit of physical excellence, the practice featured the finest in gym equipment, an elaborate big screen Wii-Fit system and a pool. Hi-low tables were in every room and there was a lap top provided for every therapist. We had a steady stream of patients who were impressed with the look, feel and size of the facility. Overall, a fine kingdom for a Rehab Muse.

> Notice if you are attracted or averted to this kingdom. Notice if you began to compare this kingdom to yours? Visualize your work kingdom and again employ all of your senses in the process. Is there any natural light? Any plants? What does it smell like? Is it cluttered or open; quiet or noisy? As you picture yourself in your kingdom, what shape does your body take? What happens to your breath? Do you have a sense of energy expansion, or one of contraction? If you like, make some notes about the felt sense of your workplace/kingdom as a place that stimulates your imagination? How can you enhance the environment of your kingdom to invite more imagination? Environment impacts our access to inspiration and imagination.

On the morning the Rehab Muse appeared, I was doing an initial evaluation with a woman in her sixties who was presenting with complaints of chronic low back pain and a milieu of symptoms suggesting health compromise in all body systems. You know this "composite" patient story all too well. Taking the history was like running the gauntlet because the woman talked incessantly. Her referring diagnosis was chronic low back pain and lumbar DDD with Fibromyalgia? Co-morbidities included Obesity, Hypertension, Type 2

Diabetes, Coronary Artery Disease and repeated bouts of Depression. The medications list was extensive. Diet was poor, sleep was disturbed, elimination was sluggish and her energy was, not surprisingly, very low.

This woman was a "frequent flier" at our practice. She was not a spinal surgery candidate, therefore she had not only received multiple episodes of care in physical therapy, but also had received her allotment of injections to the spine as well as viscosupplement injections for her knee OA. She had attended the local hospital class for education in Type 2 Diabetes on more than one occasion, but did not follow their suggestions. She had attended Weight Watchers, but always regained weight. She had been given multiple free one-month gym trials after each bout of physical therapy at our practice, but had never continued to exercise. Her list of reasons for not being able to follow through with any self-care was extensive. As is often the case in this composite patient scenario, this person was also not particularly happy with marital life, had a limited social circle and no time or energy to engage in service to others. The only thing "physically excellent" was her vocal chords, from telling her story of suffering over and over and over…. Did her physician realize how many times he had referred this woman to PT despite no meaningful change for her complaints and no clinically significant outcomes? What was the whopping price tag for her medical bills over the past five years? What would the PT owner of the practice say if the plan of care was no more physical therapy? This patient is a classic example of how a small percent of consumers with chronic illnesses, particularly chronic pain, typically consume a majority of health care resources.

Notice if you have joined me in feeling your energy drain, or your breath shrink or your stomach tense. Do you experience "chi sucking" as you identify with this "composite patient"? Has your visualization of the kingdom changed? Seeing a castle moat filled with crocodiles? Are you still feeling like meeting a muse is a possibility for you? Notice the sensitivity of your creative energy.

After running the gauntlet of this patient's history, I allowed myself compassion for starting my clinical day in this room with yet another "non-complaint/failed patient." (Like many of you seasoned clinicians may notice, a disproportionate amount of this type of patient appears on your schedule when you are good at what you do. Yes, my hair is grey, but apparently "a nice grey" that looks great on me.) I let out a very long breath to relieve my chest tension, to purposefully make some space for empathy in hope for stimulating a tide of compassion to send in this woman's direction. My heart could then look behind the eyes for the positive potential in this fellow human being.

Truth be told, I had not thought about a muse until the very moment she flew out of my mouth. I simply heard myself tell this patient that what she obviously needed was a muse! This muse would clear away all of the excuses she had just articulated for why she could not find the motivation to make the necessary lifestyle changes she needed to improve her health status. The muse would do the job of revealing to her that SHE possessed the power to heal…it was not MY job, or anyone else's, to rehabilitate her! Viva la freedom. A moment of stunned silence naturally ensued for both of us. In the next moment, it was obvious that she expected ME to pull a muse out of my pocket and hand it over….the usual medical model.

Open your mind and imagination to meet your Rehab Muse.

Close, or lower your eyes and softly use all five senses to deeply notice your present environment. Soften your facial expression, especially the eyes. Notice how vision changes when your eyes are soft. Moisten your lips and invite a soft smile. What do you smell, hear and taste? How is your breath stretching your skin? Now use all five senses to imagine a Rehab Muse……..Here are a few questions to get you started. Is your muse wearing spandex and tennis shoes, or a Greek gown? Does it have wings? A wand? What might the muse share with you? Does the muse speak?

What messages does your muse have to impart about whether your mind is open or closed to new concepts? (In case you are wondering, my Rehab Muse was dressed in yoga gear, had a satchel of books on Buddhism, was carrying a bow and arrow and the muse dust tasted like sweet tarts.)

The Rehab Muse sprinkled magic dust and, poof, I boarded a bio psychosocial thought train. My muse whispered, "Aren't you supposed to be the expert in movement here? What could be? As you know, "what could be" is a fundamental creative question. Poof, more muse dust. What could be……If her back pain were relieved, how could her story change? If she recovered the spinal support she needed, could she be less fearful and therefore act less angry? (Fear is often the hidden emotion that elicits anger. FABQ and anger are associated with chronic LBP) *How could spinal support and release of fear change her movement quality?* If her spine could move from a solid and centered foundation, could she learn to stand her ground and shift out of the role of victim? *How could feeling centered and able to stand her ground affect her balance?* If she realized she had the power to modify her brain and learn resilience, could her chronic stress be alleviated? *How could a sense of resilience be expressed in the plyometric quality of her movement patterns?* Could "lightening up" with a 40 lbs. weight loss biomechanically resolve her knee pain- or is fear also weakening her knees? *What does unburdened movement look like?* If her energy improved from good nutrition, her food choices reflecting an understanding that she literally re-creates her tissues out of the food she eats, could she be more active, and perhaps reverse her hypertension and her Type 2 Diabetes? *How is vitality expressed in movement?* Could her self-image change even if her body reshaped via a 40 lb. weight loss? Where was the joy in the woman's life? Could she learn to love herself so that she could feel loved by others? *How could she literally move through the world if she could be inspired to transform herself in these ways? More importantly, could therapeutic exercises be directed toward movement qualities that would inspire her to the lifestyle changes she needs for health and well-being?*

My limited beliefs about how movement is habitually used in rehabilitation instantaneously dropped. Rehabilitating rehabilitation is about empowering patients to access their innate healing power. They have simply forgotten about it. We all have a Rehab Muse! I did not have to hand it over to her but instead show her the way in to her own. Fostering creativity in rehabilitation means finding ways to "re-member" these patients who, as I have described above, have become disintegrated or dismembered from their embodiment and human capacity for healing. As Matt Taylor is fond of saying, to truly "re-habilitate" we must "re-create" a place fit to live in. Recreate body as temple and refuge and source to move through life joyfully. *Movement tells a story and can help us re-write our story*. This was my inspiration! I sincerely hope you enjoyed the story.

What "could be" in rehabilitation if YOU imagine movement from a new perspective? Get up and play with YOUR perspective. How do you move within a vision of: Transforming society by optimizing movement to improve the human experience? (The updated vision statement for the APTA. I was in the House of Delegates representing Arizona when Vision 2020 was created. This is a much better statement, but I wonder if the perspective on the scope of optimizing movement... could be unbounded?)

Refer to the qualities of movement table below that Matt Taylor and I created in 2010. I offer this simply as a "what could be?")

Kosha	Movement Quality	
Physical Body	Positive	Negative
	Flexible	Limited
	Smooth	Crepitation
	Centered	Malaligned
	Balanced	Imbalanced
	Coordinated	Uncoordinated
	Accurate	Inaccurate
	Purposeful	Random
	Stable	Unstable
	Strong	Weak
Energy Body	Vital	Dull
	Free	Blocked
	Powerful	Suppressed
	Fluid	Stagnant
	Pulsating	Erratic
	Radiating	Trapped
Emotional Body	Open	Protective
	Free	Burdened
	Light	Heavy
	Excited	Lethargic
Witness Body	Aware	Unaware
	Alert	Asleep, Dull
	Observant	Distracted
	Present	Past or Future
Spiritual Body	Blissful and flowing in Unity	Distraught and disjointed in Separation

EPILOGUE: MOVING CREATIVE INSPIRATION INTO FORM

"Do all that you can, with all that you have,
in the time that you have, in the place where you are." ~ Nkosi Johnson.

After using my workplace at the time as a rich sounding board for ideas and hearing resounding limitations that were focused more on concern for the reimbursement system that supported the kingdom than the patients in the kingdom, I took the retreat I recommended to you earlier in the chapter. This retreat allowed the creative inspiration I received that day to form into a clear vision that has shaped my therapeutic practice today, Health In Motion LLC. Needing a new kingdom led to the creation of the movement arts studio, Body Language

Studio that has become an extension my practice as a source of rehabilitation for my community. It is now four years after the Rehab Muse inspired me. Body Language Studio trains the public in yoga, fitness and martial arts and offers instruction in drawing, clay building and creative writing. In essence, I have combined all of the things I value under one roof. I have chosen to provide all of the studio services outside of the insurance arena. I firmly believe that part of the uncovering of our Rehab Muse involves reaching into our own pockets to pay for what we value. I make my services accessible and affordable in a variety of ways as I am located in a town with a median family income of $32,000.

We are social animals, so I focus a lot on group therapeutic exercise at the studio. My studio is full of people who have been "discharged from rehabilitation" but have not "re-membered". They are not moving well enough to function successfully in most public group exercise classes and did not get inspired by their health care to re-create their health. In a group senior stretch and tone class, what happens when you give an 88 year old with throat cancer, emphysema and multi-level spinal fusion a cowboy hat to wave around in one hand as he works balance when his stated goal is to lose the cane and get his swagger back? How about when you offer an overweight woman a tiara and a magic wand as she sweats off some calories for weight loss while working her hip strength and balance on the ballet bar to relieve her knee pain. Or encourage the shy woman with a sunken chest a bedazzled belly dancing scarf for her scapular range of motion. What if you invite "free" dance to some favorite tunes? Add statements of affirmation for the qualities of movement we are working on during? What happens is that rehabilitation becomes a lot more playful. I also teach a chair assisted yoga class populated by joint replacement and post spinal fusion patients and those with MS. Make no mistake-I am offering rehabilitation, and this is taking place outside of the health system. People are paying small fees out of pocket for it because they value what is happening for them. What if more rehab centers offered something like this model for a few months after discharge, to help people re-engage socially?

Sustaining into the fourth year of fine tuning my methods for teaching people to access their Rehab Muse for health and healing has required all the talents and skills in creative thinking that I knew I had and quite a few that I have had to acquire. Along the way, my attractions and aversions have been clearly revealed! Space sharing the studio with related businesses that offer martial arts, dance training and other performing arts has been congruous with the studio mission and beneficial to financial sustainability. Bringing in other practitioners who offer related wellness services broadens the client base. This includes massage and facial services and life coaches. Offering "karma"/service classes in exchange for help with operations has proved both convenient and cost effective. Offering what people want as well as what they need is key. Conventional group fitness classes at a low price bring people in the door. Once the relationship is formed, I invite them to broaden their horizons into the mindful movement arts. Networking continuously in the community with the Chamber of Commerce and writing blogs for the community newspaper keeps the topic of health promotion in the public eye and keeps me associated with the topic. Hosting health and well-being educational talks, events around mindful eating, healthy meal preparation, and clothing exchanges attracts my largely female client base. Being aware of my own appearance, energy and conduct in my community also requires steady attention to role modeling.

Finally, feeding my own intellect through ongoing studies of yoga and integrative health, keeps me fresh. At this writing I am in the first class of allied health professionals to go through an Integrative Health program offered by pioneering Center for Integrative Medicine at the University of Arizona. The nature of everything is impermanent, so the process of creation and re-creation is a continuous one. Much love and nurturance is needed to balance work and play. My greatest blessing is a supportive family who loves me dearly!

May you joyfully foster creativity in rehabilitation!

In: Fostering Creativity in Rehabilitation
Editor: Matthew J. Taylor

ISBN: 978-1-63485-118-3
© 2016 Nova Science Publishers, Inc.

Chapter 23

CAREER TRANSITIONS AND NEW HORIZONS

Jerry Gillon, PT, ATC, OCS

Betty and Bobo's Bakery, Cedar Rapids, IA, US

A progressive decision to leave our 20-year-old practice became a reality when a long time employee wanted to become an owner/partner. It was my opinion another owner wasn't needed; but a fresh, younger, energetic owner would be a benefit to the continued success of the clinic. Allowing him to take the reins provided him an opportunity to exercise his creativity and me to lean toward another, undetermined direction. This is not to say I have been on a steady, direct course. I feel I am still moving toward a final destination as I learn from my current bread baking experience. Each undertaking, each experience provides knowledge and wisdom for a yet unknown opportunity to "serve somebody"

WHAT CHALLENGES AND OPPORTUNITIES ARE SPECIFIC TO YOUR PROFESSION?

Any and all professions have challenges and opportunities. The challenges may represent the true opportunities and the opportunities can be challenges. The profession that I was educated for was an outlet for me to be exposed to both. It was my chosen method for doing what all of us know we must do; and that is to, as Bob Dylan says, "Serve somebody." Physical therapy was and continues to be a career I enjoy and practice daily, but I have channeled my need for creativity in a gentler, friendlier direction.

My challenges are now simpler, the opportunities less grandiose but enjoyable and equally important to my sense of contributing and bringing pleasure to others.

WHAT DID/ARE YOU DO/DOING?

I entered the physical therapy profession as the result of a series of gradual choices beginning in 9th grade, which to this day are the result of others gently guiding me.

Their wisdom, insight, and willingness to invest themselves in me at those various points in my life was significant. And to them, I am eternally grateful. I began my career away from my hometown working in a private clinic owned by pioneers in the field of private practice known then as "Tetrad" but now known as Therapeutic Associates. Today they are celebrating 60 years as privately-owned clinics. Later returning to my home, I created an outpatient clinic for a group of orthopedists (Yes, a POPTS it was and one that recognized the importance of honesty and accountability in providing service to their patients). In that position, I created a Sports Injury Clinic and a network of high school and local college athletic trainer services. When I had done what I felt needed to be done there, I left and created the first onsite industrial physical therapy clinic at our largest employer in the city. Almost immediately I recognized our moral compasses were not pointing the same direction and we parted ways. During this time my wife (also a physical therapist) opened her clinic and I quickly joined her. That clinic continues today with former employees as the new owners. Along the way I taught four years at the University of Iowa, teaching courses in orthopedic physical therapy, surface anatomy, administration, and musculoskeletal therapeutics. I was also involved in the creation of a network of contract physical therapy services to rural hospitals providing staff and clinical direction. I continued in our clinic until deciding it was a good time to let it be.

I entered my 2nd career more as an outlet for creativity and a desire to share what my wife and I have always enjoyed as well, which is to provide something that someone actually paid for at the time. It does become trying in the field of physical therapy to observe the progressive erosion of the monetary value of your services. This is particularly difficult when you feel you are charging appropriately, providing cost-effective treatment, running a smoothly operating, efficient clinic in an appropriately sized and appointed space. Once again, I was gently nudged in the direction by others and am also grateful to them.

But in both of these outlets for service and creativity, physical therapy and bread baking, I exceeded my expectations of my abilities. My chosen outlets have not been financially lucrative, nor have I gained a position of authority or professional stature, which are certainly common and appropriate goals. However, what I have gained and continue to gain is "unsolicited testimonials" from those whose paths I have crossed in providing my service or product to them or a family member. They will look me in the eye and thank me for being someone they could trust, who was there to help them in their time of need, someone who brought a smile to their face when in pain or when they were feeling the effects of injury, illness, disease, or aging. Now, as I bake bread, I provide them with honest goodness in a product whose taste, texture, and aroma transport them to another time, another place as they remember themselves in grandma's kitchen with a bread they thought they would never taste again. And I get to see the joy in their face, and the tear in their eye. As I sat here writing this, a friend, a healthcare peer, and a bakery customer came up to me and relayed her bread story to me. She said that she stopped in midbite when she realized this taste was exactly the same taste as the bread her Mother made.

WHERE DID YOUR IDEAS/DESIRE COME FROM?

Where all of our ideas come from; observation, openness, honesty, and desire.

WHAT SUPPORTED YOUR PROCESS?

Gradual reconfirmation of a chosen direction over time. Always looking for the holes in my plan, but at the right moments having someone or something placed in front of me showing me that I am doing what is right for me and others at that point in time.

WHAT INHIBITED IT?

Myself when I would allow it.

DO YOU HAVE ANY PERSONAL PRACTICES THAT YOU THINK SUPPORT YOUR CREATIVITY OR WORLD VIEWS?

My world view is simple. We create it all; our accomplishments and our problems. As a person, a community, a society, a nation, and a planet. If we create it, we can control it. Whatever it may be, it may eventually escape our grasp and our ability to keep it in balance with our needs and the greater good. My personal practice to support my creativity is to do as we all know to do and have been told to do in many ways by many people. "Clear your head", "Get your mind off it", "Step away", "It will come to you", "Listen to your heart", "Meditate", Take a walk". In essence, getting out of your head and into your soul to find the support, insight, and guidance one always needs. One of my chosen methods, or should I say the method chosen by my life and business partner, is walking. In my working and leisure life, I pursue an activity or skill of interest until I have it mastered at its maximum useful level where it becomes a source of enjoyment to myself and fulfills a need of others. I become consumed in the process with little regard to all else around me. That personal trait along with my attention deficit disorder (never diagnosed by anyone but my wife) transports me into many, fascinating rabbit holes from which I conceivably could remain in forever. Recognizing this reality and the need to maintain a life balance as well as recharge my creativity, we began to walk: across Spain and France. With a lightly loaded backpack, we walk 20 miles a day, 30 days. One foot in front of the other, day after day after day, year after year after year. Eleven years of allowing the rhythm to surface, allowing yourself to join with it, allowing it to consume and direct you.

Doing this in countries where the culture and social landscape is different provides us with a fresh perspective on many things. It is an opportunity to share, learn, and even use our physical therapy skills for walkers from all parts of the world feeling the effects of the hills and trails. Among the many benefits, it allowed us to reconnect. Reconnect with ourselves, each other, and humanity in an arena apart from healthcare academics, and home.

This process helps me maintain a focus on what I feel is important. If allowed to run unchecked, I would still be in a rabbit hole somewhere.

How Has the Experience Influenced Your Current Creativity?

It has shown me anyone can do anything if they have a desire to, the energy and time to commit themselves to it. Everything that I have wanted to do, I have done. I wanted to bake bread and have a bakery with my only experience being my home baking. I now bake the best bread in our city and bake more than 20 kinds of bread. I am only stopped by recognizing the need for balance in my life and the desire to keep things simple.

Describe Your Experience with Creating,…Is It a Steady Process? Episodic? Manic? Drought?

Creativity is cyclical; recognize when you're at the top of your creative cycle and accept it when you're not. Interaction with others is an important factor to facilitate your internal motivation to channel your creativity; but beware; it can also be a factor that may try to crush your creativity.

Does It Feel Like it Comes from "You" or Elsewhere?

It comes from elsewhere but is funneled, distilled, and enriched by me.

How Do You Nurture or Nurse Fledgling Ideas?

I spend a good deal of time thinking through each step and what the ultimate value and cost may be to the completed idea.

What Roles Does/Did Your Community/Colleagues ' Play in Your Creative Experience?

Positive reinforcement and facilitating decisions of expansion/contraction.

What Would You Do Differently?

Move more slowly and definitively.

WHAT'S NEXT?

It hasn't arrived.

WORDS OF WISDOM/INSPIRATION?

Observe and evaluate what you see and what is said to you and around you as you consider your creative ideas and goals. What you see and hear may represent the wisdom to change course or the inspiration to carry on. You need to be willing to heed that which you prefer to ignore; or to ignore that which you hear. But remember, your soul is here to serve somebody and that somebody may not be you.

In: Fostering Creativity in Rehabilitation
Editor: Matthew J. Taylor

ISBN: 978-1-63485-118-3
© 2016 Nova Science Publishers, Inc.

Chapter 24

THE WORK BEGINS

Matthew J. Taylor, PT, PhD

Director, Matthew J. Taylor Institute, Scottsdale, AZ, US

ABSTRACT

This chapter is an invitation to the silence that has been mentioned in so many chapters and with it, silence's effective surprise. Our western culture has been biased to "doing" first as both a value and as part of the patriarchal dominator system earlier described. The postnormal times of uncertainty hint at the wisdom of restoring balance between doing and being/silence. Following a brief discussion of this rationale, there are exercises to enact and explore silence in preparation for Chapter 25's "Domain Practices for Priming Creativity." The exercises are only a few of the many long rich traditions of human inquiry and this is not intended to be an exhaustive treatment of the topic of silence.

INTRODUCTION

"Effective surprises ... seem rather to have the quality of obviousness about them when they occur, producing a shock of recognition following which there is no longer astonishment. ...AND

The main paradox of such combinatorial creation, however, is that effective surprise is almost always followed by "the exercise of technique" — in other words, creativity requires the fusion of inspiration and technique, which appear at first to be opposite in spirit: one spontaneous, the other derived from repeated deliberate practice."

~ Jerome Bruner "On Knowing: Essays for the Left Hand" [1962]

The theory is done. The stories have been told. Now it's time to write the new chapters of how rehabilitation will continue to rehabilitate. Julie and so many others are counting on us. As we begin, remember we move forward together with our patients, no longer alone as the expert. From now on when the silence of "not knowing" arises, there is no need to hurry to fill it with activity or "certainty'. Rather, with the patient, we both pick up our brushes and begin the first small strokes onto that blank canvas. Shrouded in a spirit of exploration, compassion and deep caring….creativity emerges for us both, and in doing so, we are both healed and our lives made more *fit to live in.*

These last four chapters are a complex interwoven whole as depicted in Figure 1. Our division of these into four separate chapters is merely a linear constraint of the written word having to be ordered. Each chapter will touch the others and be frequently tied back to the rest of the text as a result. Your deliberate practice that will generate effective surprises begins now.

SPACE MAKING

Montuori and Purser (1997) wrote that the existence of alternative approaches and questions can provide an extremely useful form of self-knowledge, as we see ourselves and our assumptions questioned by the existence of different approaches. This chapter is about our clinical mastery development not just from a "head-oriented" conceptual thinking about our assumptions. These new approaches will allow us to more deeply explore our assumptions and our perspectives that are colored by those assumptions. As we explore new approaches to clinical mastery practice, we often experience reactions to our existing practices. In doing so we often define new perspectives in opposition to what was our normal way of being and acting in the world. This is the process of deconstructing, or making space, and it is the "destruction as the first step of creativity" hinted at several times now in this book. Slowly through this critical inquiry we examine each normal times brick of certainty and through the practice, literally transform our knowing and being in the world.

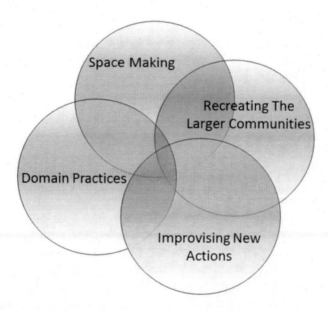

Figure 1. Action Steps to Foster Creativity.

The space making exercises are important for our small, local ordinary creativity to emerge. They take on even greater importance at the organizational level. Efforts to initiate rehabilitation practices from patient-centered or interprofessional team-based methods without taking into account the many differences between all of the parties participating are bound to fail. This is because in our culture dependence/partnership are not typically considered virtues and for Americans, surrendering independence/autonomy is considered a fate almost worse than death (Slater, 1991). If we merely view the desired conceptual collaborative practices of care as 'tools' that can be borrowed in a decontextualized manner it will be highly problematic and would reflect our North-American tendency to discount culture and historicity (Hampden-Turner & Trompenaars, 1993). This frustration will be especially evident when trying to move from the normal times "patient dependent on provider for rehabilitation expertise" to creating together with the patient as an interprofessional team.

Therefore, we begin to make space by deconstructing. There will be other deconstructing exercises in the ensuing chapters too, but these first few will begin to bring down our unseen walls of certainty. Adopting these new metaperspectives is required to correct misperceptions and bring forth new understanding to prime our creativity as both individuals and various communities. These metaperspectives will release our trap of a singular view that limits our understanding and generates at best only a partial, if not actually an inaccurate view. As Ceruti (1986, 1989) has shown so clearly, this broader awareness of complexity is tied to our shift from a normal times representational epistemology to a postnormal times epistemology of construction. In order to construct, we must hone our skill in the post-normal times to be able to deconstruct. After these deconstructions below, there will be some simple embodied practices to bring more space realized via our somatic, mental and emotional quieting practice.

EXERCISES

The Disclaimer: *As health professionals, please keep in mind your own health and contra-indications to doing any of these activities. They are all extremely gentle, but if you have any discomfort or unpleasant response to one or more of them, stop immediately and seek professional consultation before continuing.*

You can begin anywhere in these exercises. Take your time. Do the exercises vs. just reading about them. Return to them again once you have completed the book to plan what mix of practices might create your best palette to prime creativity based on your preference and goals.

Berwick's Steps

In the Preface, Donald Berwick was quoted and he later contends that in addition to the beginning of this new healthcare design being *"vastly further from the current design of care than we may at first wish it to be, or believe it to be..."* and that it must come from the inside of us, not from somewhere outside of us (Weeks, 2014). That is, we own the key to the new design and it begins with these introspective steps that include deconstruction. Get comfortable, pull out some paper to write down your answers (don't just think them), write without filtering, and most of all, have fun deconstructing reality!

1. Reconsider your view of health: what is the matter with healthcare now? What matters to you most in healthcare? What is fun? What tires you? What about health would make you spring out of bed in the morning? What part of your profession needs rehabilitation? What part could be better utilized to change health?

2. Reconsider the form and function of what you do control. What things do you do out of obligation but not inspiration? Why? Could they be done differently? Could technology, delegation or innovation change any what you do control? Dig deep into the tiniest details from how you greet colleagues first thing to how you say farewell to your most difficult patient. Pick through a mental video of your entire day, pulling out single frames and asking, what assumptions drive this behavior/technique or process? No activity is sacrosanct.

3. Take account of what tools you have beyond health care boundaries. List all the talents, passions and abilities you have that are not being utilized in your current edifice of practice. Yes, your ability to identify birds in the field, cross stitch or imitate the Simpson characters….no filters, list them all.

4. Bring systems thinking to rehabilitation. Mindmap all the systems you can think of that affect you, your work environment, your patients, their communities, etc. Just label each in a circle and start linking the circles with lines to the others, creating a huge web of the complexity of the human experience. There's nothing to do with this but keep a running tab on it over a couple weeks as you tear down and discover new ones to add to the web.

5. Re-establish faith in and use of relationship/connectedness as what matters most in healthcare. What have you been told that says otherwise? Is it true? When do you have the most reward at work? What do patients or students say mattered most to them? Who comes back to say thanks and what is it they thank you for? If you were going to be bold and audacious in your use of connectedness, what would you start doing differently tomorrow… no holds barred?

6. Remember, embrace and celebrate loving kindness. Similar to the last exercise, but also grounded in our working definition of creativity in rehabilitation being tied to compassion: for self and the other. What things do you do now that aren't rooted in loving kindness? Could they be changed and if so, how? What things are? What could you do more of to show loving kindness? Why wouldn't you? Have you surrendered control of some of this to someone or some position that doesn't warrant it? What would it feel like to exercise more from a sense of celebrating loving kindness? (For the research-evidence-only holdouts you might know, the literature says it matters for our and other's health outcomes too.)

Find an old file folder, label "Me" and put your answers in there for your eyes only. Cycle back to this exercise again when new insights emerge or real world encounters add to your lists.

Rotation of Consciousness

Assume a comfortable seated position with your back straight and supported, and your eyes closed. Your feet should be on the ground, knees slightly wider than hip-width apart, and hands resting softly on your lap or thighs. This somatic awareness exercise quiets the central nervous system while enhancing bodily perception to make space for new awareness.

Starting with your right thumb, name that body part silently to yourself "right thumb", then sense that part without moving it, then move to each finger on the right hand, wrist, forearm, etc., saying the part name silently and sensing it. From the right shoulder, head down the right side of the trunk naming rib cage, abdomen, back, front of the hip, and so forth all the way down the front of the right leg and across the toes, then back up the sole of the foot and the back of the leg name/sensing each area. Once done on the right, repeat on the left side of the body. After the left side is finished, then do the same for the right side of the head being very detailed and then the left side of the head, finishing with sensing your entire body. Rest several minutes in the silence that follows, keeping your attention directed to just feeling the soft, natural sensation of your resting breathing.

After opening your eyes, if you had any insights, emotional responses or other ideas that aren't easily categorized, jot some notes for your folder to archive the experience.

Alternate Nostril Breathing... The Balanced Breath

This simple breathing exercise can be done in the same position as the Rotation of Consciousness. Start with just 2-3 minutes of practice, and gradually add a minute every couple sessions. The breath should be natural, neither pushing or pulling the breath faster or harder. The rules are to begin with an inhalation in the left nostril, then switch to the other nostril every time you are filled with breath, and when finishing, do so on a left nostril exhalation.

- Cover right nostril with an index finger, inhale (I) left nostril.
- Switch finger to close left, exhale(E) out of right nostril.
- Inhale right, switch finger to close right nostril.
- Exhale left nostril, (E) left.
- Inhale left, switch finger to close right nostril, and so on.

After you finish, sit quietly for a couple minutes paying attention to your experience with your eyes closed. When you open your eyes, record any impressions or experiences for your folder.

Focused Breathing

- Gently rest tip of tongue on the center of the roof of your mouth.
- Mouth closed; Breathe in and out of the nose naturally without pushing or pulling the breath, keeping tongue connected but soft.

- Imagery: Imagine breathing "through" the tongue…both on the in and out breath.
- Repeat for 3-5 minutes, eyes stay soft.

After completing, record any insights or experiences you may have had for your folder.

Soham Mantra

The repetition of a sound, even just imagining the sound without audibly making it, creates deep quieting of the central nervous system. This mantra of Soham, a Sanskrit term meaning "I am that" is a simple but powerful tool for staying present to the moment. When used this way, "Soham" serves to control one's breathing pattern, to help achieve a deeper, natural breath, and to gain concentration. It also builds a thicker insula between your dorsal prefrontal cortex and limbic system...but not for this book!

- Sooooo... is the sound of inhalation, and is remembered in the mind along with that inhalation.
- Hummmm... is the sound of exhalation, and is remembered in the mind along with that exhalation.
- Repeat for 3 minutes or so. Then for one minute do only the "hummmm" on the exhale, remaining silent on the inhale.
- Then stay silent on both the inhale and exhale for one minute.

After completing, record any insights or experiences you may have had for your folder.

Guided Imagery Exercise on Inspiration (Courtesy Cheryl Van Demark)

Experience the sensations of inspiration by recalling the last time you felt inspired about anything, big or small. Take some long, slow exhales of the breath. Try a shush sound. Request your brain to access the memory of being inspired. Shush……. As you access the memory, notice the feelings and sensations of inspiration that accompany your next few inhalations of the breath. Let the physical sense of expansion of your body with your inhalations represent possibility without limitation. Notice whatever thoughts and feelings arise for you, and then watch them pass away and be replaced by new flows of thoughts and feelings. It is generally a bustling scene!

Allow your mind to wander into a pleasant state similar to a daydream, so you remain awake. Day dreams are not rushed. Enjoy yourself. Continue to notice what thoughts arise, how they pass, and what new thoughts arise as you breathe in deepening sensations of inspiration.

Direct the ever-changing thoughts and feelings into a vision of a flowing narrow stream. Release your memory of inspiration into the stream, but keep the sensations and feelings of inspiration. As the banks of the stream widen, watch the flow gradually slow.

Visualize the banks of the steam widening more until the stream becomes a pool wherein the waters slowly swirl. Look deeper into the pool, below the moving surface where the cloudy sediment settles into a clear bottom. There is no need to be anywhere or to do anything. Invite a present state of inspiration now for your creative participation in rehabilitating rehabilitation. Open the heart and mind to unlimited possibilities.

May you find your inspiration. May your inspiration serve the greatest good for all.

CONCLUSION

Now that you have begun to sweep clean some space, it is time to move on to the domain practices for priming creative mergence. These noncreative practices invite new behaviors, new anatomy and physiology in us via learning and neuroplasticity, and ultimately out of this silence, our collective future will emerge. Have fun, dabble as you are attracted and note especially those activities from which you are repelled or dismissive. Very often the resistance to a practice is a bellwether for pointing you to exactly what you should do and might most radically prime you to transform your life and the lives that you encounter in your rehabilitation practice.

REFERENCES

Ceruti, M. (1986). *Il vincolo e la possibilita`*. Milano, Italy: Feltrinelli. English Translation (1994). *Constraints and possibilities. The evolution of knowledge and knowledge of evolution.* New York: Gordon & Breach.

Ceruti, M. (1989). *La danza che crea. [The creative dance]* Milano: Feltrinelli.

Hampden-Turner, C. & Trompenaars, A. (1993). *The seven cultures of capitalism.* New York: Doubleday.

Montuori, A. & Purser, R. (1997). Le dimensioni sociali della creatività. *Pluriverso, 1,* 2, 78-88.

Slater, P. (1991). *A dream deferred. America's discontent and the search for a new democratic ideal.* Boston: Beacon.

Weeks, J. (2014). Hooking up: Don Berwick, Integrative medicine and his call for a radical shift to 'health creation'. *The Huffington Post.* Retrieved July 7, 2014 from http://www.huffingtonpost.com/john-weeks/don-berwick-integrative-m_b_4781105.html

In: Fostering Creativity in Rehabilitation
Editor: Matthew J. Taylor

ISBN: 978-1-63485-118-3
© 2016 Nova Science Publishers, Inc.

Chapter 25

DOMAIN PRACTICES TO PRIME FOR CREATIVITY

Matthew J. Taylor, PT, PhD
Director, Matthew J. Taylor Institute, Scottsdale, AZ, US

ABSTRACT

This chapter contains practical and more in-depth noncreative practices to prime for creative emergence in your life and practice. In Chapter 3, "A New Understanding of Creativity" we proposed these domain practices based on Halifax's (2012) heuristic model of compassion. This chapter offers a brief further explanation of each of the two domains of the three axes. The explanation is followed by practices that then prime for the emergence of creativity rooted in a compassionate perspective to relieve the suffering of both ourselves and the other. Each domain influences the other five and examples of what to attend to in order to experience this interconnection are provided.

INTRODUCTION

Creativity emerges out of context and experience, therefore no one can tell you how to be creative because they lack both your context and experience. So my job in this chapter is to point you toward practices that prime you to fully express your innate creativity. You will notice that many of the practices could just as well have been listed under other domains. The categorical assignments were based on somewhat artificial divisions for what are often multi-domain practices. Having said that, there are no specific directions or sequences to offer. While there are days when it would be nice to have someone just prescribe reps and intensities like training a muscle, in the long run the effective surprises of Bruner in the last chapter make it worth this effort. Pick and choose those that gain your attention and over time give each at least one try. Not to worry, your complex being will distribute the effects correctly no matter the sequence or intensity! Fortunately, the creative emergence is far more fun and fascinating than a mere prescription to follow any day.

APPLYING OUR NEW UNDERSTANDING OF CREATIVITY

Succinctly from Chapter 3, "A New Understanding of Creativity," we proposed that creativity is composed of noncreativity elements. At least three interdependent experiential modes that are nonlinear and coemergent appear to prime and optimize creativity. For us as rehabilitation professionals, they include the A/A Axis, giving rise to/= attentional and affective and primes/= mental balance; the I/I Axis, based in the cognitive domain that relates to the cultivation of intention and insight and primes/= discernment; and the E/E Axis, or embodied and engaged processes that prime/= enactive, ethical, and engaged responses to the presence of suffering, and give rise to eudaemonia (human flourishing/happiness), equanimity, and ethical grounding. Creativity emerges as a process having been primed by practices in:

1.) the attentional and affective domains,
2.) the intentional and insight domains, and,
3.) the embodied and engaged domains of subjective experience.

As such in this chapter you will discover what some of those practices are and be encouraged to construct a regular practice of them to prime your creativity. All of this takes place moment to moment in your personal adaptive, dynamic relationship between: Mind, Body and the Environment. The nature of complex being dictates that these domains can be reciprocal, asymmetrical, and also engender sense making. To elaborate on creativity's internal dynamics, creativity arises as an emergent process from the ground of these interrelated attentional, somatosensory, and cognitive processes that are embedded in and responsive to your individual context. As such these practices are then heuristic and will be different each time you practice one and discover anew the fruit of the practice as though for the first time.

EXERCISES DECONSTRUCTING CREATIVITY

The first exercises will have you deconstruct/reconstruct your current understanding of creativity. From there we will proceed to the domain practices.

Self Reflection Exercise: Describe your relationship with the concepts of creativity that you utilize right now before employing the remainder of the practices: ...

The Shifting Lens Drill: A valuable exercise is to intentionally reconstruct your understanding of creativity is through a variety of lens of perspective. In this exercise you will write what you know and also research online how others see through a kaleidoscope of perspectives on creativity to reconstruct your understanding of creativity. The first lens has been done for you and you can add to it as well.

Answer this question: Creativity in _____ is viewed as....

Evolutionary Biology: Complexity increases and the speed of adaptation increases. A coordinated response with the organism's environments is required to survive. Living things display responsiveness; nonliving things do not. Organisms transform material that is unlike itself into materials that are like it. Reproduction includes combining traits in unique new individuals and considerable time is invested in care prior to independent living. organisms have the ability to adapt to their environment through the process of evolution. During evolution, changes occur in populations, and the organisms in the population become better able to metabolize, respond, and reproduce. They develop abilities to cope with their environment that their ancestors did not have and that results in a greater variety of organisms than existed in previous eras. The environment influences the living things that it surrounds. Living things can alter their environment if the environment becomes difficult to live in. Neurophysiology of plasticity and learning...

The Visual Arts: ...
Business: ...
Music: …
Philosophy: ...
The Food Industry: …
Religions: ...
Ancient/Indigenous Healing Systems: ...
What other lens could you employ?

Updated Self Reflection Exercise: Describe how your relationship with the concepts of creativity have changed, if any after reading and reflecting on the above lens: ...

Personal Historical Creativity Reflection: Reflect on times you have felt creative in rehabilitation as a therapist, clinical supervisor, teacher or co-worker. Have you continued to practice that behavior? Did it change the way you behaved in other circumstances? How could it have been even better? ...

Discovering Holons Exercise: Any observed system is always described by an observing system. The observer's (our) operations and decisions intervene on several levels in the process of system construction. We trace, first of all, the boundary between system and environment, and establish the relationship between system and subsystem, between global dynamics and components. A system is always, at the same time, a subsystem and a suprasystem (the definition of a holon), and its dynamic is regulated by the constraints of the dynamics in which it participates, and in turn imposes constraints on the dynamics of the various subsystem components. Exercising a systemic approach sees this proliferation of scopes as a reflection of the plurality of perspectives generated in the study of a phenomenon, and generates the discovery of the polysystemic nature of systems. A systems approach therefore *problematizes* our understanding of phenomena by emphasizing their complexity, which becomes apparent when we observe the variety of relationships and interrelationships any system entails. That's a mouthful, but the more we practice observing, the more we breakdown the old simplified parts perspective of normal times and begin to build a richer, constructed picture of reality that primes our creative expression.

The exercise is to practice "seeing" the holons and listing them. For instance start with your dog: subatomic particle: atoms: molecules: compounds: cell structures: cells: tissues:

organs: dog: canines: mammals: vertebrates: animals: living things: the Earth: planets: solar system…. etc.

Get the idea? Now try: female patient with cancer; occupational therapy; depression; pizza; jokes; cell phones; and so forth…. have fun in your discoveries of the holons!

Professional Practice Deconstruction Exercise: What boundaries might you shift regarding what has historically been the scope of practice of your particular profession and what now could be said to be part of what your profession does but is either literally outside your legal scope of practice, or just not done as conventional care? And if you shifted your practice in such ways, what might be/has been the result? Shake up those holon boundaries a bit!

DOMAIN PRACTICES

Enjoy picking and choosing from the domains of our three axes of creativity. Most are simple pointers to practices easily explored, while others will have short descriptions if not readily apparent or available for learning about the practice.

ATTENTION

Noticing: Just begin to notice. Notice (pause momentarily) and ask, how did that happen? When a solution to a vexing problem comes to you. When you avoid an argument or resolve a conflict. When you utilize one of your favorite gadgets. When a patient asks a question or makes a statement and you suddenly know what to do next. Or when you don't know what to do next. When you find yourself wasting time with TV or the internet. Over and over, just notice and ask silently. The act of paying attention, pausing and reflecting are of course the bedrock of clinical mastery. I'm suggesting you merely redouble your practice of looking and asking, putting a novel demand on your nervous system to consider and filter in a way that is just a bit different than your habit. Noticing your noticing is critical behavior to move toward more experiences of ordinary and extraordinary creativity.

Sit still: For 10 minutes daily observing your breathing pattern, noticing when you get distracted from paying attention and return to the task of paying attention with a gentle smile.

Candle flame focus: Light a candle, time how long you can sustain your attention on the base of the flame before looking up at the dancing tongue or elsewhere. Keep track and improve!

Sit or walk slowly in nature: Let your entire body soften and receive the sounds, scents, touches, sights and changing sensations. Gently watch how your thoughts and breathing respond.

Dive deep into an art form: Allow yourself to fall deeply into the expression and lose track of time and surroundings on a regular basis. You don't have to be "good"…it is just for your engagement and to direct your attention from the treadmill of thought behind your eyebrows!

AFFECTIVE

RO-eMotions (Range of Emotions): Emotions affect learning, to include motor learning and pain perception. In the future screening for and identifying emotions around pain or dysfunction will be a part of almost every physical therapy evaluation. The current dominant perspective is that evaluation of the patient's emotions is limited to psychology as another discipline or to those obvious "psych-cases." Play with basic mindful emotional awareness exercises...sit slumped, what emotion is that? Sit tall and straight, what is that? Celebrate, what is that? Anger?....let me see it by your posture! Thoughts are movements. Change the thoughts, movement changes...ask any elite athlete or performing artist. By the same token, posture influences mood and mood is affected by posture. How many can you experience and then start to notice how many you every day.

Breath: Emotions Connection: Play with your breathing and watch your emotional state shift... breathe short and fast; now one long sigh; how about holding your breath?...try some more patterns and sense what happens to you emotionally. Then notice what your breath does when you act scared, happy, sexy, funny, curious, serious, ...keep going, what else? Pay attention with friends, at work, etc. It's literally everywhere!

Power dynamics exercise: From Garner's Chapter 6, list your many relationships both personal and professional and then rank them along the domination/partnership continuum. How about your relationship with yourself for various parts of your life? You and any loved ones? Between you and your patients? Now journal what those each feel like and how those feelings might shift if you altered the dynamic along the continuum. Use Chapter 26 to plan to make any changes that are inviting.

Bored Posture: Either socially or professionally, note your posture/breath when you feel bored. Alter one or both and note what happens.

Honestly answer "How are you?" when asked: When it is socially and professionally appropriate...and maybe sometimes when it isn't! See what happens...

Practice non-judgmental awareness with our "illness behavior" patients: Can you reach deep within yourself to extend compassion with the realization that this person is walking this path to receive a lesson necessary for their spiritual growth; whether or not they themselves are aware of it today? Where do any judgments that arise within you come from? Are they worth keeping?

Practice emotional body scans: Begin to notice where in your soma you experience various sensations when in different emotional states. If appropriate, invite your patients to notice and report back to you. There is always a somatic response. If you or they can't feel anything, you really need to practice this one!

Pets as teachers: If you have one or access to one, what do they teach you about your emotions? Query your patients about what and how their pets help them sense and experience their emotions. It is a very safe way to enter a deep level of rapport in the clinic.

Emotional media diet: Start paying attention to what emotions the various media you consume during the day create. Be selective and make sure it nurtures rather than depletes. Billions have been spent to excite and titillate you...possibly not in your best interest or actually adding to compassion fatigue if violent or graphic.

INTENTION

Create a between patient mindful ritual: Feel the water if you wash your hands. Say a prayer/set an intention for the former and/or next patient. Exhale more deeply three times while sensing the support of the floor beneath you.

Add some beauty to the space you spend a great deal of time in daily: Note how it shifts things. When do you stop noticing? What happens when you bring something new? What is acceptable ass beauty? Says who?

Metta meditation practice: Look it up. It is Buddhist in origin, but non-denominational to fit with any traditional spiritual practice. An embodied practice of holding yourself, loved ones and others in your heart and wishing them well. Good research demonstrating it facilitates heart rate variability and can teach compassionate behavior to pre-schoolers.

Prayer practices: The rosary, mala bead practice, tonglen practice, morning/evening prayer practices. All are great techniques for generating enhanced intentional awareness.

Explore Nonviolent Communication practices: Read and practice the exercises set forth by Marshall B. Rosenberg's organization, many of which are free. Excellent for personal and professional use.

INSIGHT

Develop mentor;mentee relationships: Be one of each. If you already, freshen up the relationship by sharing what you are learning here.

Read "Waking": Pick up a copy of Matthew Sanford's award-winning book, "Waking." What part's of how you meet your patients might be enhanced by meeting them at the mindbody level he so richly describes in the book?

Read across the disciplines: Once a month read a few short pieces from disciplines or perspectives that are very different from your own. Try to see things through their lens. What's your physical, respiratory, emotional response to the work? Any insights pertinent to your "world"?

Study and practice the insight meditation techniques: There are several and they are very low tech, easy to learn.

Research the contemplative practices: All major religions have them. Try one that matches your interests and see if there is a local group that practices.

Self study: Consider doing the various online tests such as Enneagram, Myers-Briggs, Disc personality inventory, etc. Again there often local study groups in metro areas if you are intrigued.

Explore intuition training: Not the "I can see the future" type, but along the lines described by Roth-Roemer in Chapter 21.

Read across disciplines: This bears repeating. Get out of your silos of perspective. Watch a different news channel. Read differing editorials. Stretch! You won't catch anything!

EMBODIMENT

Guided Imagery: There are plenty of free audiocasts of guided imageries online for healing. Listen to some, reflecting on your experience afterward and noting if there might be a place for such a practice in your own self care or to use professionally with your clients.

Yoga asanas/postures: study the meanings behind the names and see if you can sense it in your body.

Sex: The only reason we are all here. A huge part of being human but so misaligned over the past decades. If your sex life isn't enriching and deeply humanizing for you, there are quality highly trained and regulated professionals that can support your development of this critical part of being embodied.

Chapters 25 and 27: Both offer many more activities.

Develop a playful habit: Tumble, dance, try improve, acting, coloring, wood work, a craft...make it fun and no agenda other than to just be that little kid having fun with new crayons!

ENGAGEMENT

Teach Breath Awareness: Along the do one, teach one vein. Try it with a favorite, comfortable patient and get their feedback.

Increase the use of metaphor and images: In your personal and professional practices, intentionally increase your use of both to almost the uncomfortable level for you....note how the others respond and seek their feedback.

Do a half handstand with your feet against the wall: What was your initial response? What happened as you considered it? Did you research what I meant? Did you try? How is this like what you ask of your consumers? What would make it more comfortable for them to engage in the activity you propose?

Do the raisin mindfulness exercise: It's online. Easy to do. If you don't like raisins, a piece of chocolate work too. We have a bowl of chocolates with the exercise posted next to them. Most just gobble the candy!

Learn the basics of mindfulness and then apply it to your profession: It ain't rocket science. Someone else has probably already written about it in your profession. Try it out for yourself and your patients.

Try a new mindbody practice: Yoga, tai chi, dance, martial arts, pottery, tumbling, acrobatics, acupuncture, ...something that will be a new edge and watch all of your other domains kick in the act!

CONCLUSION

Avoid the temptation to feel overwhelmed. Remember this is a process, not an event. There is no end point to get arrive at on time. Rather, think of these practices and the ones ahead as new friends with which to develop a relationship over time. Some you will visit often, others maybe only once or occasionally. Some keys to keep in mind about these practices are to be patient, playful and to actively explore without expectation. Other helpful hints are to set a schedule with short, but regular practices. You can stick to just one or alternate between any you would like to try. , start small, reassess, find support or develop a buddy system, and take your discoveries out into new actions. The improvisation of the new actions into your world is the new riff Montuori encouraged in the Preface. We are on stage, the spotlight swings onto us, let it rip! ...and the band plays on.

REFERENCE

Halifax, J. (2012). A heuristic model of enactive compassion. *Curr Opin Support Palliat Care,* Vol 6, 2, 228-235.

In: Fostering Creativity in Rehabilitation
Editor: Matthew J. Taylor

ISBN: 978-1-63485-118-3
© 2016 Nova Science Publishers, Inc.

Chapter 26

IMPROVISING NEW ACTIONS

Matthew J. Taylor, PT, PhD
Director, Matthew J. Taylor Institute, Scottsdale, AZ, US

ABSTRACT

This chapter lists a variety of activities and experiential exercises based on the more theoretical content of Chapter 8, "The Implementation of Creativity." The Engagement/ Embodiment axis of the new understanding of creativity model is more fully experienced here as the noncreative activities that prime creative emergence. The mark of a clinical master is to have a discipline of not only acting in the workspace, but also a system of reflection, insight and then re-enacting based on that embodied reflection. Engaging in new actions in our environments is the experimentation phase. In doing so as professionals it enhances our ability to act from compassion and does so through tried and true methods, as well discovering/creating new ones of being with the patient.

INTRODUCTION

Now it is time for experimenting with the new insights discovered along the way through our domain practices and resting in silence. According to Govindarajan and Trimble in "Beyond the Idea" (2013), this is the very much harder half as described in Chapter 8, "The Implementation of Creativity." In this chapter the exercises are designed to ease the work of "chop wood and carry water" by sharpening your axe and making the carry just a bit more downhill. Taking our vision of what could be and then enacting it into the world is what gives juice to our lives. This chapter is being written on Labor Day morning. What better "labor" than for us to birth something that hasn't been before into the world?

We begin with just a short bit of supportive advice grounded in our past theoretical chapters. The remainder of the chapter is a series of exercises to make the prototyping of our vision even more fun. Think of the exercises as practicing scales are to the musician. Not our favorite, but with full understanding that with their mastery, along comes the enjoyment of riffing our improvisations all day long, delighting in the effective surprises that blossom as a result. Maestro?...tap, tap, tap...and a one, and a....

NEW ACTION EXERCISING GUIDELINES

Taking new action as rehabilitation professionals does sometimes include literally doing things quite differently than we did before. More often though, using our model of the practice domains will probably have you doing the very same movements but now in a very different frame of mind and intention. The new operating system of Chapter 3 often changes more the "how" than the "what" of our actions. Sure there will many times the "what" changes, especially as your skills of domain practice sharpen. For now however, begin to savor the subtle nuances in the "how's" that Sanford admonished us to develop in Chapter 2, "The Need for Creativity from the Patient's Perspective."

Be bold, but not obnoxious in trying on new actions. How stealth can you be? If we do this correctly, our engagement isn't to make us look good, but to transform the moment of suffering we are sharing with the other. When we boldly, but gently alter our past response, though it may be tortuous on our insides, if we sustain awareness and the intention to empower the other rather than leave them dependent as in normal times practice, we both heal.

Starting small is probably the best advice. One new action today and watch. Then repeat again the next day. Biting off too much change is difficult for our own personal system and really hard for the larger external systems to accept. You have the rest of your life to do this, remember? Like they often say about yoga, this process of creativity is slow medicine, but strong medicine. Just be sure to take some everyday.

Finally, be patient AND aggressive. Give things time to emerge, but also ruthlessly discard what your embodied perception guides you to eliminate. These are the rapid learning experiments of Chapter 8. When your regularly scheduled reappraisals show weak or no result, move on to some new action, but garner the learning that came from reflecting on the effort. Failure points us down the road, only getting us that much closer to success. So with an easy sense of humor about us not being so all important or responsible, enjoy these experiments in life!

NEW ACTION EXERCISES

Make a Workspace

Once you have read Allen's "Getting Things Done" (2002), set a time each week when you will review your week and plan the coming week. The book details the actions that are involved during this 20-30 minute review, but without this regular pause, the axe dulls and the path heads uphill in a hurry. This single recurring action will become the flywheel that fuels effective new actions for you. Like all flywheels it takes a good deal of effort to initiate the turning, but once underway it is a force to drive many innovative actions. As noted in

Chapter 24, something has to be destroyed to make room for this new weekly workspace. Be ruthless, but in a compassionate kind of way!

Capture Your Insights

Identify how you are going to capture new ideas in a fashion that let's you know you won't lose them. Again, Allen (2002) has a great variety of simple systems for this process. For those with smart phones there is the notepad app, audio recorder, email/text the idea to yourself... almost an endless variety to include the little tiny black book in your pocket or purse. Choose what fits you and start capturing. You will be surprised how quickly capturing new insights becomes a regular occurrence. It's my favorite collection!

Develop a Reliable System of Scheduling Actions Based on Embodiment

Consider this simple insight: In order to act, we move from our bodies. So? Well most planning systems don't take that fact into account. Typically you list all these "Someday I'll" goals and sub-tasks and then schedule them. What isn't generally mentioned is you have to be physically in the right circumstance to complete the action (i.e., "Buy diapers" is on Saturday but you are camping with the Girl Scouts that day). Allen's (2012) book details more, but suffice it to say, you need to plan according to where you literally are physically and what actions you can take. Driving cross-country prohibits you from "plant some herbs in the backyard" for instance. The embodied system really sharpens the axe when you utilize such a perspective. The system should also have a fail-safe way of notifying you of deadlines before it's too late to act accordingly. This also releases you from that nagging neurophysiological tension of "isn't there something I should be doing?" and creates more space per Chapter 24. This is far simpler than it sounds and Allen (2002) has great ways to do so, especially with e-mail. Did you order it yet?

Ask for Feedback on New Actions

Now that we're freed from the normal times illusion of having to be the perfect expert without flaws, there is a freedom to be appropriately vulnerable. When you have tried something new (i.e., asking a patient to share more, when in the past you might have passed a comment off as too messy to pursue) let the other person know that this was new for you and seek their response as to whether they found the new action helpful or not. Either way, ask specifically in what way it was or wasn't. This feedback process models for them new ways of behaving from vulnerability themselves and brings you both to a more peer-level, learning team model of our complex being. Use the feedback then to fuel the next round of action and enhance your clinical mastery. Who knew EBM could be so much fun?

Create an Appropriate Team to Support New Action

"Beyond the Idea" (2002) details the specifics and the process of assembling a "team" to implement new actions. Chapter 8 outlines the steps, but here in this exercise you actually sit down and plan accordingly. The first few times will of course be somewhat clumsy as a new action for you, but repetition makes it natural and often automatic. Move between the literal teams and the metaphoric teams based on the size of your project and the identified work ahead. Failure to address this basic conflict between maintaining all of the other things you or your organization do and implementing something new is almost guaranteed to create future suffering for someone. Note that when you honestly assess what team members you need to bring in, that invites the actions of establishing new relationships beyond your silo of experience...so ask for help and extend your network of contacts and interests with abandon. This new wider net of connections primes the emergence for effective surprises down the road. People want to help as a rule, so ask for the help you need as you build your team. I needed 15 contributing authors for this book and only one flat out refused, and the other who couldn't because of other commitments, sent me to someone that could. I also did the legwork of vetting those I didn't personally know by reviewing their publications for an ability to write and confirming from others that they were punctual in completing tasks. That extra bit of work building my team led to a 100% on-time completion of chapters. This will be time well spent as you build out your various implementation teams, to include just marshalling your own internal team of resources for personal projects. So get building your own "Dream Team" and I'll see you at the tournament of rehabilitation!

Become a Better Storyteller

Human beings are sense makers of reality. We tell each other stories and the best storytellers can inspire entire cultures and epochs. In the medical sciences this "lowest form of evidence" has been denigrated over the past century. However the literature is demonstrating that this is what patients' value and that good stories (a.k.a. patient narratives and our patient education stories) affect outcomes. So study the art and science of storytelling. This includes that constant story going on within yourself of course. Then begin to listen more deeply to other's stories. When appropriate, offer gentle, or not so gentle, edits of story to see how it affects behavior. When your story moves both the heart and mind of others, it will surpass any other treatment tool on your belt and give you as the Chapter 8 Innovation Superperson, new powers of rehabilitation. Every storyteller can improve. So pay close attention to how stories influence you and gain insight upon reflection on those stories. Then use that insight to enhance your stories in rehabilitation. For example, read and feel this single sentence story about empathy, "Another person's pain", Jamison (2014) writes, "registers as an experience in the perceiver: empathy as forced symmetry, a bodily echo". Powerful and visceral as you feel that echo, isn't it? Additionally, the team building in the prior exercise requires a good story too in order to sign on, and then an even better story to stay on, as the work gets underway. And, I'm telling you a story right now by the way. Has it moved you to behave differently in the future?

Act as If

I first remember hearing the title of this exercise on a Norman Vincent Peale self-help audiotape. The exercise has many related names such as "Fake it until you make it," or "See one, do one, teach one," and of course, Nike's "Just Do It™!" Inertia to change freezes us in our habits, both of mind and bodily action. We now understand by our complex being model of creativity that the E/E axis can drive the mental and vice versa. Our habit is to try to push from the mental into action. This exercise invites us to enact new actions from engagement to shift the mental, and do it sooner rather than later. If you wait to not feel dominated in a situation such as Garner describes so well in Chapter 6, you will probably never change that relationship. Courage isn't feeling no fear, but feeling the fear and acting anyway. We have our domain practices of affective attunement and insight to prime us to engage sooner in new actions (experiment?) and learn faster ala Govindarajan and Trimble (2013). The curtain draws back, time to improvise new action!

CONCLUSION

Remember this implementing new action is the harder half on innovation. You can begin to do so anyway as you relax into improvisation much like Rio describes in Chapter 17. The flywheel of change is indeed hard to initiate. But performing actions grounded in the science of change management insures more learning and better results in the uncertainty of our postnormal times. Keep a ready sense of humor along the way. We are all really pretty hilarious when viewed from a distance, just teetering between the Greek comedy and tragedy. Then watch how your internal and external worlds are transformed in the co-emergent creative process and enjoy the ride!

REFERENCES

Allen, D. (2002). *Getting things done: The art of stress-free productivity*. New York: Penguin Press.

Govindarajan, V. & Trimble, C. (2013*). Beyond the idea*. New York: St. Martin's Press.

Jamison, L. (2014). *The empathy exams: essays*. Minneapolis, MN: Graywolf Press.

In: Fostering Creativity in Rehabilitation   ISBN: 978-1-63485-118-3
Editor: Matthew J. Taylor   © 2016 Nova Science Publishers, Inc.

Chapter 27

RECREATING THE LARGER REHABILITATION COMMUNITY: SMALL OFFICES TO INSTITUTIONS

Matthew J. Taylor, PT, PhD
Director, Matthew J. Taylor Institute, Scottsdale, AZ, US

ABSTRACT

This final chapter offers suggestions on how our behaviors and practices are literally no longer isolated events, but inextricably woven into the larger community. The lone genius myth not only wrongly stated the source of creativity arose from the individual, but it also limited the story of our power to a small radius of influence except in the rare case of such a genius. We now understand that in order to be truly creative, the creative action must influence reality beyond the individual creator. As the new research attests, compassion and altruistic behavior are not just traits, but skills that can be trained and enhanced. We are powerful as a social species, so we can and do influence those around us to ignite ever expanding circles of emergence in Bruner's effective surprises throughout our various communities. The embodied techniques used by organizational development leaders are included as well as strategies used to influence health workers' behavior in institutions. The chapter concludes with action lists for leaders.

INTRODUCTION

"Go to the people. Live with them. Learn from them. Love them. Start with what they know. Build with what they have. But with the best leaders, when the work is done, the task accomplished, the people will say, 'We have done this ourselves."

—Attributed to Lao Tzu

"Simplicity is the key that unlocks the blocks to creativity in individuals and organizations. If you adopt a practice of cultivating creativity, then because you are part of the system, the system becomes more creative..."

It is that simple. This isn't some New Age thinking or Eastern koan, but the summation of Peter Senge, director of the Center for Organizational Learning at MIT. He stated,

"What is most systemic is most local....that's why personal cultivation is so important." - (Senge et al., 2004).

Whether you are a solo practitioner or the director of a national rehabilitation chain, our times necessitate you enhance the creativity of your area of professional rehabilitation. For this chapter we will reference you as the director for simplicity sake, no matter the size of your operation. To affect change and the expression of creativity in your sphere of influence will require new behaviors, but hopefully the two quotes above offer some solace for you. The postnormal times management of today actually reaches back to Lao Tzu's pre-pre normal times philosophy. Done properly your group will have created a better service and sense they did it themselves. The two quotes from "Presence" emphasize simplicity and the importance of personal practice. Chapters 24-26 have shared those techniques already. So let's set some larger context briefly, lightly review some theory regarding organizational creativity, and finish with a few more practices.

THE CONTEXT OF ORGANIZATIONAL CREATIVITY

So what are the hallmarks of the creative individual and organization? I am afraid they probably do not match the checklist of the optimal employee or department! Barron (1990) listed these as some of the characteristics for the individual, but they apply to organizations as well:

1. Independence of judgment
2. Tolerance for ambiguity
3. Moves from polarizations and oppositional thinking (either/or) to complex paradoxical thinking (both/and)
4. Androgyny (clarity on gender attributes and roles to include assertiveness, goal acquisition, nurturing and tolerance of flexible time concepts)
5. Preference for complexity of outlook, asymmetry over symmetry, and easy movement between order and disorder.

Yet, aren't these the tensions we face every day: quality care in a hurry; compassionate but firm boundaries; follow the protocol but the customer is always right, etc.? "I'm not sure....Could be...Maybe...just get it done somehow" are not the usual answers supervisors, peers, subordinates or patients are seeking. We human beings crave certainty and security, but is that something you as a director can realistically provide? We can no more proclaim certainty of clinical outcomes to the new poly-trauma patient on the ward then we can in response to subordinates' questions about funding for continuing education next year. Can we balance being firm in issuing notice about benefit cutbacks AND at the same time be compassionate and nurturing when the anger is directed back at us as bearers of the news? We know the 21st century rehabilitation director cannot afford to be disingenuous by feigning toughness and surety when it does not exist. Our associates are too savvy and too well connected for that type of rigid, rote leadership to last long. How then do you break free of old patterns and habits to adopt creative characteristics and still keep your job? Barron (1990) stated, "In the creative process there is an incessant dialectic and an essential tension between two seemingly opposed dispositional tendencies: the tendency toward structuring and integration and the tendency toward disruption of structure and diffusion of energy and attention." It is awareness of this tension of opposites that once appreciated and sustained can shift our perspectives and crack open creative insight for ourselves and our departments. It is also related to the tension between sustaining ongoing operations and implementing new activities in Chapters 8 and 26.

The good news is Barron goes on to state that the central idea to understanding creative ecosystems is that, "Simplicity leads to complexity before a new and more elegant simplicity can be achieved." That sentence bears rereading several times. The keys are 'ecosystem' and 'simplicity'. As we discussed in Chapter 3, the myth of the lone creative genius is just that, a myth (Barron, 1990; Collins, 2001; Gladwell, 2008). Creativity occurs within systems and is a systems effect. That would seem to take the pressure off of us as individuals because it's the system's fault, until we remember "we are the systems!" Darn, this creativity stuff is like being in a perpetual Zen master's presence. Not to worry though, the second word was 'simplicity.'

For those seeking a more technical and detailed exploration, I would recommend Scharmer's "Theory U" (2007) and his latest, "Leading from the Emerging Future," (Scharmer & Kaufer, 2013). These works offer great theoretical examination of the complexity involved in large scale change and creativity. They also offer inspiring examples of how this is already working which is a contrast to the steady stream of bad news usually inundating our director's inbox.

Let's repeat. Simplicity is the key that unlocks the blocks to creativity in individuals and organizations. If you adopt a practice of cultivating creativity, then because you are part of the system, the system becomes more creative. It is that simple. Of course a personal cultivation of creativity is a simple practice that can be very difficult to sustain! Allow me to give you a simple recipe to follow, and then we will break down the ingredients so you can get your creative juices cooking right now.

The Creativity Recipe: Marry over time and in silence: 1 part Suspension of Assumptions/Judgments; 1 part Awareness and Suspension of the Emotional Palette; 1 part Visioning Your Best Possible Future; and, 1 part Resiliency and Persistence. Season with passion and sprinkle in plenty of robust humor.

Suspension of Assumptions/Judgments: As directors it is our responsibility to creatively direct and lead. Can you say out loud and with conviction, "I am creative!"…try it. Did you mean it? What else did you 'hear' in saying it? That's why the silence is important. In your practice, say 10 minutes per day, in complete silence, develop the skill of observing your self judgments and assumptions about the situation you want to solve creatively. When working in a group, cultivate the ability to step back as a group and ask in silence, what are our assumptions about this situation? The exercise can yield new perspectives and previously unrealized barriers. The difficult part is both you and any group you lead has to be OK with the discomfort of being silent and 'listening,' as our cultural judgment is silent introspection is synonymous with doing nothing or wasting time. Studies suggest otherwise and the act of setting aside for the moment these assumptions and judgments, to include "I am not creative", is the essential first step in the process of cultivating creativity.

Awareness and Suspension of the Emotional Palette: Simultaneously in the silence you will discover this second ingredient presents as an immediate and often varied set of emotional responses about the situation. The recipe requires those involved to note the various emotional experiences tied to the situation. Note them all, from anger, frustration, grief to joyful exuberance, and then simply set them aside for the time being. As a systems process the emotions themselves will generate new insights around the first ingredient, and those insights new emotions, and so forth in a recursive cyclical system. Become aware and suspend. This 'doing nothing' gets very busy fast!

Visioning Your Best Possible Future Situation: After allowing the first two ingredients to stew, there usually comes a natural stillness or quieting. At this point you ask yourself /the group to envision in great detail what the best possible future situation would look like. No limits and any judgments, assumptions or emotions are to cycle back into the awareness and suspension category. Just allow the best to come forward. There may not be big a-hah's at that precise moment, but the practice seems to open the door to more frequent fresh insights and perspectives at the most surprising times. "Trust the process" becomes the creative cook's mantra.

Resiliency and Persistence: The first three ingredients generate an alchemy of insight and renewed zeal to take what seemed to have been hopeless disorder and begin to apply small shifts in dealing with the situation. What comes forward is a willfulness driven by a clear passion based on that spark that started you into your rehabilitation career in the first place. That spark is a love for being of service, being in meaningful relationship, and making a useful contribution. Senge (2004) wrote, "When we are used as an instrument to serve something other than life, we lose our feelings and our capacities to sense. We just go through the motions." This practice restores the flames of what we care most about and motivates us to act. It also fosters a freedom to laugh again at the absurdity of the many situations life presents to us both at work and at home.

Recipe Disclaimer: Step out of the kitchen if you don't want to change now. This simple recipe has changed individual lives for thousands of years and is this moment changing Fortune 100 companies (Senge et al., 2004; Scharmer, 2007). This process is what led me to move to a competitive metropolitan market and open a private PT practice where I didn't have a single referral source, had never billed insurance, and have no physical therapy equipment in the practice, save an old ultrasound unit. I thought I could have a busy practice with no modalities and some empty rooms! (and I do.)

That best future will continue to emerge for us on a daily basis. Greater yet then my local practice results is the fact that I took these ideas to the Courage Center of Minneapolis MN as I report below where I led research that demonstrated an entire organization can be more creative and a become a more fulfilling place to work as a full-service, multiple facilities, in and outpatient rehabilitation center. Every parameter we examined yielded statistically significant positive results.

THE COURAGE STUDY

In 2008, Matthew Sanford and I led a two year study at the Courage Center Rehabilitation facility in Golden Valley, MN (Flynn & Olson, 2009). Rather than just teach providers yoga, I suggested we try some of these embodied creativity domain practices to see if we might affect the consciousness and creativity of the entire organization. Utilizing a collaborative inquiry methodology, we worked with all levels of the organization inviting them to a daily practice of simple awareness combining mindfulness, restorative yoga postures, Theory U and corporate narrative work. The results were encouraging and presented at a national rehabilitation conference in 2010. Unfortunately the '08 economic downturn exhausted funding and the research had to be terminated. In addition to the many positive benefits for the staff and the transference of behavior to patients, we also discovered that when the domain practice are utilized in an organization, there must be adaptations by the institution. When the individual members began to sense across their entire being, it also gives them a voice for change. This results in participants speaking up for what isn't healthy and demanding change from their discoveries within the practice. While the changes were accepted at some levels, other times members discovered their need to change employment and in one instance, career. Leaders need to appreciate that creativity enhancement is not just keeping the troops calm, but a powerful igniter of change that often includes destruction of the status quo along the way as part of the growth. Now for some personal practices for you as a director.

PRACTICES FOR DIRECTORS

The following are activities to explore that others have found helpful in directing. Use them as they appeal to you or simply try one a week.

Finding the Fire in Your Mission

- Do you really expect your patients and staff to change if you won't?
- Commit to *a* program of personal growth through a mindbody practice…this is applied neuroplasticity.
- Don't look to the herd for ideas
- Look inside…daily
- Meet and get to know: Judgment, Cynicism and Fear in your personal self talk.
- Take the media junk food out of your "diet": TV, radio, news, net, & neighbors.
- You can sleep when you're dead…this is hard work…or could it be play?

Fostering New Relationships

- Identify your needs and passions…what wakes you up happy with ideas at 3 a.m.?
- Do yours match those in your practice?
- Do you get pulled to work or pushed?
- How are you at failing?...is it OK?
- When's the last time you did something that really bombed?
- If nothing has bombed, was there ever a risk?

- When did an associate last take a risk or offer to take a risk?

5 Action Steps

1. Make space for creative thinking after body-based practice
2. Repeat step # 1 daily
3. Monthly breakfast/lunch with a mastermind colleague(s).
4. Write clear, measurable goals: i.e., One new PT service in place by 010116
5. Volunteer your service somewhere meaningful.
6. Create Accountability: ...Hire a business coach if you are serious.
7. *Hey...that's 6 steps! ....get used to it...the baker's dozen is the new standard.*

Finding the Resources

- Life's short...get professional help on your team per Chapter 8.
- Reward innovation/systems enhancements immediately upon demonstrated effectiveness.
- Focus and stay on message...over and over and over
- Eliminate what doesn't feed you...people, programs and patients...that's what makes the new space.
- Tell your story to who will ever stand still.
- Meet with your mentor (s).
- Be fearless and don't be so serious.
- Ask for help...from patients, friends, colleagues

Those are but a few actions, but incorporated with the others, should be more than enough to get you and your organization underway to new creativity. Come back over and over to the silence. That was the results we found in Minnesota and that I hear from those I consult with around the country. Silence first. Doing arises out of that silence.

CONCLUSION

Consciousness is said to be our next frontier. As directors we can be well positioned to lead such an exploration not just within the individual, but the consciousness of human institutions. It is incumbent for us as the vanguard of bringing creativity into institutions that we quicken the pace of our own evolution, broadening our context to match our culture and our skills to include those touched on above. The benefits for the individual, institution and greater community are all in great need right now. The same fervor that fueled our early rehabilitation study now needs to spread into becoming culturally competent to discover and deliver practices that incorporate the best of the above practices and also create innovative systems of delivery not even imagined today. How do we do this? Within the complexity of our circumstance lies the simplicity of the of modern day organizational change: we practice daily. Again, Senge wrote in response to the question of how do we change organizational consciousness, "What is most systemic is most local....that's why personal cultivation [practice] is so important." (Senge et al., 2004). It is that simple. This is our charge to step up and foster the next unfoldment of this art and science of rehabilitation we have dedicated our lives to sharing. We stand on the shoulders of the great professionals, only to become the shoulders for the next generations to climb upon. Have fun rehabilitating rehabilitation!

REFERENCES

Barron, F. (1995). *No rootless flower: An ecology of creativity: Perspectives on creativity research*. Creskill, NJ: Hampton Press.

Collins, J. (2001). *Good to great: Why some companies make the leap... and others don't*. NewYork: Harper Collins.

Flynn, N. & Olson, N. (2009). "New Age" Solutions to Age Old Problems in Rehabilitation: Staff Retention and Stress Reduction Notes from presentation, AMRPA, San Antonio, TX Oct. 2009.

Gladwell, M. (2008). *Outliers: The story of success*. Boston: Little, Brown and Co.

Scharmer, O. (2007). *Theory U: Leading from the future as it emerges*. Boston: SOL.

Scharmer, C. O. & Kaufer, K. (2013). Leading from the emerging future: From ego-system to eco-system economies. San Francisco, CA: Berrett-Koehler Publishers.

Senge, P., et al. (2004). *Presence: Human purpose and the field of the future*. Cambridge, MA: SOL.

Editor's Contact Information

Matthew J. Taylor, PT, PhD
Scottsdale AZ Founder and Director
Matthew J. Taylor Institute
10213 N. 92nd Street Suite 102
Scottsdale, AZ 85258
E-mail: matthew@matthewjtaylor.com

INDEX

#

20th century, x, 23, 67
21st century, ix, x, xi, 23, 41, 67, 82, 86, 107, 258
9/11, 153

A

abuse, 50, 157
academia, xiv, 13, 59, 60, 61, 62, 64, 65, 66, 67, 68, 69, 148, 150, 189, 190
access, 4, 16, 17, 37, 49, 53, 76, 77, 80, 92, 95, 96, 97, 139, 156, 157, 191, 199, 200, 223, 225, 227, 240, 247
accessibility, 12
accountability, 76, 84, 230
accounting, 32, 157, 201
accreditation, 62, 63, 64, 68, 151
action research, 53
actuality, 181
acupuncture, 68, 120, 124, 209, 249
adaptation(s), xv, 10, 51, 130, 245, 261
ADHD, 139
administrators, 64, 142, 147
adulthood, 129, 140
adults, 16, 125
advancement, 5, 9, 15, 49
advocacy, 82
aesthetic(s), 27, 35
affective, 37, 38, 39, 41, 104, 105, 107, 108, 218, 244, 255
affirming, 126, 180
age, x, xvi, 5, 32, 45, 48, 80, 95, 120, 127, 132, 134, 137, 138, 140, 142, 151, 180, 212, 216
ageing population, 128
agencies, 64

aggression, 74
AIDS, 120, 121, 126
alternative medicine, 126
alternative treatments, 72
altruistic behavior, 39, 257
American culture, 6
amputation, 117
amygdala, 149
anatomy, xi, 39, 41, 128, 135, 192, 199, 230, 241
ancestors, 245
anger, 134, 207, 218, 225, 258, 260
ankles, 20
anorexia, 154, 155
antagonism, 29
anus, 209
anxiety, 142, 147, 149, 155, 194, 212, 216
appetite, 97
appointments, 84
aptitude, 24
arithmetic, 61
arousal, 38
artery, 185
articulation, xvi, 23
aspiration, 34
assertiveness, 74, 258
assessment, 7, 25, 49, 126, 127, 132, 135
asymmetry, 9, 35, 258
asymptomatic, 131, 132
athletes, 187, 188, 194
atmosphere, 75, 81, 206, 209
atoms, 245
attachment, 38
attentional, 37, 38, 244
attitudes, 3, 74, 171, 212
audition, 176
authenticity, 81, 194
authority, 49, 210, 211, 230

autism, 137, 139

autonomy, 6, 8, 10, 38, 80, 115, 147, 209, 237

avoidance, 38

awareness, xviii, 7, 15, 16, 19, 20, 28, 29, 30, 31, 32, 37, 38, 48, 55, 92, 93, 94, 96, 98, 103, 127, 156, 158, 177, 191, 198, 209, 210, 218, 219, 237, 239, 247, 248, 252, 259, 260, 261

axes, 17, 35, 36, 37, 38, 39, 40, 43, 100, 105, 243, 246

axiology, 33

axis, 17, 36, 37, 38, 39, 102, 103, 251, 255

B

back pain, 73, 103, 122, 129, 131, 198, 223, 225

banks, 240

bargaining, 134

barriers, 30, 38, 76, 80, 89, 145, 259

base, xi, xiv, xvi, 13, 18, 31, 34, 37, 48, 72, 78, 90, 198, 227, 246

behaviorists, 141

behaviors, xvii, 9, 10, 12, 13, 38, 41, 42, 55, 56, 81, 91, 101, 102, 108, 157, 207, 210, 241, 257, 258

benefits, xiii, 106, 114, 156, 173, 190, 192, 231, 261, 263

Bhutan, 171

bias, 3, 6, 8, 49

Bible, 96

Big Bang, 42

biomechanics, 128, 135, 192

biomedical paradigm, 73

birds, 220, 238

births, 72

bisociation, 9

blame, 12, 63, 105

blank canvas, xiii, 13, 26, 57, 108, 236

blends, 106

blind spot, 8, 31, 56, 92, 96, 98

blogs, 5, 54, 227

blood, 202

blood flow, 202

blueprint, 86

body image, 156

bonds, 182

bone(s), 35, 37, 38, 39, 103, 127, 128, 129, 130, 131, 132, 133, 135, 217

bone marrow, 217

bone marrow transplant, 217

bone mass, 127, 130, 132, 133

boredom, 42

bounds, 91

bowel, xiii

brain, 9, 12, 25, 27, 28, 37, 42, 83, 95, 98, 139, 141, 149, 156, 190, 193, 195, 219, 220, 225, 240

brain activity, 25, 42

brain imagery, 9

brainstorming, xvi, 7, 26, 34, 43

breakdown, 245

breast cancer, 124

breathing, 6, 56, 189, 201, 220, 239, 240, 246, 247

Buddhism, 225

bulimia, 155

bullying, 84

burn, 103, 133

burnout, x, 12, 51, 119, 123, 134, 161

business model, 51, 155

businesses, 153, 176, 227

Butcher, 85

C

cancer, 120, 121, 122, 124, 215, 227, 246

capitalism, 45, 76, 241

care model, 51

caregivers, 15, 16, 18, 19, 20, 46, 72, 185

caricature, 207

cascades, 134

case studies, 199

case study, 105, 129

cash, 104, 133, 201

casting, 28

catalyst, xiv, 13, 48, 90

catharsis, 181

catheter, 215

cattle, 167

causality, 30, 31, 54, 104

causation, 92

cell phones, 246

central nervous system, 95, 239, 240

cerebral cortex, 156

cerebral palsy, 129

certainty, x, 9, 10, 23, 28, 49, 50, 57, 67, 69, 236, 237, 258

certification, 133, 156, 198

challenges, xiii, xiv, xv, xvii, 4, 13, 23, 24, 28, 35, 43, 47, 48, 53, 54, 79, 82, 94, 104, 113, 119, 122, 129, 131, 137, 138, 139, 140, 144, 147, 148, 149, 161, 168, 172, 176, 187, 188, 200, 202, 203, 205, 206, 207, 216, 217, 229

Chamber of Commerce, 227

chaos, 45, 54, 107, 120, 181, 183, 205, 207, 209, 210

checks and balances, 76

chemotherapy, 124

Chicago, 45

childcare, 184

childhood, 52, 141, 149, 153, 211
children, 75, 86, 95, 103, 104, 106, 122, 124, 125, 138, 141, 149, 168, 172, 178, 184, 207, 212
China, 120
chopping, 100
chronic diseases, 82, 121, 122
chronic illness, 89, 96, 126, 224
cities, 122, 157, 158
citizenship, 79, 80
City, 98, 130, 157, 169
civilization, 8
clarity, 9, 37, 97, 107, 108, 120, 144, 195, 199, 258
classes, 60, 64, 154, 162, 163, 197, 198, 202, 203, 227
classification, 34, 206
classroom, xviii, 81, 101, 116, 125, 140, 141, 172, 177
clients, 79, 101, 114, 117, 137, 138, 139, 140, 141, 142, 143, 144, 153, 162, 176, 179, 181, 182, 184, 188, 189, 190, 191, 193, 195, 205, 206, 207, 208, 209, 210, 249
climate, 36, 188
climate change, 36
clinical application, 36
clinical interventions, 40
clinical judgment, 138
clinical mastery, xv, 4, 7, 8, 13, 25, 26, 27, 30, 31, 32, 38, 41, 42, 47, 49, 51, 54, 55, 56, 57, 63, 91, 94, 106, 119, 207, 236, 246, 253
Clinical Prediction Rules, 50
clinical trials, 28, 116, 122
clothing, 157, 227
coaches, 189, 227
Cochrane Collaboration, 49
coding, 19
coffee, 168
cognition, 35, 39, 137
cognitive dimension, 38
cognitive dissonance, 55
cognitive flexibility, 144
cognitive perspective, 38
cognitive process, 244
collaboration, xvi, 10, 26, 43, 49, 71, 73, 77, 81, 82, 83, 84, 113, 144, 185, 201, 205, 206
collage, 163
collective unconscious, 164, 166
collectivism, 32
college campuses, 61
college students, 45, 95, 177
colleges, 61, 62, 159, 188
collisions, 9
color, 27, 157, 163, 167
coma, 15, 177

communication, 46, 56, 79, 96, 137, 139, 140, 141, 180, 193, 205, 208, 209
communication skills, 56, 139, 140
communication systems, 138
communities, xiv, xvii, 71, 79, 82, 85, 121, 139, 157, 158, 194, 195, 205, 237, 238, 257
community, xi, xvii, 6, 23, 30, 32, 47, 52, 53, 65, 78, 79, 82, 86, 102, 121, 122, 141, 142, 143, 145, 151, 152, 153, 155, 158, 168, 176, 177, 181, 182, 183, 187, 188, 194, 198, 199, 200, 219, 227, 231, 257, 263
community support, 121, 158
compassion, 12, 23, 27, 33, 34, 35, 38, 39, 41, 45, 51, 55, 63, 74, 76, 78, 92, 93, 94, 97, 99, 104, 105, 106, 109, 120, 122, 178, 180, 201, 206, 208, 211, 216, 220, 224, 236, 238, 243, 247, 250, 251, 257
compensation, 12, 18
competition, 26, 43, 74, 81, 167, 179, 188
competitors, 100
compilation, 49
complement, 24
complex being, 28, 30, 31, 33, 35, 36, 38, 40, 41, 102, 243, 244, 253, 255
complexity, x, 9, 11, 28, 29, 30, 31, 32, 33, 41, 45, 47, 50, 53, 55, 104, 142, 147, 182, 205, 217, 237, 238, 245, 258, 259, 263
composers, 178
compounds, 206, 245
comprehension, 216
compression, 127, 128, 129, 130
compression fracture, 127, 128, 129, 130
computer, 27, 43, 107, 220
conception, 17
conceptualization, 18
conditioning, 6, 38, 73, 74, 85, 95
conference, 87, 102, 106, 189, 215, 261
configuration, 31
conflict, 43, 83, 100, 105, 106, 107, 108, 149, 246, 254
conformity, 9, 12
connectivity, xviii
consciousness, xviii, 16, 44, 92, 152, 180, 212, 261, 262
construction, 28, 104, 237, 245
constructivism, 25, 27, 33
consulting, 153, 217
consumers, ix, 10, 51, 224, 249
consumption, 52, 90
continuing education, xiv, 3, 68, 69, 131, 132, 202, 203, 258
controlled trials, 82
controversial, 131

convention, 25
conversations, ix, 124, 205, 208, 211, 212
conviction, 259
cooking, 143, 259
cooperation, 215
COPD, 132
coping strategies, 123, 161
correlation, 49, 190
cortex, 156
cost, 11, 48, 76, 77, 97, 148, 207, 227, 230, 232
counseling, 154, 207
Courage Center, 106, 260, 261
course content, 161
creative abilities, 79
creative potential, 72, 74, 76, 79, 80
creative process, xiv, xvii, 8, 9, 43, 45, 57, 71, 89,
    90, 93, 94, 122, 144, 149, 151, 165, 166, 168,
    178, 181, 182, 197, 205, 208, 209, 219, 220, 255,
    259
creative thinking, 144, 145, 227, 262
creatives, x, 9, 180
creep, 43
critical thinking, 51, 69
critical value, 17
criticism, 163, 166, 181
crop, 157
crossing over, 108
C-section, 72
CT, 82
cultivation, 34, 35, 81, 93, 244, 258, 259, 263
cultural beliefs, 76
cultural competence, 71
cultural differences, 6
cultural tradition, 32
cultural transformation, 79, 83, 85
culture, xvi, xviii, 6, 7, 8, 12, 45, 57, 73, 74, 79, 80,
    83, 86, 101, 120, 125, 137, 179, 184, 206, 211,
    212, 231, 237, 263
cure, 120
current limit, 3, 32, 47
curriculum, 61, 62, 68, 119, 123, 138, 139, 140, 141,
    143, 148, 149, 150, 151, 152, 221
customers, 100
cycles, 36, 37, 199

D

dance(s), xiii, 38, 44, 56, 106, 107, 167, 171, 181,
    184, 185, 206, 211, 212, 217, 227, 241, 249
dancers, 167, 168
danger, 121
dark matter, 40
data gathering, 50

data processing, 53
database, 49
deconstruct, 74, 141, 237, 244
deconstruction, 28, 238
deficit, 231
dehumanization, 72
delirium, 215
dementia, 175, 183, 185
demonstrations, 89
denial, 94, 134
Department of Education, 70
depression, xiii, 149, 155, 184, 215, 246
depth, 11, 51, 79, 190, 243
derivatives, 9
despair, 124, 184
destruction, 13, 103, 108, 236, 261
developmental process, 10
deviation, 10
devolution, 89
dichotomy, 17, 48
diet, 247, 261
diffusion, 259
digital television, 56
dignity, 4, 11
directives, 76
directors, x, 259, 262
disability, 16, 95, 120, 171
disclosure, 205
discomfort, 31, 142, 202, 237, 259
discrimination, 84, 85, 121
disease rate, 82
diseases, 67, 123
disorder, 42, 45, 154, 155, 156, 157, 158, 159, 231,
    258, 260
disorienting dilemma, 54
disposable income, 155
distance education, 80
distress, 213
distribution, 17
diversity, 29, 31, 41, 95, 104
doctors, 10, 16, 17, 18, 77, 80, 209
domain practices, 55, 100, 102, 103, 105, 108, 241,
    243, 244, 251, 255, 261
dominator, xvi, 50, 74, 76, 77, 81, 82, 83, 84, 235
drawing, 52, 162, 163, 165, 166, 227
dream, 14, 134, 135, 163, 164, 165, 166, 167, 168,
    169, 199, 200, 241
drought, 162, 166
drugs, 5
DSM, 139
dynamic systems, 34
dynamism, 36
dysregulated, 37

E

earthquakes, 89
Easter, 95
eating disorders, 154, 155, 156, 157, 158
EBM, xiv, xvi, 11, 13, 27, 31, 39, 42, 44, 47, 48, 49, 50, 51, 52, 53, 54, 55, 56, 57, 63, 97, 253
ecology, 14, 44, 45, 263
economic downturn, 261
economic systems, 93
economics, 86
ecosystem, 93, 96, 259
education, ix, xiv, 3, 10, 11, 12, 13, 33, 43, 44, 60, 61, 62, 64, 67, 68, 69, 70, 80, 81, 83, 85, 86, 87, 97, 131, 132, 135, 147, 148, 158, 176, 179, 184, 190, 192, 194, 202, 203, 211, 216, 218, 224, 254, 258
education reform, 81
educational experience, 61
educational programs, 65
educational system, 67, 184
educators, 52, 141, 143
effective surprises, 236, 243, 252, 254, 257
effort level, 220
egalitarian, 78, 80
elaboration, 79
electives, 148
elementary school, 139
e-mail, 91, 253
embodied, xviii, 13, 15, 34, 35, 37, 39, 41, 43, 52, 55, 56, 69, 102, 103, 105, 107, 108, 237, 244, 248, 249, 251, 252, 253, 257, 261
emergency, 72
emergent, 30, 31, 34, 42, 99, 244, 255
emotion, 178, 191, 225, 247
emotional experience, 260
emotional reactions, 37
emotional responses, 6, 239, 260
emotional state, 191, 247
empathy, 37, 39, 51, 55, 63, 66, 67, 74, 78, 93, 104, 123, 181, 224, 254, 255
emphysema, 227
employees, ix, 102, 145, 201, 230
employment, 200, 261
enact, xiv, 35, 39, 41, 102, 105, 235, 255
encouragement, 6, 154, 164, 177, 212
endurance, xvi, 121, 134, 192
end-users, 51
enemies, 211
energy, 20, 89, 90, 91, 93, 96, 98, 124, 133, 157, 158, 164, 166, 173, 184, 200, 201, 202, 209, 210, 212, 217, 223, 224, 225, 227, 232, 259

engaged, 4, 11, 17, 18, 35, 37, 40, 56, 83, 96, 102, 182, 244
England, xi
environment(s), xv, xvi, 4, 12, 30, 31, 34, 36, 39, 42, 56, 57, 79, 80, 84, 91, 92, 93, 99, 132, 134, 138, 139, 142, 147, 148, 163, 166, 172, 173, 200, 207, 208, 209, 210, 216, 223, 225, 245, 251
environmental influences, 40
epidemic, 82, 122, 134
epidemiology, 49, 58
epigenomics, 40
epistemology, 7, 11, 27, 28, 29, 32, 33, 237
equilibrium, 35
equipment, 103, 121, 223, 260
equity, 76, 83
erosion, 230
essence, xv, 18, 91, 120, 126, 163, 195, 227, 231
ethics, 38, 39, 43, 80, 132, 205, 208
Europe, 5, 60, 61
everyday life, x
evidence, ix, xvi, 9, 11, 24, 25, 34, 35, 47, 48, 49, 50, 51, 52, 53, 55, 57, 58, 64, 72, 73, 82, 87, 122, 128, 133, 134, 137, 138, 140, 145, 147, 152, 189, 223, 238, 254
evidence-based medicine, xvi, 25, 47, 48, 58, 73
evolution, xiii, xiv, 13, 14, 31, 44, 48, 74, 144, 151, 152, 207, 241, 245, 263
examinations, 8
exclusion, 25, 28
execution, xvii, 99
executive function, 139
executive functioning, 139
exercise, 24, 25, 26, 48, 50, 54, 56, 73, 97, 107, 114, 120, 122, 126, 127, 128, 129, 131, 132, 133, 134, 135, 149, 150, 151, 164, 165, 168, 169, 180, 189, 194, 224, 227, 229, 235, 238, 239, 244, 245, 247, 249, 254, 255, 259
expertise, 11, 26, 29, 42, 49, 52, 55, 57, 77, 81, 87, 135, 237
exposure, 54, 155
extensor, 129

F

Facebook, 194
facial expression, 225
faculty, 59, 60, 61, 62, 64, 65, 66, 67, 68, 129, 148, 150, 190
faith, 177, 193, 199, 216, 218, 222, 238
families, 20, 60, 61, 77, 78, 121, 137, 138, 148, 156, 157, 172, 205, 209, 212
family income, 227
family life, 18, 102

family members, 77, 120, 123, 167, 178
family therapy, 155
fear(s), 4, 20, 40, 55, 81, 84, 90, 97, 101, 134, 144,
    160, 179, 184, 206, 212, 216, 217, 218, 221, 225,
    255
feelings, 16, 77, 149, 165, 173, 240, 247, 260
femininity, 76
ferret, 7
fights, 80
filters, 238
financial, 5, 12, 51, 74, 76, 100, 134, 171, 201, 206,
    212, 227
fine arts, 63, 179
fine tuning, 227
fires, 89, 96
fitness, 102, 197, 227
flame, 99, 184, 185, 246
flaws, 253
flex, 133
flexibility, 7, 12, 137, 138, 188, 197, 205
flooding, 139, 164
floods, 89
flourishment, 105
flowers, 165, 211, 212
fluid, x, 15, 24, 25
food, xvii, 154, 156, 159, 166, 173, 225, 261
force, 47, 61, 104, 120, 122, 159, 189, 206, 252
forecasting, 48
foreign language, 215
formal education, 69, 141, 177
formula, 181
foundations, ix, 7
fractures, 132, 133, 134
France, 231
freedom, 6, 33, 65, 91, 98, 123, 126, 134, 178, 188,
    189, 200, 206, 209, 210, 224, 253, 260
freedom of choice, 6, 33
freezing, 156
Freud, xi
friendship, 173, 176, 205
fruits, 135
functional MRI, 96
funding, 4, 33, 70, 121, 122, 176, 208, 258, 261
funds, 103
fusion, 227, 235

G

Ganesha, 30, 105
GDP, 76
gender differences, 33
gender equity, 74
generative learning, 12

genitals, 209
genomics, 51
geometry, 61
Gestalt, 218
gifted, 139, 140, 182
ginger, 71
global economy, 86
global scale, 95
goal-setting, 107
God, 26, 217
GPA, 62, 63, 67
GPS, 44
grades, 65
graduate program, 63
graduate students, xiv, 62, 119, 123, 126
grants, 66, 115, 121
grass, 11, 179
grassroots, 16, 213
Greeks, 90
grounding, 20, 38, 39, 164, 172, 244
group interactions, 8
group therapy, 207
growth, xiii, 50, 61, 70, 121, 144, 148, 153, 162,
    164, 165, 172, 173, 194, 198, 200, 206, 247, 261
guessing, 39
guidance, 17, 92, 128, 143, 216, 231
guidelines, 47, 56
guilt, 208

H

hair, 224
Haiti, 120
happiness, 98, 115, 171, 244
Hawaii, 114
head and neck cancer, 124
healing, 3, 15, 16, 18, 19, 29, 30, 55, 56, 57, 74, 77,
    79, 90, 93, 96, 98, 120, 122, 124, 129, 147, 148,
    149, 150, 151, 152, 155, 158, 159, 175, 201, 207,
    208, 209, 216, 217, 219, 225, 227, 249
health care, 44, 50, 71, 72, 73, 74, 76, 77, 78, 79, 80,
    81, 82, 83, 84, 85, 86, 87, 98, 113, 114, 120, 123,
    126, 132, 173, 187, 190, 206, 213, 224, 227, 238
health care professionals, 76, 77, 78, 81, 113, 126,
    190
health care programs, 81
health care system, 72, 73, 76, 82, 85, 132
health promotion, 79, 227
health status, 73, 95, 97, 224
heart disease, 97
heart rate, 248
height, 129, 132, 155, 194
hemianopsia, 172

hemiparesis, 130

heuristic, 36, 45, 109, 243, 244, 250

hierarchical, 73, 78, 81, 83

high school, 95, 103, 129, 139, 141, 142, 154, 158, 159, 176, 187, 216, 217, 230

high school grades, 176

higher education, 65, 70

hiring, 60, 121, 201

history, xv, 3, 4, 5, 10, 23, 24, 31, 48, 54, 60, 61, 70, 86, 104, 113, 127, 131, 138, 153, 155, 157, 176, 183, 190, 223, 224

HIV, 120, 121, 122, 125, 126

HIV/AIDS, 121

holism, 152

holistic, 32, 74, 84, 113, 121, 148, 151, 158, 176, 199

holons, 245, 246

honesty, 202, 230, 231

hospice, 120, 148, 176, 212

hospitality, 80

hospitalization, 129, 155, 156

host, xvi, 155, 187, 188, 209

House, 226

human activity, xviii

human body, 92, 135, 208

human condition, 212

human dignity, 11, 121

human experience, ix, 51, 95, 128, 135, 180, 197, 198, 206, 226, 238

human health, xv

human interactions, xviii, 27, 53, 57

human nature, 14, 16, 45

human resources, 157

human right(s), 95

hurricanes, 89

husband, 72, 124, 157, 164, 172, 200, 201, 212

hypertension, 225

hypothesis, 108

I

ideal(s), 14, 76, 200, 241

identification, 49

identity, 10, 30, 82, 161, 166

illumination, 9

illusion, 33, 99, 100, 253

imagery, 163

images, 163, 249

imagination, 42, 45, 63, 90, 91, 92, 162, 169, 209, 210, 223, 225

imbalances, 57, 105

imitation, 63

immune system, 27

immunologist, 28

impairments, 139

implementation, xvii, 89, 100, 101, 102, 103, 104, 105, 106, 107, 108, 109, 123, 148, 254

improvements, 16, 66

improvisation, 177, 182, 185, 250, 255

improvising, 178

impulses, 105, 156, 157

impulsivity, 157

income, 66

incongruity, 48

incubator, xvii

independence, 9, 100, 113, 131, 216, 237

Independence, 258

independent living, 245

Index Medicus, 49

individualism, 6, 32

individuality, 144

individuals, x, xvi, 5, 7, 8, 9, 16, 29, 30, 49, 57, 62, 77, 101, 114, 121, 122, 123, 140, 141, 142, 153, 154, 157, 158, 161, 163, 171, 176, 200, 205, 206, 207, 211, 212, 213, 221, 237, 245, 257, 259

individuation, 162, 163, 165, 169

industrialization, 61

industries, 61

industry, 153, 157, 161

inefficiency, 108

inequality, 95

inequity, 74

inferences, 141

inflation, xiv, 13

infrastructure, 36

ingredients, 9, 12, 27, 43, 259, 260

inhibition, 179

inhibitor, 179

injections, 73, 224

injuries, 18, 133, 139, 189, 194

injury, 15, 17, 18, 72, 82, 113, 129, 217, 230

inner world, 178, 180

innovation, ix, x, xi, xvii, 10, 32, 43, 44, 45, 47, 59, 62, 70, 71, 73, 81, 99, 100, 104, 105, 130, 138, 205, 207, 238, 255, 262

innovator, xvii, 130

insecurity, 194

insight, xvii, 16, 26, 36, 37, 38, 39, 41, 44, 51, 55, 56, 69, 97, 100, 102, 104, 105, 107, 108, 124, 134, 172, 198, 205, 212, 216, 218, 230, 231, 244, 248, 251, 253, 254, 255, 259, 260

inspiration, xvii, 90, 92, 94, 97, 98, 99, 109, 120, 151, 162, 172, 182, 203, 211, 223, 225, 226, 233, 235, 238, 240, 241

institutions, xvii, xviii, 28, 42, 65, 69, 98, 184, 188, 190, 205, 257, 263

insurance policy, 121
integration, 18, 19, 156, 192, 202, 259
integrity, 76
intellect, 105, 181, 228
intelligence, 96, 145
intention, 23, 37, 38, 39, 41, 89, 90, 93, 102, 104, 105, 106, 107, 108, 157, 178, 244, 248, 252
interdependence, 32
interest groups, 54
interference, 45, 193
internist, 156
internship, 177, 199, 216
interpersonal conflict, 26
interpersonal neurobiology, 40
interpersonal relations, 79
interpersonal relationships, 79
interpersonal skills, 138
interprofessionalism, 12, 32, 33
interrelatedness, 122
intervention, xviii, 54, 65, 83, 116, 120, 129, 175, 180
intimacy, 201
intimidation, 83
intrinsic motivation, 43
intrinsic value, 121
introspection, 25, 42, 56, 124, 177, 207, 259
intuition, 50, 51, 120, 123, 212, 216, 217, 218, 219, 220, 221, 248
Iowa, 230
isolation, 13, 25, 27, 28, 32, 35, 38, 42, 82, 151, 184
issues, xvii, 17, 29, 32, 89, 106, 119, 129, 140, 145, 147, 148, 187, 188, 209, 217
Italy, xi, 14, 44, 241

J

joints, 20
jumping, 54, 120
justification, 4

K

kill, 73
knees, xiii, 129, 225, 239

L

lack of confidence, 179
lactation, 181
landscape, 16, 79, 219, 231
language skills, 140, 141
Lao Tzu, 257, 258

laws, 24
LCAT, vi, 161
lead, 38, 52, 54, 61, 83, 93, 105, 116, 119, 124, 128, 135, 159, 171, 178, 179, 259, 262
leadership, 70, 73, 78, 79, 81, 82, 83, 85, 87, 179, 259
learned helplessness, 208
learners, 139
learning, 12, 18, 20, 43, 60, 82, 90, 91, 93, 98, 99, 101, 102, 106, 108, 120, 137, 138, 139, 140, 141, 142, 143, 148, 149, 153, 171, 172, 177, 178, 182, 184, 192, 212, 215, 217, 221, 241, 245, 246, 247, 248, 252, 253, 255
learning disabilities, 141
learning environment, 138
learning organizations, 82
learning process, 142
learning skills, 140, 141
legend, 77, 101
legs, 16, 17, 19
leisure, 171, 172, 173, 231
leisure time, 172
lens, x, 5, 18, 30, 31, 50, 56, 85, 89, 137, 139, 199, 244, 245, 248
level of education, 115
liberation, 91, 93
liberty, 200
life experiences, 90, 162, 165, 205
lifelong learning, 81
lifestyle changes, 97, 224, 225
lifetime, 35, 127, 135
ligament, 18
light, 24, 29, 47, 90, 97, 123, 165, 183, 184, 197, 200, 203, 210, 223
limbic system, 240
literacy, 77, 80, 85
local community, 142
locus, 83
lone genius, x, xi, xvi, 6, 25, 38, 76, 257
loneliness, 151
love, 13, 26, 93, 97, 98, 115, 116, 119, 148, 160, 164, 166, 172, 202, 209, 211, 212, 216, 221, 225, 228, 260
lumbar spine, 102
lying, 103, 177, 210

M

machinery, 9
magazines, 190
magnitude, 57, 95
majority, 6, 16, 67, 184, 202, 224
mammals, 246

man, 4, 39, 51, 86, 92, 94, 108, 139, 159, 164, 240, 260

management, 49, 87, 99, 100, 102, 107, 123, 127, 129, 130, 131, 132, 133, 153, 206, 255, 258

manic, 116, 166

marital life, 224

marketing, 5, 36, 121, 157, 200

marketing strategy, 121

marriage, xi, 29, 102, 207, 217

martial art, 189, 227, 249

mass, 5, 86

mass communication, 86

materials, 101, 165, 245

maternal care, 72

matrix, 27

matter, 26, 33, 63, 92, 106, 167, 168, 191, 211, 238, 243, 258

media, 5, 32, 53, 121, 139, 158, 162, 165, 247, 261

median, 227

medical, ix, xv, 10, 16, 18, 26, 50, 61, 70, 72, 80, 81, 83, 86, 102, 113, 122, 123, 127, 130, 133, 134, 137, 148, 153, 156, 172, 173, 176, 189, 190, 197, 198, 209, 216, 217, 224, 254

medical care, 123, 134

medical science, 254

Medicare, 201

medicine, xi, xvi, 25, 47, 48, 49, 53, 58, 61, 69, 70, 73, 74, 80, 82, 83, 84, 87, 95, 96, 97, 116, 122, 124, 126, 130, 169, 189, 197, 241, 252

memory, 16, 182, 184, 240

memory loss, 182

mental capacity, 128

mental health, 10, 17, 46, 114, 141, 143, 145, 155, 157, 158, 219

mental health professionals, 10, 145, 219

mental state, 37

mentor, 56, 94, 139, 144, 154, 179, 182, 199, 248, 262

mentoring, 182

mergers, 123, 187, 188

messages, 154, 156, 184, 225

metaphor, 40, 90, 92, 95, 96, 100, 107, 156, 185, 249

methodological implications, 6

methodology, 31, 32, 144, 261

Mexico, 163, 169

military, 208

mind-body, 15, 16, 17, 18, 19, 20, 122

mindfulness, 10, 37, 46, 91, 93, 94, 96, 123, 124, 125, 126, 179, 193, 208, 218, 249, 261

Minneapolis, 45, 158, 255, 260

minorities, 61

misconceptions, 17, 23, 52

mission, 97, 107, 157, 158, 178, 211, 227

models, xiv, 10, 13, 33, 61, 74, 93, 99, 253

modern science, 57

modernity, x

modifications, 128

molecules, 245

momentum, 121, 125, 169

morality, 5

motivation, 4, 19, 43, 97, 104, 138, 182, 224, 232

MSW, vi, 205

multiple factors, 101

multiple sclerosis, 132

murder, 193

muscle contraction, 132

muscles, 18, 202

musculoskeletal, 194, 230

muse, 80, 95, 224, 225

music, xi, 5, 27, 61, 155, 163, 168, 175, 176, 177, 178, 179, 180, 181, 182, 183, 184, 185, 191, 211, 212

music therapy, 155, 175, 176, 177, 178, 180, 182, 183, 184, 185

musicians, 178, 182, 188, 191

mutual respect, 75, 81

mythology, 101

N

naming, 239

narratives, 45, 96, 106, 254

natural pregnancy, 72

negative consequences, 81

negative effects, 68

negative experiences, 81

negotiating, 76

nervous system, 102, 192, 194, 246

Netherlands, 45

neti neti, 25, 26, 38, 41, 42

networking, 153, 154

neural connection, 219

neurobiology, 40

neurons, 95

neuropathy, 122, 124

neuroplasticity, 39, 40, 41, 96, 219, 241, 261

neuroscience, 83, 98

neutral, 8

next generation, 263

nightmares, 206

noncreative practices, 100, 241, 243

North America, 6, 9, 70, 126

noticing, 36, 48, 123, 140, 246, 248

nurses, 20, 54, 80, 147, 148, 149, 151, 152

nursing, 44, 61, 86, 147, 148, 149, 151, 152, 168, 176, 181, 182

nursing care, 147
nursing home, 182
nurturance, 228
nurture, 116, 151, 166, 168, 177, 193
nutrition, 62, 153, 154, 155, 159, 225

O

obedience, 12
objectivity, 33
obstacles, 30, 57, 94, 95, 101, 176
occupational therapy, 61, 113, 246
OCD, 155
OCS, vi, xvii, 229
offenders, 182
oil, 47, 90
old age, 135
ontology, 11, 27, 33
open spaces, 52
openness, 216, 218, 231
operating system, 27, 33, 43, 252
operations, 32, 101, 105, 106, 108, 227, 245, 259
opportunities, 8, 9, 28, 29, 52, 81, 97, 102, 113, 134,
    147, 148, 149, 155, 159, 161, 162, 172, 173, 176,
    177, 181, 187, 188, 206, 207, 208, 211, 213, 229
oppression, 147
ordinary creativity, 7, 11, 23, 27, 40, 41, 106, 237
organism, 245
organizational development, 53, 83, 257
organize, 195, 211
organs, 246
osteoarthritis, 122
osteoporosis, 127, 128, 129, 130, 131, 132, 133, 134
outpatient, 114, 130, 154, 156, 157, 158, 159, 200,
    230, 260
outreach, 122, 159
overlap, 218
overtime, 100
overweight, 227
ownership, 97

P

pain, xiii, 3, 11, 12, 17, 18, 27, 28, 54, 72, 95, 121,
    123, 124, 129, 131, 132, 177, 199, 206, 210, 217,
    224, 225, 227, 230, 247, 254
pain management, 54, 72, 121, 131
pain perception, 247
paints, 163, 167
pairing, 48
palate, 120, 138
palpation, 202

pancreas, 15
paradigm, 16, 17, 26, 45, 48, 74, 79, 82, 141, 198,
    199
paradigm shift, 74, 79, 141, 198
parallel, 156
paralysis, 17, 18
parenthood, 90
parents, 63, 142, 143, 212
parole, 208
participants, 53, 77, 101, 206, 221, 261
partnership, 44, 50, 74, 75, 76, 77, 78, 79, 80, 81, 82,
    83, 84, 85, 86, 103, 107, 237, 247
pathologist, 137
patient care, 48, 49, 50, 71, 72, 73, 119, 130, 131,
    133, 199, 201
payroll, 102
peace, 122, 177, 179
peak experience, 181
pedagogy, 10, 81
peer group, 177
peer review, 59, 65, 66, 70
pelvic floor, 202
pelvis, 192, 199, 202
perfectionism, 212
performers, 60, 179, 187, 188, 189, 191, 192, 193,
    194
performing artists, 188
permission, 123, 163, 167
perseverance, 40, 99
persistence, 101, 130
personal choice, 83
personal development, 184
personal history, 211
personal life, 131
personal relations, 159
personal relationship, 159
personality, 25, 42, 44, 128, 132, 143, 173, 248
personality type, 25, 42
personnel costs, 108
phenomenology, 46
phonograph, 5
photographs, 163
physical activity, 122
physical health, 17
physical therapist, xiii, 10, 90, 129, 130, 131, 132,
    185, 188, 198, 219, 223, 230
physical therapy, xvi, 3, 34, 51, 61, 62, 64, 70, 86,
    90, 102, 103, 126, 127, 128, 130, 132, 133, 134,
    135, 187, 190, 195, 197, 198, 200, 202, 224, 230,
    231, 247, 260
physicians, 73, 74, 76, 81, 132, 200, 219
physics, 51, 69, 135
physiology, 39, 41, 241

piano, 176, 178
Picasso, x, xi, 90
pitch, 106
placebo, 54
planets, 246
plants, 35, 165, 166, 173, 223
plasticity, 245
platform, 96, 124
Plato, 60
playing, 167, 177, 178, 182, 188, 191, 212
pleasure, 35, 229
pluralism, x
poetry, 151
polarity, 148, 149
polarization, 48
policy, 50, 72, 73, 77, 80, 83, 86
policy makers, 50
political meeting, 179
pollination, 194
pollution, 184
population, 13, 60, 120, 121, 122, 125, 126, 131,
    132, 139, 158, 208, 245
positive relationship, 164
postnormal times, x, xi, 23, 45, 48, 50, 53, 54, 55,
    59, 63, 66, 67, 68, 69, 70, 100, 235, 237, 255, 258
potential benefits, xiv
poverty, 95
poverty line, 95
practical knowledge, 67, 188
prayer, 56, 151, 153, 209, 248
predictability, x, 11, 24, 27, 39, 48, 50, 57
prediction models, 11
prefrontal cortex, 83, 240
pregnancy, 73, 199, 205
prejudice, 121
preparation, 9, 227, 235
preschool, 184
prescription drugs, 72
presence, 12, 17, 19, 37, 39, 43, 72, 122, 127, 147,
    149, 167, 244, 259
president, 103, 105
prestige, 187
prevention, 122, 148
prime, xiv, xvii, 4, 23, 24, 26, 35, 37, 38, 39, 40, 96,
    218, 237, 241, 243, 244, 251, 255
priming, 39, 96, 102, 104, 208, 241
principles, xiv, 6, 16, 31, 49, 107, 127, 128, 129,
    130, 133
prior knowledge, 81
private practice, xvii, 84, 121, 130, 133, 137, 153,
    154, 155, 176, 187, 188, 206, 221, 223, 230
problem solving, 43, 77, 184
problem-solving, 172, 175

professional development, xvi
professional growth, 138
professionalism, 80, 81, 85, 86
profit, xv, 16, 93, 158, 201
profitability, 87
prognosis, 79
programming, 155
project, xv, 70, 100, 101, 107, 108, 116, 122, 138,
    154, 191, 212, 254
proliferation, 40, 66, 176, 245
proposition, 5
prosperity, 77, 157
protection, 95, 122
prototypes, 93, 94
psychiatrist, 156
psychiatry, 82, 141
psychologist, 28, 142, 215, 217
psychology, 7, 8, 14, 17, 32, 53, 61, 63, 141, 177,
    216, 217, 218, 247
psychotherapy, 155, 156, 162, 177, 208, 210
PTSD, 155, 207, 209
public awareness, 158
public health, 77, 80, 86
publishing, 60, 66

Q

qualitative research, 53
quality improvement, 41
quality of life, 3, 77, 85, 120, 134, 171, 172
quantitative research, 183
questioning, xv, 143, 205, 210
quieting, 56, 237, 240, 260

R

race, x, 93, 98
racing, 43
radio, 5, 158, 261
radius, 200, 257
rate of change, x
reactions, 38, 128, 236
reactivity, 41
reading, xvi, xvii, 6, 24, 26, 35, 54, 90, 102, 106,
    116, 122, 135, 139, 140, 141, 157, 189, 190, 191,
    193, 213, 237, 245
reading comprehension, 139, 140, 141
real income, xiv, 13
real time, 40, 55, 57
realism, 11, 33, 53
reality, xvii, 5, 6, 7, 9, 16, 27, 28, 29, 33, 36, 37, 48,
    51, 53, 54, 59, 65, 90, 92, 95, 99, 100, 104, 105,

106, 132, 145, 151, 198, 199, 229, 231, 238, 245, 254, 257
reasoning, 54
recall, 91, 96
recalling, 240
recession, 106, 176
recognition, 8, 9, 30, 138, 149, 235
recommendations, 86, 95
reconstruction, xiii
recovery, 17, 18, 19, 129, 157, 158, 180, 182, 216, 219
recreation, 150, 171, 172, 173, 176
recreational, 18, 171, 172, 173
recruiting, 106
recurrence, 131
reductionism, 32
reductionistic, 6, 7, 25
reflexes, 200
reform, 85
refugees, 182
regeneration, 30
regression, 54
regulations, 83, 159
rehabilitation program, 42, 67
reinforcement, 232
relationship, xvi, 5, 11, 15, 16, 17, 18, 19, 29, 31, 34, 35, 36, 39, 41, 42, 50, 56, 63, 64, 67, 71, 72, 73, 74, 76, 77, 79, 80, 81, 82, 84, 90, 105, 128, 143, 158, 159, 164, 175, 178, 179, 181, 205, 206, 207, 208, 227, 238, 244, 245, 247, 248, 249, 255, 260
relatives, 176
relativity, 29
relaxation, 149, 150, 151, 211
relevance, xviii, 49
relief, xiii, 31, 47, 57, 128, 129, 131, 132
religion, 60, 98, 179
rendition, xi
rent, 155
representational, 27, 28, 33, 237
reproductive education, 12, 33, 63
reproductive organs, 199
reputation, 207
requirements, xiv, 13, 66, 89, 156, 162
research evidence, ix, 11, 47, 49, 51, 52, 128, 134
research funding, 106
research online, 244
researchers, 33, 52, 53, 113, 138, 173
resilience, 16, 94, 120, 124, 126, 149, 225
resiliency, xiv, 11, 13, 16, 19, 216, 217
resistance, 40, 83, 89, 105, 126, 208, 241
resolution, 56
resources, 4, 13, 33, 37, 49, 54, 57, 86, 90, 99, 100, 101, 106, 107, 206, 224, 254

response, xv, 4, 11, 12, 23, 27, 34, 37, 38, 39, 41, 48, 54, 72, 94, 107, 108, 121, 128, 149, 151, 175, 177, 207, 212, 216, 237, 245, 247, 248, 249, 252, 253, 258, 263
responsiveness, 245
restrictions, 159, 206
restructuring, 11
retirement, 103
revenue, 100
rhetoric, 61, 85
rheumatoid arthritis, 17, 217
rhythm, 220, 231
riff, xi, 211, 250
rights, 49, 80
rings, 54, 74
risk(s), 38, 42, 51, 52, 55, 62, 68, 73, 100, 121, 128, 134, 180, 206, 262
root(s), x, xvii, 11, 41, 43, 93, 98, 156, 179, 209, 218, 219
routines, 91, 97
rules, xv, 18, 107, 163, 239

S

sacrifice, 95, 103, 109
sadness, 218
safety, 11, 128, 130, 132, 134, 156, 164, 166, 183, 218
scarce resources, 100
schema, 201
scholarship, 65, 66
school, ix, xiv, xvi, 6, 10, 13, 59, 60, 61, 62, 63, 64, 65, 66, 67, 68, 70, 114, 127, 128, 129, 130, 137, 139, 140, 142, 144, 145, 150, 151, 155, 156, 165, 166, 172, 176, 177, 178, 182, 184, 187, 189, 194, 197, 198, 199, 206, 208, 216, 217, 218
schooling, 63, 198, 199
science, x, xi, xv, xviii, 16, 32, 39, 40, 44, 45, 49, 55, 61, 62, 63, 86, 96, 99, 106, 107, 126, 129, 138, 149, 152, 154, 159, 172, 179, 182, 249, 254, 255, 263
scientific method, 24, 49, 138
scope, 30, 138, 206, 226, 246
second language, 56
security, 178, 180, 258
sediment, 241
seed, xvi, 35
self-awareness, 92, 93, 94, 123
self-care, 19, 46, 100, 119, 123, 148, 149, 151, 152, 161, 164, 179, 224
self-concept, 6
self-confidence, 194
self-consciousness, 212

self-discovery, 203
self-doubt, 220
self-efficacy, 73, 79, 83
self-employed, 72
self-esteem, 81
self-image, 225
self-knowledge, 236
self-portrait(s), 163
self-reflection, 125, 177
seminars, xiii, 127, 128, 130, 133, 134, 178
sensation(s), 16, 17, 18, 19, 20, 39, 195, 239, 240, 246, 247
senses, 91, 96, 135, 194, 210, 223, 225
sensing, ix, 12, 28, 92, 191, 206, 239, 248
sensitivity, 56, 80, 190, 224
sensory experience, 178
separateness, 100
services, ix, xiv, xv, 10, 44, 51, 76, 77, 80, 97, 105, 140, 155, 156, 161, 171, 176, 201, 227, 230
sex, 249
shame, 206, 218
shape, 8, 53, 67, 92, 130, 163, 168, 223
shock, xi, 235
shoot, 194
shortage, 147, 151, 152
shortfall, 7
showing, 105, 203, 206, 231
siblings, 212
side effects, 120, 122
signals, xiii
signs, 32, 206
silence, xiii, xviii, 12, 20, 24, 31, 41, 43, 51, 55, 97, 102, 103, 104, 123, 191, 212, 224, 235, 236, 239, 241, 251, 259, 260, 262
simulation, 95
skeleton, xv, 5, 35, 36, 40
skills base, 105
skin, 114, 225
snippets, 150
sobriety, 158
social anxiety, 139, 155
social behavior, 140, 141
social circle, 224
social cognition, 139, 141
social construct, 76
social context, xviii
social contract, 81
social environment, 8, 25
social exclusion, 28
social interactions, 37
social justice, 179
social learning, 140, 141, 142, 143
social organization, 29

social phobia, 139
social policy, 77
social psychology, 44
social sciences, 32, 53, 175
social skills, 139, 140, 141, 143
social support, 199
social thinking, 140, 141, 143
social workers, 176, 205, 206, 207, 219
socialization, 73, 76
society, ix, xi, xiv, xvii, xviii, 3, 4, 5, 10, 12, 13, 32, 68, 74, 76, 77, 79, 86, 91, 92, 114, 121, 128, 135, 171, 189, 190, 226, 231
socioeconomic status, 98
sociology, 32
software, 49
solar system, 246
solitude, 42, 212
solution, xiii, 18, 19, 192, 203, 246
South Africa, 120, 125, 126
space making, 237
Spain, 231
specialists, 121, 176, 199
species, 4, 92, 257
speech, 62, 137
spending, 76, 150, 173
spinal cord, xvi, 15, 16, 17, 18
spinal cord injury, xvi
spinal fusion, 227
spinal stenosis, 131, 132
spine, xiii, 19, 20, 133, 198, 224, 225
spirituality, 98, 153, 189, 218
Spring, 103, 126
stability, x, 37, 157, 180
stabilization, 158
staff members, 157
staffing, 4
stakeholders, 82, 83
standardization, 10
stars, 123
starvation, 156
state(s), ix, xv, 28, 33, 37, 39, 48, 55, 56, 57, 68, 77, 78, 81, 90, 91, 100, 102, 103, 114, 126, 157, 173, 180, 193, 199, 203, 240, 241, 259
statistics, 63, 95
stigma, 121, 179
stigmatized, 74, 76
stimulation, 177
stomach, 224
storytelling, 219, 254
stress, 46, 89, 96, 109, 119, 123, 126, 147, 148, 149, 153, 183, 194, 217, 225, 255
stress response, 149
stretching, 225

stroke, 115, 117
strong force, 133
structure, xviii, 10, 39, 43, 46, 74, 75, 107, 143, 178,
    181, 182, 259
structuring, 259
struggle, xvii, xix, 57, 80, 89, 90, 94, 95, 100, 101,
    155, 156, 157, 162, 164, 184, 216
style, 83, 157
subjective experience, 92, 244
substance abuse, 155, 157, 158
substance addiction, 155
success rate, 121
suffering, xviii, 3, 12, 16, 19, 20, 34, 37, 38, 39, 40,
    57, 95, 96, 98, 104, 105, 107, 148, 151, 158, 200,
    206, 207, 211, 224, 243, 244, 252, 254
suicide, 95
suicide rate, 95
supervisor(s), 135, 245, 258
suppression, 70
survival, 104
susceptibility, 37
sustainability, xvii, 51, 89, 90, 96, 100, 104, 227
sweat, 208
Sweden, 163, 188, 189
Switzerland, 87
symbolism, 210
symmetry, 12, 254, 258
symptoms, 50, 55, 72, 131, 133, 199, 202, 223
systems, ix, xiii, xiv, xvi, xvii, xviii, xix, 4, 8, 11, 12,
    13, 24, 27, 28, 29, 30, 31, 34, 35, 41, 42, 51, 52,
    57, 66, 67, 69, 70, 73, 82, 83, 86, 87, 89, 91, 93,
    97, 98, 100, 101, 102, 103, 107, 108, 113, 137,
    184, 223, 238, 245, 252, 253, 259, 260, 262, 263

T

takeover, 120
talent, xvii, 24, 25, 42, 81, 179, 194
target, 95
task performance, 37
teacher training, 154, 155
teachers, 16, 134, 140, 142, 154, 156, 184, 190, 199,
    247
teaching evaluation, 172
teaching experience, 189
teaching strategies, 143
team members, 106, 108, 215, 254
teams, 78, 81, 107, 137, 139, 188, 254
techniques, xviii, 8, 10, 20, 34, 68, 99, 102, 109, 123,
    156, 162, 202, 248, 257, 258
technological developments, 53
technology, x, 4, 5, 16, 28, 53, 54, 96, 98, 134, 182,
    238

teens, 141
telephone, 127, 134
tempo, 191
tenants, 96
tension(s), 6, 10, 20, 27, 31, 48, 82, 105, 210, 224,
    253, 258, 259
tenure, 64, 65, 66, 115, 130, 150, 182
territory, 101
test scores, 176
testing, 46, 72, 137
textbook(s), xiii, xiv, 49, 64, 65, 105, 192
texture, 210, 230
therapeutic goal, 206
therapeutic practice, 227
therapeutic process, 49, 207, 210
therapeutic relationship, 15, 16, 206, 207
therapeutic touch, 209
therapeutics, 230
therapist, 51, 57, 79, 90, 114, 121, 130, 131, 132,
    133, 135, 139, 154, 157, 159, 161, 162, 164, 165,
    166, 172, 175, 176, 177, 182, 183, 188, 200, 203,
    206, 207, 223, 245
therapy, 37, 51, 57, 61, 68, 73, 90, 114, 116, 128,
    133, 155, 156, 158, 159, 161, 162, 163, 164, 165,
    168, 169, 171, 172, 173, 175, 176, 177, 179, 182,
    183, 185, 189, 191, 194, 195, 198, 200, 201, 202,
    206, 209, 210, 211, 216, 218, 224, 229, 230
thoughts, 18, 26, 30, 38, 39, 61, 69, 90, 91, 92, 94,
    96, 124, 125, 140, 157, 165, 190, 197, 206, 211,
    217, 219, 221, 240, 246, 247
threats, 83
time constraints, 96
time pressure, 187, 188
tin, 15
tissue, 12, 189
top-down, 33, 74
traditions, xi, 10, 12, 32, 93, 176, 179, 235
training, x, 3, 6, 16, 19, 40, 46, 61, 62, 69, 81, 92,
    108, 119, 120, 123, 141, 156, 159, 161, 176, 177,
    183, 188, 189, 191, 194, 195, 198, 202, 227, 243,
    248
training programs, 159
traits, 9, 10, 12, 63, 74, 75, 76, 85, 140, 245, 257
trajectory, 123
transcendence, 20, 95
transdisciplinary, xvi, 3, 13, 81, 86
transference, 261
transformation, ix, 74, 93, 148, 149, 198, 201, 205
transformational learning, 54
translation, 29
transport, 230
trauma, 16, 20, 199, 206, 258

treatment, xiii, xv, 10, 11, 16, 29, 50, 51, 54, 72, 100, 105, 120, 122, 126, 127, 128, 131, 137, 138, 139, 140, 141, 142, 154, 155, 156, 157, 158, 159, 171, 188, 189, 203, 217, 219, 230, 235, 254
trial, 50, 53, 55, 122, 179, 181
tuition, 64
turnover, 84

U

ultrasound, 72, 260
uncertainty, x, 12, 24, 28, 29, 37, 41, 48, 49, 50, 55, 63, 67, 68, 100, 104, 125, 207, 235, 255
unconditional positive regard, 206, 208
unhappiness, 194
uninsured, 72
United Kingdom, xi, 81
United States, 6, 48, 76, 82, 171
universe, 40, 41, 149, 150, 160, 207, 220
universities, 61, 62, 70, 159, 177
urban, 77
USSR, 87

V

vacuum, 57
validation, 77
valuation, 12
variables, 7, 43, 55, 67, 73, 138, 189
variations, 6
variety of domains, 101
vehicles, 92
vein, 195, 249
versatility, 53
vertebrates, 246
Vietnam, 5
violence, 29, 75, 84, 105, 147
vision, ix, xiv, xvi, xix, 12, 48, 49, 69, 76, 82, 83, 85, 96, 97, 104, 121, 123, 128, 155, 195, 205, 225, 226, 227, 240, 251
visualization, 90, 224
vocabulary, 218
vocational training, 69
Volunteers, 69

voting, 179
vulnerability, 124, 126, 184, 253

W

waking, 163
walking, 18, 56, 173, 210, 215, 231, 247
war, 5, 75
Washington, 86
waste, 108
water, 95, 99, 109, 159, 164, 248, 251
weakness, 128
wealth, 56, 85, 86, 163
web, xix, 153, 238
weight loss, 225, 227
welfare, 92
well-being, xiv, 77, 79, 130, 131, 171, 172, 225, 227
wellness, 74, 121, 123, 126, 156, 176, 179, 183, 184, 202, 221, 227
wellness coaching, 123, 126
western culture, 210, 235
wilderness, 209
Wisconsin, 86
wood, 99, 249, 251
word processing, 27
work environment, 238
work ethic, 94
workers, 61, 205, 206, 209, 257
workforce, 184
workload, 61, 64, 96, 161, 164, 169
workplace, 76, 78, 79, 147, 177, 184, 223, 226
World Health Organization (WHO), 81, 87, 95
World War I, 130
worldview, 7, 27, 31, 38, 43, 48, 85, 179
worldwide, 49, 95
worry, 167, 243, 259
wrestling, 106
wrists, 15
writing process, 151

Y

yield, xvii, 53, 54, 259
young women, 179